Communications in Computer and Information Science **881**

Commenced Publication in 2007
Founding and Former Series Editors:
Alfredo Cuzzocrea, Xiaoyong Du, Orhun Kara, Ting Liu, Dominik Ślęzak,
and Xiaokang Yang

More information about this series at http://www.springer.com/series/7899

Nathalia Peixoto · Margarida Silveira
Hesham H. Ali · Carlos Maciel
Egon L. van den Broek (Eds.)

Biomedical Engineering Systems and Technologies

10th International Joint Conference, BIOSTEC 2017
Porto, Portugal, February 21–23, 2017
Revised Selected Papers

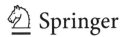 Springer

Editors
Nathalia Peixoto
George Mason University
Fairfax, VA
USA

Margarida Silveira
Instituto Superior Técnico (IST)
University of Lisbon
Lisbon
Portugal

Hesham H. Ali
University of Nebraska at Omaha
Omaha, NE
USA

Carlos Maciel
University of Sao Paulo
Sao Carlos, SP
Brazil

Egon L. van den Broek
Utrecht University
Utrecht
The Netherlands

ISSN 1865-0929   ISSN 1865-0937   (electronic)
Communications in Computer and Information Science
ISBN 978-3-319-94805-8   ISBN 978-3-319-94806-5   (eBook)
https://doi.org/10.1007/978-3-319-94806-5

Library of Congress Control Number: 2018947372

Printed on acid-free paper

This Springer imprint is published by the registered company Springer International Publishing AG
part of Springer Nature
The registered company address is: Gewerbestrasse 11, 6330 Cham, Switzerland

Preface

The present book includes extended and revised versions of a set of selected papers from the 10th International Joint Conference on Biomedical Engineering Systems and Technologies (BIOSTEC 2017), held in Porto, Portugal, during February 21–23, 2017. BIOSTEC is composed of five co-located conferences, each specialized in a different knowledge area, namely, BIODEVICES, BIOIMAGING, BIOINFORMATICS, BIO-SIGNALS, and HEALTHINF.

BIOSTEC 2017 received 297 paper submissions from 56 countries, of which only 6% are included in this book. This reflects our care in selecting contributions. These papers were selected by the conference chairs on the basis of a number of criteria that include the classifications and comments provided by the Program Committee members, the session chairs' assessment, and the program chairs' meta-review of the papers that were included in the technical program. The authors of selected papers were invited to submit a revised, extended, and improved version of their conference paper, including at least 30% new material.

The purpose of the BIOSTEC joint conferences is to bring together researchers and practitioners, including engineers, biologists, health professionals, and informatics/computer scientists. Research presented at BIOSTEC included both theoretical advances and applications of information systems, artificial intelligence, signal processing, electronics, and other engineering tools in areas related to advancing biomedical research and improving health care.

The papers included in this book contribute to the understanding of relevant research trends in biomedical engineering systems and technologies. As such, they provide an overview of the field's current state of the art.

We thank the authors for their contributions and Monica Saramago for process management. In particular, we express our gratitude to the reviewers, who helped to ensure the quality of this publication.

February 2017

Nathalia Peixoto
Margarida Silveira
Hesham H. Ali
Carlos Maciel
Egon L. van den Broek

Organization

Conference Co-chairs

Ana Fred	Instituto de Telecomunicações/IST, Portugal
Hugo Gamboa	LIBPHYS-UNL/FCT - New University of Lisbon, Portugal
Mário Vaz	INEGI LOME, FEUP, Portugal

Program Co-chairs

BIODEVICES

Nathalia Peixoto	Neural Engineering Lab, George Mason University, USA

BIOIMAGING

Margarida Silveira	Instituto Superior Técnico (IST), Portugal

BIOINFORMATICS

Hesham Ali	University of Nebraska at Omaha, USA

BIOSIGNALS

Carlos Maciel	University of São Paulo, Brazil

HEALTHINF

Egon L. van den Broek	Utrecht University, The Netherlands

BIODEVICES Program Committee

Azam Ali	University of Otago, New Zealand
Mohammed Bakr	CCIT-AASTMT, Egypt
Steve Beeby	University of Southampton, UK
Hadar Ben-Yoav	Ben-Gurion University of the Negev, Israel
Dinesh Bhatia	North Eastern Hill University, India
Efrain Zenteno Bolaños	Universidad Católica San Pablo, Peru
Luciano Boquete	Alcala University, Spain
Carlo Capelli	Norwegian School of Sport Sciences, Norway
Vítor Carvalho	IPCA and Algoritmi Research Centre, UM, Portugal
Hamid Charkhkar	Case Western Reserve University, USA
Wenxi Chen	The University of Aizu, Japan
Mireya Fernández Chimeno	Universitat Politècnica de Catalunya, Spain
Youngjae Chun	University of Pittsburgh, USA

James M. Conrad	University of North Carolina at Charlotte, USA
Albert Cook	University of Alberta, Canada
Maeve Duffy	NUI Galway, Ireland
Paddy French	Delft University of Technology, The Netherlands
Juan Carlos Garcia	University of Alcala, Spain
Javier Garcia-Casado	Universitat Politècnica de València, Spain
Bryon Gomberg	Geyra Gassner IP Law, Israel
Miguel Angel García Gonzalez	Universitat Politècnica de Catalunya, Spain
Klas Hjort	Uppsala University, Sweden
Toshiyuki Horiuchi	Tokyo Denki University, Japan
Leonid Hrebien	Drexel University, USA
Sandeep K. Jha	Indian Institute of Technology Delhi, India
Eyal Katz	Tel Aviv University, Israel
Michael Kraft	University of Liege, Belgium
Ondrej Krejcar	University of Hradec Kralove, Czech Republic
Ning Lan	Shanghai Jiao Tong University, China
Jung Chan Lee	Seoul National University, South Korea
Chwee Teck Lim	National University of Singapore, Singapore
Mai S. Mabrouk	Misr University for Science and Technology, Egypt
Jordi Madrenas	Universitat Politècnica de Catalunya, Spain
Jarmo Malinen	Aalto University, Finland
Karen May-Newman	San Diego State University, USA
Joseph Mizrahi	Technion, Israel Institute of Technology, Israel
Raimes Moraes	Universidade Federal de Santa Catarina, Brazil
Umberto Morbiducci	Politecnico di Torino, Italy
Antoni Nowakowski	Gdansk University of Technology, Poland
Eoin O'Cearbhaill	University College Dublin, Ireland
Mónica Oliveira	University of Strathclyde, UK
Abraham Otero	Universidad San Pablo CEU, Spain
Gonzalo Pajares	Universidad Complutense de Madrid, Spain
Sofia Panteliou	University of Patras, Greece
Nancy Paris	British Columbia Institute of Technology, Canada
Lionel Pazart	CHU, France
Nathalia Peixoto	George Mason University, USA
Marek Penhaker	VŠB, Technical University of Ostrava, Czech Republic
Dmitry Rogatkin	Moscow Regional Research and Clinical Institute MONIKI, Russian Federation
Wim L. C. Rutten	University of Twente, The Netherlands
Seonghan Ryu	Hannam University, South Korea
Ashutosh Sabharwal	Rice University, USA
V. V. Raghavendra Sai	IIT Madras, India
Chutham Sawigun	Mahanakorn University of Technology, Thailand
Michael J. Schöning	FH Aachen, Germany
Mauro Serpelloni	University of Brescia, Italy
Dong Ik Shin	Asan Medical Center, South Korea

Alcimar Barbosa Soares	Universidade Federal de Uberlândia, Brazil
Filomena Soares	Algoritmi Research Centre, UM, Portugal
Akihiro Takeuchi	Kitasato University School of Medicine, Japan
Gil Travish	Adaptix Ltd., UK
John Tudor	University of Southampton, UK
Renato Varoto	University of Campinas, Brazil
Pedro Vieira	Faculdade de Ciências e Tecnologia, Universidade Nova de Lisboa, Portugal
Bruno Wacogne	FEMTO-ST, France
Huikai Xie	University of Florida, USA
Sen Xu	Merck & Co., Inc., USA
Hakan Yavuz	Çukurova Üniversity, Turkey

BIOIMAGING Program Committee

Sameer K. Antani	National Library of Medicine, National Institutes of Health, USA
Peter Balazs	University of Szeged, Hungary
Grégory Barbillon	EPF-Ecole d'Ingénieurs, France
Alpan Bek	Middle East Technical University, Turkey
Mads Sylvest Bergholt	Imperial College London, UK
Obara Boguslaw	University of Durham, UK
Alberto Bravin	European Synchrotron Radiation Facility, France
Tom Brown	University of St. Andrews, UK
Enrico G. Caiani	Politecnico di Milano, Italy
Rita Casadio	University of Bologna, Italy
Alessia Cedola	CNR, Institute of Nanotechnology, Italy
Heang-Ping Chan	University of Michigan, USA
James Chan	University of California Davis, USA
Dean Chapman	University of Saskatchewan, Canada
Guanying Chen	Harbin Institute of Technology and SUNY Buffalo, China/USA
Jyh-Cheng Chen	National Yang-Ming University, Taiwan
Christos E. Constantinou	Stanford University, USA
Edite Maria Areias Figueiras	National Physical Laboratory, Portugal
Dimitrios Fotiadis	University of Ioannina, Greece
Patricia Haro Gonzalez	Universidad Autonoma Madrid, Spain
P. Gopinath	Indian Institute of Technology Roorkee, India
Dimitris Gorpas	Technical University of Munich, Germany
Alberto Del Guerra	University of Pisa, Italy
Tzung-Pei Hong	National University of Kaohsiung, Taiwan
Kazuyuki Hyodo	High Energy Accelerator Research Organization, Japan
Shu Jia	Stony Brook University, USA
Ming Jiang	Peking University, China
Xiaoyi Jiang	University of Münster, Germany

Pluim Josien	Eindhoven University of Technology, The Netherlands
Patrice Koehl	University of California, USA
Adriaan A. Lammertsma	VU University Medical Center Amsterdam, The Netherlands
Sang-Won Lee	Korea Research Institute of Standards and Science, South Korea
Rainer Leitgeb	Medical University Vienna, Austria
Ivan Lima	North Dakota State University, USA
Xiongbiao Luo	XMU-TMMU, China
Modat Marc	University College London, UK
David McGloin	University of Dundee, UK
Aidan D. Meade	Centre for Radiation and Environmental Science, Dublin Institute of Technology, Ireland
Erik Meijering	Erasmus University Medical Center, The Netherlands
Israel Rocha Mendoza	Centro de Investigación Científica y de Educación Superior de Ensenada, (CICESE), Mexico
Kunal Mitra	Florida Institute of Technology, USA
Christophoros Nikou	University of Ioannina, Greece
Joanna Isabelle Olszewska	University of West Scotland, UK
Kalman Palagyi	University of Szeged, Hungary
Joao Papa	UNESP, Universidade Estadual Paulista, Brazil
Tae Jung Park	Chung-Ang University, South Korea
Gennaro Percannella	University of Salerno, Italy
Ales Prochazka	University of Chemistry and Technology, Czech Republic
Jia Qin	University of California/University of Washington, USA
Wan Qin	University of Washington, USA
Miroslav Radojevic	Erasmus MC, Biomedical Imaging Group Rotterdam, The Netherlands
Joseph Reinhardt	University of Iowa, USA
Giovanna Rizzo	Consiglio Nazionale delle Ricerche, Italy
Bart M. ter Haar Romeny	Eindhoven University of Technology (TU/e), The Netherlands
Emanuele Schiavi	Universidad Rey Juan Carlos, Spain
Jan Schier	The Institute of Information Theory and Automation of the Czech Academy of Sciences, Czech Republic
Leonid Shvartsman	Hebrew University, Israel
Chikayoshi Sumi	Sophia University, Japan
Chi-Kuang Sun	National Taiwan University, Taiwan
Pablo Taboada	University of Santiago de Compostela, Spain
Xiaodong Tao	University of California, Santa Cruz, USA
Pécot Thierry	Medical University of South Carolina, France
Kenneth Tichauer	Illinois Institute of Technology, USA
Eric Tkaczyk	Vanderbilt University, USA
Arkadiusz Tomczyk	Lodz University of Technology, Poland

Carlos M. Travieso	University of Las Palmas de Gran Canaria, Spain
Benjamin M. W. Tsui	Johns Hopkins University, USA
Vladimír Ulman	Masaryk University, Czech Republic
Gözde Ünal	Istanbul Technical University, Turkey
Sandra Rua Ventura	School of Allied Health Technologies/Escola Superior de Saúde do Porto, Portugal
Yuanyuan Wang	Fudan University, China
Quan Wen	University of Electronic Science and Technology of China, China
Hongki Yoo	Hanyang University, South Korea
Habib Zaidi	Geneva University Hospital, Switzerland

BIOIMAGING Additional Reviewers

| Xiaoli Qi | Johns Hopkins University, USA |
| Qinqin Zhang | University of Washington, USA |

BIOINFORMATICS Program Committee

Tatsuya Akutsu	Kyoto University, Japan
Jens Allmer	Izmir Institute of Technology, Turkey
Sameer K. Antani	National Library of Medicine, National Institutes of Health, USA
Marco Antoniotti	Università degli Studi di Milano Bicocca, Italy
Joel Arrais	Universidade de Coimbra, Portugal
Rolf Backofen	Albert-Ludwigs-Universität, Germany
Lucia Ballerini	University of Edinburgh, UK
Ugur Bilge	Akdeniz University, Turkey
Leonardo Bocchi	Università di Firenze, Italy
Ulrich Bodenhofer	Johannes Kepler University Linz, Austria
Luca Bortolussi	University of Trieste, Italy
Andrea Bracciali	University of Stirling, UK
Giulio Caravagna	University of Edinburgh, UK
José Pedro Cerón Carrasco	Universidad Católica San Antonio de Murcia, Spain
Claudia Consuelo Rubiano Castellanos	Universidad Nacional de Colombia, Bogota, Colombia
Santa Di Cataldo	Politecnico di Torino, Italy
Wai-Ki Ching	The University of Hong Kong, SAR China
Mark Clement	Brigham Young University, USA
Netta Cohen	University of Leeds, UK
Federica Conte	National Research Council of Rome, Italy
Antoine Danchin	Institute of Cardiometabolism and Nutrition, France
Sérgio Deusdado	Instituto Politecnico de Bragança, Portugal
Richard Edwards	University of Southampton, UK
Fabrizio Ferre	University of Rome Tor Vergata, Italy
António Ferreira	Universidade de Lisboa, Portugal
Giulia Fiscon	National Research Council of Rome, Italy

Alexandre P. Francisco	Instituto Superior Técnico, Universidade de Lisboa, Portugal
Dario Ghersi	University of Nebraska at Omaha, USA
Arndt von Haeseler	Center of Integrative Bioinformatics Vienna, MFPL, Austria
Christopher E. Hann	University of Canterbury, New Zealand
Ronaldo Fumio Hashimoto	University of São Paulo, Brazil
Shan He	University of Birmingham, UK
Volkhard Helms	Universität des Saarlandes, Germany
Song-Nian Hu	Chinese Academy of Sciences, China
Jari Hyttinen	Tampere University of Technology, Finland
Sohei Ito	National Fisheries University, Japan
Bo Jin	MilliporeSigma, Merck KGaA, USA
Giuseppe Jurman	Fondazione Bruno Kessler, Italy
Yannis Kalaidzidis	Max Planck Institute Molecular Cell Biology and Genetics, Germany
Michael Kaufmann	Witten/Herdecke University, Germany
Natalia Khuri	Stanford University, USA
Sami Khuri	San José State University, USA
Inyoung Kim	Virginia Tech, USA
Toralf Kirsten	University of Leipzig, Germany
Jirí Kléma	Czech Technical University in Prague, Czech Republic
Peter Kokol	University of Maribor, Slovenia
Malgorzata Kotulska	Wroclaw University of Technology, Poland
Ivan Kulakovskiy	Engelhardt Institute of Molecular Biology RAS, Russian Federation
Yinglei Lai	George Washington University, USA
Carlile Lavor	University of Campinas, Brazil
Matej Lexa	Masaryk University, Czech Republic
Antonios Lontos	Frederick University, Cyprus
Shuangge Ma	Yale University, USA
Pawel Mackiewicz	Wroclaw University, Poland
Thérèse E. Malliavin	CNRS/Institut Pasteur, France
Elena Marchiori	Radboud University, The Netherlands
Andrea Marin	University of Venice, Italy
Majid Masso	George Mason University, USA
Petr Matula	Masaryk University, Czech Republic
Claudine Médigue	CEA/Genomic Institute/Genoscope and CNRS, France
Ivan Merelli	ITB CNR, Italy
Armin Mikler	University of North Texas, USA
Paolo Milazzo	University of Pisa, Italy
Saad Mneimneh	Hunter College CUNY, USA
Pedro Tiago Monteiro	INESC-ID/IST, Universidade de Lisboa, Portugal
Vincent Moulton	University of East Anglia, UK
Chad Myers	University of Minnesota, USA
Jean-Christophe Nebel	Kingston University, UK

Nazar Zaki	United Arab Emirates University, UAE
Helen Hao Zhang	University of Arizona, USA
Leming Zhou	University of Pittsburgh, USA
Zexuan Zhu	Shenzhen University, China

BIOINFORMATICS Additional Reviewers

Roberta Gori	Universitá di Pisa, Italy
Artem Kasianov	VIGG, Russian Federation

BIOSIGNALS Program Committee

Marko Ackermann	FEI University, Brazil
Jean-Marie Aerts	M3-BIORES, Katholieke Universitëit Leuven, Belgium
Robert Allen	University of Southampton, UK
Sergio Alvarez	Boston College, USA
Sridhar P. Arjunan	RMIT University, Australia
Ofer Barnea	Tel Aviv University, Israel
Eberhard Beck	Brandenburg University of Applied Sciences, Germany
Egon L. van den Broek	Utrecht University, The Netherlands
Guy Carrault	University of Rennes 1, France
Maria Claudia F. Castro	Centro Universitário da FEI, Brazil
Sergio Cerutti	Polytechnic University of Milan, Italy
Bruno Cornelis	Vrije Universiteit Brussel, Belgium
Jan Cornelis	Vrije Universiteit Brussel, Belgium
Adam Czajka	University of Notre Dame, USA
Bruce Denby	Université Pierre et Marie Curie, France
Gordana Jovanovic Dolecek	Institute INAOE, Mexico
Petr Dolezel	University of Pardubice, Czech Republic
Pier Luigi Emiliani	Italian National Research Council, Italy
Pedro Encarnação	Universidade Católica Portuguesa, Portugal
Poree fabienne	Université de Rennes 1, France
Luca Faes	Università degli Studi di Trento, Italy
Dimitrios Fotiadis	University of Ioannina, Greece
Arfan Ghani	Coventry University, UK
Inan Güler	Gazi University, Turkey
Thomas Hinze	Friedrich Schiller University Jena, Germany
Roberto Hornero	University of Valladolid, Spain
Jiri Jan	University of Technology Brno, Czech Republic
Tzyy-Ping Jung	University of California San Diego, USA
Theodoros Kostoulas	University of Geneva, Switzerland
Dagmar Krefting	Berlin University of Applied Sciences, Germany
Vaclav Kremen	Czech Technical University in Prague, Czech Republic
Lenka Lhotska	Czech Technical University in Prague, Czech Republic
Julián David Arias Londoño	Universidad de Antioquia, Colombia
Ana Rita Londral	Universidade de Lisboa, Portugal
Harald Loose	Brandenburg University of Applied Sciences, Germany

Carlos Maciel	University of São Paulo, Brazil
Hari Krishna Maganti	Saga, UK
Armando Malanda	Universidad Pública de Navarra, Spain
Pramod Kumar Meher	Nanyang Technological University, Singapore
Jirí Mekyska	Brno University of Technology, Czech Republic
Roberto Merletti	Politecnico di Torino, Italy
Mihaela Morega	University Politehnica of Bucharest, Romania
Percy Nohama	Pontifícia Universidade Católica do Paraná, Brazil
Andres Orozco-Duque	Instituto Tecnológico Metropolitano, Colombia
Krzysztof Pancerz	University of Rzeszow, Poland
Gennaro Percannella	University of Salerno, Italy
Vitor Pires	Escola Superior de Tecnologia de Setúbal, Instituto Politécnico de Setúbal, Portugal
Ales Prochazka	University of Chemistry and Technology, Czech Republic
Heather Ruskin	Dublin City University, Ireland
Tomasz Rutkowski	The University of Tokyo, Japan
Andres Santos	Universidad Politécnica de Madrid, Spain
Roberto Sassi	Università degli studi di Milano, Italy
Edward Sazonov	University of Alabama, USA
Gerald Schaefer	Loughborough University, UK
Christian Schmidt	University of Rostock, Germany
Reinhard Schneider	Fachhochschule Vorarlberg, Austria
Lotfi Senhadji	University of Rennes 1, France
Samuel Silva	Universidade de Aveiro, Portugal
Alan A Stocker	University of Pennyslvania, USA
Nicola Strisciuglio	University of Groningen, The Netherlands
Asser Tantawi	IBM, USA
António Teixeira	University of Aveiro, Portugal
João Paulo Teixeira	Polytechnic Institute of Bragança, Portugal
Carlos Eduardo Thomaz	Centro Universitário da FEI, Brazil
Carlos M. Travieso	University of Las Palmas de Gran Canaria, Spain
Pedro Gómez Vilda	Universidad Politécnica de Madrid, Spain
Gert-Jan de Vries	Philips Research Healthcare, The Netherlands
Yuanyuan Wang	Fudan University, China
Quan Wen	University of Electronic Science and Technology of China, China
Kerstin Witte	Otto von Guericke University Magdeburg, Germany
Didier Wolf	Research Centre for Automatic Control, CRAN CNRS UMR 7039, France
Pew-Thian Yap	University of North Carolina at Chapel Hill, USA
Chia-Hung Yeh	National Sun Yat-sen University, Taiwan
Rafal Zdunek	Wroclaw University of Technology, Poland
Li Zhuo	Beijing University of Technology, China

HEALTHINF Program Committee

Anurag Agrawal	CSIR Institute of Genomics and Integrative Biology, Center for Translational Research in Asthma and Lung, India
Hesham Ali	University of Nebraska at Omaha, USA
Adil Alpkocak	Dokuz Eylul University, Turkey
Flora Amato	Università degli Studi di Napoli Federico II, Italy
Francois Andry	Philips, France
Wassim Ayadi	LERIA, University of Angers, France and LaTICE, University of Tunis, Tunisia
Bert-Jan van Beijnum	University of Twente, The Netherlands
Patrick Boissy	Université de Sherbrooke and Research Centre on Aging, Canada
Sorana D. Bolboaca	Iuliu Hatieganu University of Medicine and Pharmacy, Cluj-Napoca, Romania
Alessio Bottrighi	Universitá del Piemonte Orientale, Italy
Andrew D. Boyd	University of Illinois at Chicago, USA
Egon L. van den Broek	Utrecht University, The Netherlands
Berry de Bruijn	National Research Council, Canada
Federico Cabitza	Università degli Studi di Milano-Bicocca, Italy
Eric Campo	LAAS CNRS, France
Guillermo Lopez Campos	The University of Melbourne, Australia
Marc Cavazza	University of Kent, UK
Philip K. Chan	Florida Institute of Technology, USA
Taridzo Chomutare	University Hospital of North Norway, Norway
Mihail Cocosila	Athabasca University, Canada
Miguel Coimbra	IT, University of Porto, Portugal
Emmanuel Conchon	XLIM, France
Carlos Costa	Universidade de Aveiro, Portugal
Andre Dekker	MAASTRO Clinick, The Netherlands
Chrysanne DiMarco	University of Waterloo, Canada
Liliana Dobrica	University Politehnica of Bucharest, Romania
Stephan Dreiseitl	Upper Austria University of Applied Sciences at Hagenberg, Austria
José Fonseca	UNINOVA, Portugal
Daniel Ford	Dell Research, USA
Christoph M. Friedrich	University of Applied Sciences and Arts Dortmund, Germany
Ioannis Fudos	University of Ioannina, Greece
Henry Gabb	University of Illinois at Urbana-Champaign, USA
Hugo Gamboa	New University of Lisbon, Portugal
Mauro Giacomini	University of Genoa, Italy
Laura Giarré	Università degli Studi di Palermo, Italy

Jan Sliwa	Bern University of Applied Sciences, Switzerland
George Spyrou	The Cyprus Institute of Neurology and Genetics, Cyprus
Jan Stage	Aalborg University, Denmark
Vicente Traver	Universidad Politécnica de Valencia, Spain
Mohy Uddin	King Abdullah International Medical Research Center, Saudi Arabia
Gary Ushaw	Newcastle University, UK
Aristides Vagelatos	CTI, Greece
Sumithra Velupillai	KTH, Sweden and King's College, UK
Sitalakshmi Venkatraman	Melbourne Polytechnic, Australia
Francisco Veredas	Universidad de Málaga, Spain
Justin Wan	University of Waterloo, Canada
Szymon Wilk	Poznan University of Technology, Poland
Janusz Wojtusiak	George Mason University, USA
Clement T. Yu	University of Illinois at Chicago, USA
Xuezhong Zhou	Beijing Jiaotong University, China
André Zúquete	Universidade de Aveiro, Portugal

HEALTHINF Additional Reviewers

Koundinya Desiraju	Institute of Genomics and Integrative Biology, Mall Road, Delhi, India
Angela Locoro	Università degli Studi di Milano-Bicocca, Italy
Imen Megdiche	IRIT, France
Sebastian Rauh	Heilbronn University of Applied Sciences, Germany
Kateryna Sergieieva	Heilbronn University of Applied Science, Germany

Invited Speakers

Bart M. ter Haar Romeny	Eindhoven University of Technology (TU/e), The Netherlands
Kristina Höök	Royal Institute of Technology, Sweden
Bethany Bracken	Charles River Analytics Inc., USA
Hugo Plácido da Silva	IT, Institute of Telecommunications, Portugal

Contents

Bioinformatics Models, Methods and Algorithms

Bio-inspired Systems and Signal Processing

Health Informatics

Biomedical Electronics and Devices

An Electronic-Engineered Sensory Sternal Retractor Aimed at Post-sternotomy Pain Reduction

Giovanni Saggio[1(✉)], Alessandra Bianco[2], Giancarlo Orengo[1],
Giuseppe Tancredi[1], Costantino Del Gaudio[2], and Jacob Zeitani[3]

[1] Department of Electronic Engineering, University of Rome "Tor Vergata",
Rome, Italy
saggio@uniroma2.it
[2] Department of Enterprise Engineering, INSTM Res. Unit,
University of Rome "Tor Vergata", Rome, Italy
[3] German Hospital Tirana, Tirana, Albania

Abstract. The median sternotomy can rise in rib and/or sternum micro/macro-fractures and/or brachial plexus injuries, which can even evolve in chronic pain with significant impact on patient's quality life. Post-sternotomy chronic pain is recognized as a multifactorial complex issue, and it has been assessed that sternum retraction forces, applied by the surgeons, can be considered one of these factors. In order to investigate the behavior of these forces, we developed a reliable and sterilizable system, to monitor the retraction forces along the hemisternums. Therefore, a Finochietto sternal retractor was instrumented by means of ultra-thin force sensors interfaced with ad hoc electronic circuitry. Two different sets of sensors were adopted, one of which able to support autoclave operating conditions. In-vitro tests were performed by means of a made on purpose dummy. The instrumented retractor allows monitoring the force exerted on both the arms during the opening procedure. Force versus time patterns were acquired and stored, and so we determined how the forces are distributed in terms of their mean, maximum and plateaus. Results demonstrate the reliability of the instrumented retractor in measuring forces, up to 400 N. Cost-effectiveness and feasibility can be considered further additional values of the proposed instrumented retractor.

Keywords: Chronic chest pain · Retractor · Median sternotomy
Force sensor

1 Introduction

The first median sternotomy has been performed in 1897, to remove lymph nodes. Since then, only six decades after, the median sternotomy has become the standard approach to the mediastinum, following Julian's report [1] where the superiority over thoracotomy was described underlining its less time-consuming, and higher tolerability by the patients.

© Springer International Publishing AG, part of Springer Nature 2018
N. Peixoto et al. (Eds.): BIOSTEC 2017, CCIS 881, pp. 3–18, 2018.
https://doi.org/10.1007/978-3-319-94806-5_1

Briefly, to access the mediastinum through the median sternotomy, a skin incision is made, approximately 2 cm under the sternal notch and extended below the xiphoid. The exact midline over the sternum is marked with electrocautery to avoid faulty sternotomy. Before the sternum incision is made, a pathway is create above the suprasternal ligament and then continued beneath the manubrium and finally, performed as well under the xiphoid to guarantee the separation of the mediastinum structures from the posterior sternum bone.

Although, in comparison to extensive thoracotomy, midline sternotomy is less traumatic, persistent postoperative pain remain the Achilles' heel, affecting negatively early postoperative respiratory function, delayed hospital discharge and increasing costs [2–4]. The process of pain is difficult to assess [5], anyway the pain is considered chronic when localized in the surgical site and persist over three months. In a prospective study, a number of independent predictors for persistent thoracic pain following sternotomy were identified, including urgent surgery, and re-sternotomy [6]. In this study, at one year, 42 (35%) patients reported chronic thoracic pain. Similarly, another work reported the prevalence of post-operative pain as high as 39.3% at the mean time of 28 months after surgery [7]. In 2001, Mazzeffi and Khelemsky [8] estimated a 28% overall incidence of non-cardiac pain one year after surgery. Several studies assessed that women are substantially more likely to suffer early and chronic postoperative pain than men [6, 9], and that the prevalence of post-sternotomy chronic pain decreases with age [6, 8]. These studies highlight the negative impact on daily life of the population who experienced sternotomy and suffer postoperative pain. In fact with the introduction of less invasive surgical procedures to treat cardiac pathologies, although with limited surgical field, surgeons who are in favor claim that it is not only cosmetic, but guaranteeing better and faster post-operative recovery.

Chronic post-sternotomy pain can be related to patient's age, gender and degenerative process like osteoporosis. It can be also related directly to the surgical procedure, including secondary sternal osteomyelitis and/or sternocostal chondritis, incomplete bone healing. If the internal thoracic arteries are harvested in myocardial revascularization, the different retractors, used to facilitated vessel exposure, add additional trauma. In this contest the way of harvesting and the use of ellectrocautery might affect wound healing and persistence pain.

To access to the mediastinum, retractors are being used to allow adequate surgical field. Hemi-sternums separation extent of the force impressed during sternum opening might lead to rib fracture, eventually associated to brachial plexus injury (BPI) [10–14]. Thus, there is an actual clinical need to provide to the surgeons suitable instrumented retractors able to monitor in real time the forces exerted on the two halves during the sternum opening procedure. In this way, by monitoring forces applied on the sternum, it will be possible to find the balance between adequate surgical field and excessive trauma to the chest. By evaluating major risk factors, width chest opening can be tailored to the patients. For example if female gender is prone to chronic pain, chest separation should be reduced to minimum.

Furthermore, with the increasing interest of shifting the cardiac surgery procedures from full to partial sternotomy, including the "J" and "T" incisions, the proposed study might be useful to evaluate and compare the forces applied on the sternum in the various surgical approaches to determine the best access, allowing at the same time the optimal surgical view and successively good quality of life.

Only few data are available for the actual value of the forces exerted by a retractor on the skeletal cage, dummy reproduced [15], or of corpses or animal models [16]. Aigner et al. [17] pointed out that data obtained from human patients are not presently available in the literature probably due to the lack of an instrumented sternal retractor readily suitable for the translation to surgery.

For this purpose, we designed and realized a sterilizable system based on a commonly adopted straight sternal retractor (Finocchietto) equipped with ultrathin force sensors and conditioning electronic circuitry. The forces experienced during the retraction were monitored in real-time by means of a home-made dummy.

The idea is to acquire data on the intensity and distribution of exerted retraction forces during hemi-sternums separation in view of future challenging clinical studies aimed to reduce the risk of chronic post-sternotomy pain.

2 Materials

A commonly adopted straight sternal retractor, Finochietto type (Fig. 1a), was equipped with both ultra-thin force sensors (Fig. 1b and c) and electronic circuitry. The resulting electronic-engineered "sensory retractor" was tested by means of a home-made dummy.

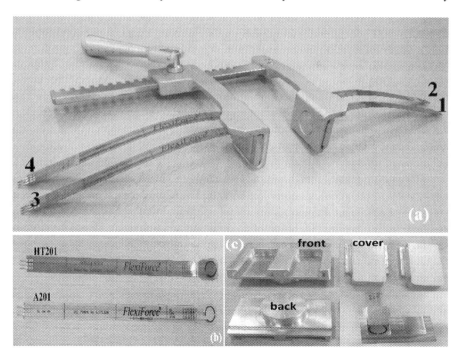

Fig. 1. (a) The Finochietto retractor equipped with the four sensors placed in positions designed from 1 to 4 according to the figure. (b) The ultra-thin force sensors, HT201 (top) and A201 (bottom) types. (c) Aluminum sensors' housings: front, back and cover [15].

2.1   Ultra-Thin Force Sensors

We considered two different types of commercial piezo-resistive flexible ultra-thin (0.203 mm, 0.008 in.) off-the-shelf force sensors, the FlexiForce® A201 (these according to [17]) and the FlexiForce® HT201 (both types by Tekscan, Boston, USA), having a circular sensing area of 9.53 mm (0.375 in.) in diameter, on one edge, connected through a silver strip to the electric contacts, on the other edge (Fig. 1b). The A201 type, with a polyester substrate, can measure forces up to 440 N, within a temperature operating range of −9 °C to +60 °C (15 °F to 140 °F). The HT201 type, with a polyimide substrate, can measure forces up to 445 N, within −9 °C to +204 °C (15 °F to 400 °F).

2.2   Sensor Testing

To assess sensor characterization under known forces, we used a universal tensile test machine (LRX, by Lloyd Instruments, Berwyn, PA, US), showed in Fig. 2a. It is a single column digital machine able to provide a constant compression/extension force, up to 2500 N depending on the used load cell (Fig. 2b and c). Several parameters can be set, in particular the fall and rise speed, used to measure the repeatability and reproducibility of measurements, and the load cell sensibility. Machine operations are controlled by the NEXIGEN software, which can simultaneously analyze the test results sampled @1 kHz and acquired through the RS232 interface.

One sensor sample at a time was positioned under the load cell.

The used load cell was an electronic component (transducer), made of an elastic hard metal (e.g. stainless steel) to which is connected a Wheatstone bridge, with four strain gauges varying their resistance under traction, which generates a voltage signal depending on the cell deformation.

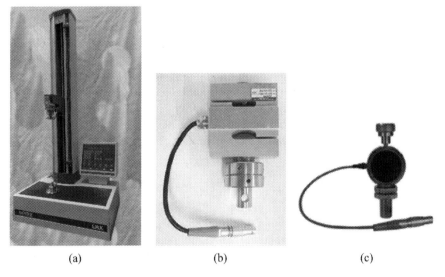

(a)   (b)   (c)

Fig. 2. (a) LRX (Lloyd Instrument) testing machine used for sensor characterization under compression, (b) and (c) Load cells used for sensor characterization.

In such a way, the electric voltage value is referred to the force applied. The voltage signal is amplified, calibrated and compensated with temperature, then processed by an algorithm to correct the device nonlinearity. Consequently, the value of the applied force was determined, taking into account deformation and material characteristics. Two load cells of 50 N and 500 N, respectively (Fig. 2a and b) were used for sensor characterization.

2.3   Data Acquisition

The electrical resistance values (outputs of the sensors) were converted into voltages by means of voltage dividers. Those voltage signals fed an electronic circuitry, based on an Arduino-compatible microcontroller board, which operated 10 bit digital conversions and sent data to a personal computer via USB port. The following data process was handled by ad-hoc home-made LabView (by National Instruments, TX, USA) and Matlab (by MathWorks, Massachusetts, USA) routines.

Front-End Electronics. The front-end electronic circuit was developed on the basis of a previous one, which was made to interface flex and electromyography sensors [18]. In particular, the electrical resistance values (outputs of the sensors) were converted into voltages by means of voltage dividers (Fig. 3a), differently with respect to the inverting operational amplifier recommended by the manufacturer (Fig. 3b). This was to reduce the circuit size rather than provide signal amplification. Moreover, the inverting amplifier needs a double supply, whereas this circuit shares the same +5 V bias supply of the following microcontroller board, taken from the USB cable connecting to the personal computer (PC). The front-end circuit is a simple voltage divider, where the sensor is represented by the series resistor. A shunt capacitance of 100 nF was used to filter noise coming from the bias supply (Fig. 3a). When the force applied to each sensor increases, the sensor resistance decreases, and the corresponding output voltage, accordingly to Eq. (1), proportionally increases.

$$V_{OUT} = V_{BIAS} \frac{R_P}{R_{SENS} + R_P} \qquad (1)$$

The values of each shunt resistors RP was determined taking into account some needs. In particular, RP has to protect each sensor against excessive currents, and has to guarantee the largest-as-possible output voltage swing so to allow adequate resolution for the following digital conversion. With a force value ranging from 1 to 400 N, the sensor resistance span of 1 MΩ roughly. Since the maximum allowable current for the sensor is 2.5 mA, when the sensor is in short circuit, the RP value must be higher than

$$R_P > \frac{5\,V}{2.5\,mA} = 2\,k\Omega \qquad (2)$$

but correctly determined as the geometric mean of the extreme sensor resistance values, in accordance with the findings in [19].

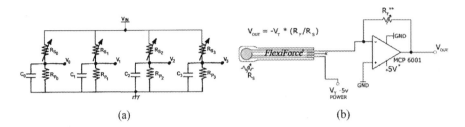

Fig. 3. (a) Adopted front-end circuits for the four FlexiForce A201 and HT201 sensors, (b) front-end circuit for the FlexiForce A201 and HT201 sensors recommended by Tekscan.

The digital conversion is made by a 10 bit analog to digital converter (ADC), to which corresponds a voltage resolution given by Eq. (3)

$$V_{LSB} = \frac{5\,\text{V}}{2^{10} - 1} \simeq 4.9\,\text{mV} \tag{3}$$

The minimum voltage from the front-end circuit, in case of zero applied force, calculated by Eq. (1) with $R_{SENS} = 1\,\text{M}\Omega$, should be greater than V_{LSB}

$$V_{OUTmin} = 5\,\text{V}\frac{R_P}{1\,\text{M}\Omega + R_P} > 4.9\,\text{mV} \tag{4}$$

which implies $R_P > 1\,\text{k}\Omega$. Finally, the selected value was $R_P = 47\,\text{k}\Omega$.

Digital Processing. The voltage signals fed an electronic board circuitry, based on Arduino Uno, which operated 10 bit digital conversions and sent data to a personal computer via USB port at a sampling rate of 175 Hz. Afterwards, the Arduino Uno board was replaced with Luigino328 (an Arduino-compatible microcontroller board based on an ATMega328 MCU). This was because Luigino328 allows switching the bias supply to an external one, without overcharge the USB port of a Personal Computer (PC), which could be damaged for supply current greater than 500 mA, whereas in Arduino the supply from the USB port has the highest priority. Luigino328, in fact, has also a small microcontroller (PIC16F) for the following tasks: (1) to handle the voltage selector, (2) to disconnect the serial port when programming the board, without remove shields using the serial port and (3) to exclude the SmartReset function, avoiding to reset the board every time a serial port is connected, allowing the running program to go on independently. This device allowed interfacing the LabView integrated development environment (IDE) without the sudden resets which occur in Arduino. Finally, the Luigino328 is equipped with the LM1117 voltage regulator, which is more reliable than the MC33269D of Arduino, especially for high supply currents.

Two software routines were realized for the ATMega328, the former to read the output of only one sensor, to perform its characterization, the latter to read simultaneously the four sensors on the sternal retractor, to register its strength on the body.

Serial Communication. To start a serial communication, it is possible to select the transmission speed (baud rate) in bit per second (bps), within 300–115200 bps. The standard rate is 9600, whereas we used 19200 bps. The default data length is 8 bit, no parity and one stop bit. We adopted the RS-232 as standard communication protocol, reduced to 9 pin (usually COM), virtually implemented on a USB port, being COM ports unavailable on up-to-date PC.

The ADC converts the analog sample in a 10 bit digital string. For serial communication, however, the 10 bit string is divided into two bytes (8 bit). Three token bytes (all 1's) were inserted before each data sample. Actually, two bytes would be enough for the token string, because the data bits cannot be all 1's, coming from a 10 bit ADC, six bits are definitely 0's. We added one more token byte to make the system more reliable with strong EM interferences. Considering the start (0) and stop (1) bit before and after each byte, the string length for each acquisition is 50 bit, as represented in Table 1. When the acquisition system reads simultaneously the four sensor applied to the sternal retractor, the three token bytes are transmitted only once, then two bytes for each sensor, for a total number of 110 bits, according to the scheme in Table 2.

Table 1. Serial packet transmission for data acquisition from a single sensor device.

0	Byte	1	0	byte	1	0	byte	1	0	byte	1	0	byte	1
	3 token bytes (30 bits)							2 data bytes (20 bits)						
	50 bits													

Table 2. Serial packet transmission for simultaneous data acquisition from four sensor devices.

3 token bytes	sensor 1 2 bytes	sensor 2 2 bytes	sensor 3 2 bytes	sensor 4 2 bytes
30 bits	20 bits	20 bits	20 bits	20 bits
110 bits				

2.4 Sternal Retractor

An aluminum straight Finochietto retractor (by Tekno-Medical Optik-Chirurgie GmbH Tuttlingen, Germany) was equipped with an array of four force sensors. Two sensors were placed on the blade of the mobile arm and two on the blade of the fixed arm (Fig. 1a), the size of the blade being 44.4 mm (1.75 in.) in length and 30.9 mm (1.22 in.) in width. The sum of the single detected forces on each blade yielded the total force for both the fixed and the mobile arm. The ultra-thin force sensors were placed in ad-hoc smooth aluminum housings (Fig. 1c).

2.5   In-vitro Test

In-vitro tests of the instrumented Finochietto retractor were performed by means of a made-on-purpose dummy built up with four gas pistons (manufactured by Team Pro, Italy), two for each side, laterally anchored to a wooden shell (Fig. 4a). Different set of gas pistons were evaluated, i.e., 150 N, 100 N and 80 N. On the basis of several opening/closing cycles performed by three different surgeons, the dummy equipped with the 80 N pistons offered the most realistic feeling with respect to the clinical practice. However, pistons can be easily replaced. The instrumented retractor, equipped with the four force sensors, was positioned into the dummy (Fig. 4b).

The Authors are aware that the mechanics of the proposed dummy is very simple with respect to the complex biomechanics of the rib cage. Anyway, the idea was to realize a dummy able to support the test of the device and not meant to be taken as a biomechanical model of the rib cage.

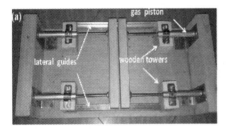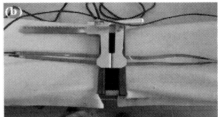

Fig. 4. (a) The home made dummy built up using four gas pistons fixed to a wooden skeleton, the compressible parts positioned outward in a face-to-face configuration. In vitro tests: (b) the instrumented Finochietto retractor positioned into the dummy equipped with the four force sensors (S1, S2, S3, S4).

3   Methods

3.1   Sensor Characterization

In this section the selected methods for static and dynamic characterization of the force sensors will be deeply described. Both of them were accomplished with the LRX testing machine with two load cells for compression up to 5 N and 500 N, respectively. Due to the sensor thinness, the sensor sample was placed on a stainless steel platform, and a 10 mm diameter steel disk was placed on the active area of the sensor, to achieve the required pressure on device during the jack fall down. References on sensor location help to replace the sample measurement in the same conditions.

Static Characterization. In the static characterization the descent rate of the jack was set to 5 mm/min and the static measurements were acquired @5 N, 10 N, 20 N, 30 N and 40 N with the 50 N load cell, and from 40 N to 400 N, step 40 N, with the 500 N load cell. Two minutes break were set before each step to acquire measurements, through the LabView-Arduino interface.

Considering a baud rate of 19200 bps for 2 min or 120 s, 50 bit for each sensor sample, the acquired resistance samples are $(19200/50) \cdot 120 = 46080$. Waiting 52 s, when the sensor response was considered enough stable, 3000 resistance samples were considered for a duration of almost 7 s, of which the average and the standard deviation were calculated. In the same time interval, 30 samples of the force magnitude were considered among the only 384 samples stored by the test machine acquisition system in 120 s, because the sampling frequency is much smaller than that of Luigino/LabView interface.

Figure 5a and b shows the characterization of the HT201 and A201 devices, respectively. The sensor resistance is represented as the average and standard deviation among eight sensor samples as a function of the average compression force at each step. Ultrathin flexible force sensors HT201 and A201 both showed exponential resistance decay with the impressed force. Plots demonstrate the same behavior for A201 and HT201 sensors, but in the force range 30–440 N standard deviations are very small (7–42 kΩ, 8–51 kΩ respectively), whereas in the range 5–30 N standard deviations become high (96–482 kΩ, 47–1000 kΩ respectively).

In order to investigate if HT201 sensors can effectively support autoclaving conditions, these sensors were also characterized following the same procedure after five cycles of autoclave treatment (VaporMatic 770, Asal Srl, Milan, Italy). HT201 sensors did not show a significantly different behavior after five cycles of autoclave conditioning, which is a reasonable result since these sensors have been specifically designed for high temperature applications (up to 400 °F, approximately 200 °C). In any case, in the occurrence of degradation in performances, those sensors can be easily and conveniently replaced.

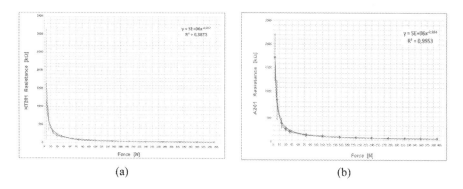

(a)   (b)

Fig. 5. (a) Measured resistance versus force (R vs. F) for different sensor (a) HT201 type, (b) A201 type.

Dynamic Characterization. Dynamic characterization was made to verify repeatability of a single sensor sample and check whether the static and dynamic behaviors are similar. We set the same force range but four descent rate for the jack: 1 mm/min, 5 mm/min, 30 mm/min and 60 mm/min. The machine repeated 5 iterations forward and back for each speed rate, each time increasing and decreasing at a constant rate the traction force from 0 N to 400 N and down again to 0 N. The repetition period depends on the descent rate of the jack.

Results for the average sensor resistance against increasing force with different speed, superimposed for comparison with two equal and symmetrical static characteristics in Fig. 6a and b show A201 sensors behave with lower repeatability than HT201 counterparts, changing the variation rate of the applied force.

Dynamic characterization was also repeated after five cycles of autoclave treatment for HT201 sensors, and characteristics do not show a significantly different behavior after treatment, as in the static case (so results are not presented for sake of brevity).

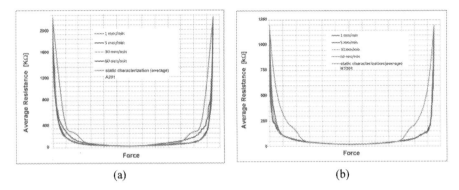

        (a)   (b)

Fig. 6. Average sensor resistance against increasing force with different speed, superimposed for comparison with two equal and symmetrical static characteristics for A201 (a) and HT201 (b) devices.

3.2   In-vitro Test

In the limited literature concerning the measurement of sternal forces, both on animals and corpses, a standard protocol to regulate the data acquisition and processing is missing, therefore it is impossible to compare the performance of systems developed by different research teams, because measurements results were obtained in different conditions, such as the speed, the aperture number and points, the human or animal subject under test. For this purpose, a statistical approach was applied [20] to sensory sternal retractor assessments, to compare different systems by evaluating mean, range and standard deviation tables for each tested subject. Since typical sternal apertures in cardiac surgery range from 5 to 10 cm, the standard conditions set out for the test applied to sternal force measurements are:

(1) 5 cm wide aperture (rest position)
(2) 10 cm wide aperture (operating position)

Moreover, to assure the same conditions in different measurement sessions, special references were inserted on the dummy to make the retractor positioned always in the same way.

Test procedure consisted in four opening/closing cycles of the dummy by means of the instrumented retractor up to two different fixed widths, i.e. 5 cm (1.97 in.) and 10 cm (3.94 in.). On the basis of the feeling/practice of the surgeons, each opening/closing cycle was performed at a roughly constant rate of 2 s/cm, that is 10 s for 5 cm (1.97 in.) and 20 s for 10 cm (3.94 in.). The two final positions (5 cm, 1.97 in. and 10 cm, 3.94 in.) were held for 60 s so to evidence response decay, if any. The response of all the sensors in terms of force (F) versus time (t) was real-time acquired. Then, mean force (F_{mean}), maximum force (F_{max}) and plateau force ($F_{plateau}$) were evaluated, the last as the mean value of the force recorded during 60 s in the final rest position. The distribution of the forces exerted along the two halves of the dummy was also determined.

4   Results and Discussion

4.1   Recent Findings

The investigated range of force (i.e., 5–400 N) includes the values reported by Bolotin et al. [21] and by Aigner et al. [17]. In more details, Bolotin et al. reported the first known successfully attempt to employ an instrumented retractor to monitor forces during cardiothoracic surgery. They equipped stainless steel curved profile retractor blades with strain gauges to measure applied forces during retraction, and reported results for lateral thoracotomy and median sternotomy on cadavers and sheep. The average force applied during force-controlled retraction was (77.88 N ± 38.85 N) and the maximum force displayed during force-controlled retraction (323.99 N ± 127.79 N).

Aigner et al. equipped a straight (SSR) (MTEZ 424 735; Heintel GmbH, Vienna, Austria) and a curved retractor (CSR) (Dubost Thoracic Retractor DC30000-00; Delacroix-Chevalier, Paris, France), with FlexiForce sensors, A201 type (Tekscan Inc). The blade of the mobile arm of the SSR (length 6.5 cm and width 4.5 cm) was equipped with two arrays of 4 sensors, and the mobile arm of the CSR (length 9.7 cm, width 4.8 cm, curvature radius 21 cm) was equipped with two arrays of 5 sensors. The sum of the single sensor forces yielded the total force. Force distribution, total force and displacement were recorded to a spread width of 10 cm in 18 corpses (11 males and 7 females). For every corpse, 4 measurement iterations were performed for both retractors; each retraction was performed in 14.3 s ± 6.2 s to reach 10 cm widespread. The Authors concluded that the shape of sternal retractors considerably influences the force distribution on the sternal incision. On the other side, it is reported that the total mean retraction force was not significant different between SSR and CSR (222.8 N ± 52.9 N versus 226.4 N ± 71.9 N). Nevertheless, the recorded mean total force was remarkably dependent on the gender. For the first retraction, it was 256.2 N ± 43.3 N for males and only 174.9 N ± 52.9 N for females.

Moreover, in the case of SSR the forces on the cranial and caudal sternum are significantly higher than in the median section. For SSR the maximum total force for full retraction was 349.4 N ± 77.9 N, while force distribution during the first retraction for the cranial/median/caudal part of the sternum was 101.5 N ± 43.9/29.1 N ± 33.9/63.0 N ± 31.4 N.

Aigner et al. assessed that the force distribution did not change significantly for the other 3 retractions, for the different investigated spread widths (i.e. 5, 7.5, and 10 cm) and was not gender dependent. The maximum force for full retraction was 493.6 N, whereas the smallest maximum force was 159.0 N.

4.2   Finochietto In-vitro Results

Our results obtained for HT201 sensors are resumed in Table 3 and the typical force (N) versus time (s) patterns are presented in Fig. 7. In all cases, a high stability of the response to a fixed exerted force was evidenced. In fact, the value of $F_{plateau}$ showed a mean standard deviation as low as 0.33 N ± 0.16 N. Some valuable information can be obtained from the acquired data.

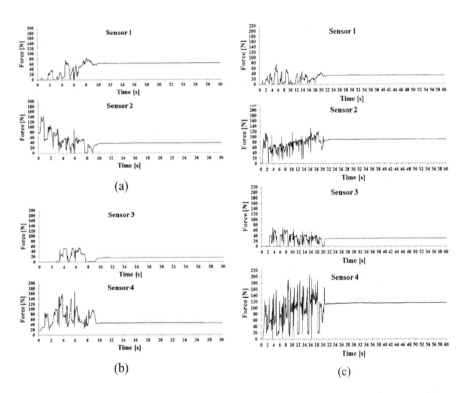

Fig. 7. (a) and (b) Response of the four sensors (housed as shown in Fig. 1a) in terms of force [N] versus time [s] during the 5 cm opening procedure. (c) Response of the four sensors (housed as showed in Fig. 1a) in terms of force [N] versus time [s] during the 10 cm opening procedure.

For example, the total average force for the mobile blade ranged between 60.1 N ± 6.0 N for 5 cm spread and 98.0 N ± 36.5 N for 10 cm spread, as expected for a dummy built-up with 80 N gas pistons. The deviation with respect to this value is also expected and is to be attributed to the uneven pressure distribution onto the circular sensors due to the rough surface finishing of the contact area i.e. wood in the dummy.

It is interesting to observe during the retraction, the Finochietto experienced along the mobile arm a total F_{max} (sensor#4 + sensor#3) that exceeded 200 N, ranging from 219.1 N $\pm$ 9.7 N for 5 cm spread and 266.6 N $\pm$ 25.4 N for 10 cm spread.

The force distribution along the retractor blade is also particularly interesting. In fact, in all cases, the highest maximum force (F_{max}) was detected by sensor #4 positioned on the mobile arm in proximal (cranial) position (Fig. 1a), the value ranged between 156.4 N $\pm$ 12.5 N for 5 cm spread and 199.7 N $\pm$ 21.2 N for 10 cm spread. The lowest F_{max} values were 62.7 N $\pm$ 5.4 N for 5 cm and 66.9 N $\pm$ 4.3 N for 10 cm, registered in correspondence of sensor #3 of the mobile arm in distal (caudal) position.

Interestingly, median sternotomy in corpses performed by means of a straight sternal retractor gave a comparable force distribution [17]. This result suggests that the made-on-purpose dummy enable to perform reliable test and thus it might also be employed by surgeons in order to assess their own learning curve for each specific instrumented retractor. Furthermore, sensor #4 detected also the highest value of ($F_{max} - F_{mean}$), i.e. 114.6 N $\pm$ 12.9 N and 116.9 N $\pm$ 16.9 N, respectively, for 10 cm and 5 cm opening. For all the other sensors, this value does not exceed 75.7 N $\pm$ 21.1 N, independently from the position on the retractor.

On the basis of these results, the presented implementation system can be considered a valuable tool to evaluate intensity and distribution of retraction forces in human patients for conventional sternotomy procedures. On the basis of our knowledge, these data are not yet available in the Literature. As already previously suggested by Bolotin [16], the final goal is to develop clinical studies aimed at coherently correlating the biomechanical information obtained for a specific surgical procedure with the incidence of post-sternotomy chronic pain. In this respect, for example, the actual outcomes of cranial versus caudal positioning of the sternal retractor could be assessed. As far as we know, in the past decade such kinds of studies have not yet been performed probably due to the lack of an implemented user-friendly retractor suitable for conventional clinical sterilization process.

Moreover, the performance of this versatile design might also contribute to estimate the actual impact of minimally invasive cardiac surgery techniques. In fact, since the 1990s, these procedures are receiving an increasing interest due to a number of potential advantages with respect to traditional sternotomy, including reduced operative trauma, less perioperative morbidity along with improved aesthetic outcomes, shorter hospital stay and accelerated rehabilitation [22]. According to recent studies, the overall outcomes and costs are believed to be comparable with those of conventional sternotomy [23, 24]. It has to be considered that partial sternotomy, in minimally invasive cardiac surgery procedures, allows the displacement of only a part of the hemi-thorax, which might be subject to increased exerted forces eventually leading to excessive stress on the "dynamic" chest wall. The proposed study might be useful in the clinical setting to determine the optimal balance between surgical field and sternum separation.

The system can be considered cost-effective and potentially adaptable to different surgical retractors simply providing the appropriate housings.

Table 3. Values of the mean, maximum and plateau forces (expressed in N) measured by HT201 sensors positioned according to Fig. 1a (i.e. S1, S2, S3, S4). The related standard deviation values are reported in parentheses [15].

Spread	Force [N]	S1	S2	S3	S4	S1+S2 fixed blade	S3+S4 mobile blade
5 cm	Mean	60.8 (5.7)	39.2 (4.4)	18.3 (2.1)	41.8 (7.7)	100.1 (8.5)	60.1 (6.1)
	Max	97.3 (10.6)	115.0 (19.5)	62.7 (5.4)	156.4 (12.5)	212.2 (14.8)	219.1 (9.7)
	Plateau	63.9 (5.8)	39.4 (4.9)	17.9 (1.8)	38.3 (8.3)	103.3 (9.0)	56.3 (7.2)
	Max-mean	36.5 (8.7)	75.7 (21.1)	44.4 (4.0)	114.6 (12.9)	112.2 (12.5)	159.0 (12.6)
10 cm	Mean	37.6 (8.8)	82.5 (5.60)	15.2 (10.4)	82.8 (26.8)	120.1 (12.8)	98.0 (36.5)
	Max	79.6 (17.5)	126.3 (6.62)	66.9 (4.3)	199.7 (21.3)	205.9 (20.8)	266.6 (25.4)
	Plateau	41.2 (6.7)	89.1 (7.02)	13.1 (12.9)	84.7 (32.0)	130.2 (11.7)	97.8 (44.4)
	Max-mean	42.0 (14.1)	43.8 (6.98)	54.7 (9.4)	116.9 (16.9)	85.8 (13.6)	168.6 (26.3)

5   Conclusions

Median sternotomy is a surgical incision through the sternum, then after to allow access to the mediastinum a retractor is positioned. Wide opening of the hemi-sternum, by means of the retractor, guarantee better view and facilitate the surgical procedure. However, its increase the stress on the sternum halves and ribs, leading to partial or complete fractures and/or micro-fractures resulting in post-operative and chronic pain in a non-negligible number of patients.

By measuring the forces during different opening procedures, we demonstrated how it can be possible to understand and find the compromise between adequate surgical field and the risk for sternum and ribs fractures, aiming at improving patients postoperative coarse.

Within such a frame, this paper reports a new electronic-engineered sensory sternal retractor aimed at measuring the forces impressed by the plates when opening a dummy ribcage, so in an in-vitro median sternotomy condition.

We demonstrated that the impressed forces present "spikes", i.e. sudden changes, with peak force values meaningfully higher of the plateau values which, from a mechanical point of view, can be the reason of the cracks/micro-cracks of the ribcage, and so of the persistent postoperative pain suffered by a number of patients after the surgical procedure.

References

1. Julian, O.C., Lopez-Belio, M., Dye, W.S., Javid, H., Grove, W.J.: The median sternal incision in intracardiac surgery with extracorporeal circulation: a general evolution of its use in heart surgery. Surgery **42**, 753–761 (1957)
2. Defalque, R.J., Bromley, J.J.: Poststernotomy neuralgia: a new pain syndrome. Anesth. Analg. **69**(1), 81–82 (1989)
3. Bruce, J., Drury, N., Poobalan, A.S., Jeffrey, R.R., Smith, W.C., Chambers, W.A.: The prevalence of chronic chest and leg pain following cardiac surgery: a historical cohort study. Pain **112**(3), 413 (2004)

4. Wildgaard, K., Kehlet, H.: Persistent Postsurgical Pain Syndromes, Chronic post-thoracotomy pain—what is new in pathogenic mechanisms and strategies for prevention? Tech. Reg. Anesth. Pain Manag. **15**(3), 83–89 (2011)
5. Riillo, F., Bagnato, C., Allievi, A.G., Takagi, A., Fabrizi, L., Saggio, G., Arichi, T., Burdet, E.: Ann. Biomed. Eng. **44**(8), 2431–2441 (2016)
6. van Gulik, L., Janssen, L.I., Ahlers, S.J.G.M., Bruins, P., Driessen, A.H.G., van Boven, W. J., van Dongen, E.P.A., Knibbe, C.A.J.: Risk factors for chronic thoracic pain after cardiac surgery via sternotomy. Eur. J. Cardiothorac. Surg. **40**, 1309–1313 (2011)
7. Hazelrigg, S.R., Cetindag, I.B., Fullerton, J.: Acute and chronic pain syndromes after thoracic surgery. Surg. Clin. N. Am. **82**, 849–865 (2002)
8. Mazzeffi, M., Khelemsky, Y.: Poststernotomy pain: a clinical review. J. Cardiothorac. Vasc. Anesth. **25**(6), 1163–1178 (2011)
9. Ochroch, E.A., Gottschalk, A., Troxel, A.B., Farrar, J.T.: Women suffer more short and long-term pain than men after major thoracotomy. Clin. J. Pain **22**, 491–498 (2006)
10. Zeitani, J., Penta de Peppo, A., Moscarelli, M., Gurrieri, L., Scafuri, A., Nardi, P., Nanni, F., Di Marzio, E., Chiariello, L.: Influence of sternal size and inadvertent paramedian sternotomy on stability of the closure site: a clinical and mechanical study. J. Thorac. Cardiovac. Surg. **132**, 38–42 (2006)
11. Healey, S., O'Neill, B., Bilal, H., Waterworth, P.: Does retraction of the sternum during median sternotomy result in brachial plexus injuries? Interact. CardioVasc. Thorac. Surg. **17**, 151–158 (2013)
12. Suzuki, S., Kikuchi, K., Takagi, K., Masuda, H., Yoshizu, H., Tanaka, S., Ogata, T.: Brachial plexus injury and fracture of the first rib as complications of median sternotomy. J. Japan. Assoc. Thorac. Surg. **38**(9), 1459–1462 (1990)
13. Zeitani, J., Penta de Peppo, A., Bianco, A., Nanni, F., Scafuri, A., Bertoldo, F., Salvati, A., Nardella, S., Chiariello, L.: Performance of a novel sternal synthesis device after median and faulty sternotomy: mechanical test and early clinical experience. Ann. Thorac. Surg. **85**(1), 287–293 (2008)
14. Baisden, C.E., Greenwald, L.V., Symbas, P.N.: Occult rib fractures and brachial plexus injury following median sternotomy for open-heart operations. Ann. Thorac. Surg. **38**(3), 192–194 (1984)
15. Saggio, G., Tancredi, G., Sbernini, L., Gaudio, C., Bianco, A., Zeitani, J.: In-vitro force assessments of an autoclavable instrumented sternal retractor. In: Proceedings of the 10th International Joint Conference on Biomedical Engineering Systems and Technologies (BIOSTEC 2017) - Volume 1: BIODEVICES, pp. 25–31 (2017)
16. Bolotin, G., Buckner, G.D., Campbell, N.B., Kocherginsky, M., Raman, J., Jeevanandam, V., Maessen, J.G.: Tissue-disruptive forces during median sternotomy. Heart Surg. Forum **10**(6), 487–492 (2007)
17. Aigner, P., Eskandary, F., Schlöglhofer, T., Gottardi, R., Aumayr, K., Laufer, G., Schima, H.: Sternal force distribution during median sternotomy retraction. J. Thorac. Cardiovasc. Surg. **146**(6), 1381–1386 (2013)
18. Saggio, G., Orengo, G., Leggieri, A.: Sensory glove and surface EMG with suitable conditioning electronics for extended monitoring and functional hand assessment. In: Proceedings of the 9th International Joint Conference on Biomedical Engineering Systems and Technologies (BIOSTEC), co-located 9th International Conference on Bio-inspired Systems and Signal Processing (BIOSIGNALS), Rome, Italy (2016)
19. Saggio, G., Bocchetti, S., Pinto, C., Orengo, G.: Electronic interface and signal conditioning circuitry for data glove systems useful as 3D HMI tools for disabled persons. In: International Conference on Health Informatics (BIOSTEC-Healthinf), pp. 248–253 (2011)

20. Orengo, G., Lagati, A., Saggio, G.: Modeling wearable bend sensor behavior for human motion capture. IEEE Sens. J. **14**(7), 2307–2316 (2014)
21. Bolotin, G., Buckner, G.D., Jardine, N.J., Kiefer, A.J., Campbell, N.B., Kocherginsky, M., Raman, J., Jeevanandam, V.: A novel instrumented retractor to monitor tissue-disruptive forces during lateral thoracotomy. J. Thorac. Cardiovasc. Surg. **133**(4), 949–954 (2007)
22. Ward, A.F., Grossi, E.A., Galloway, A.C.: Minimally invasive mitral surgery through right mini-thoracotomy under direct vision. J Thorac Dis. **5**(6), 673–679 (2013)
23. Reser, D., Holubec, T., Caliskan, E., Guidotti, A., Maisano, F.: Left anterior small thoracotomy for minimally invasive coronary artery bypass grafting, Multimed. Man. Cardiothorac. Surg. 1–5 (2015). https://www.ncbi.nlm.nih.gov/labs/articles/26420246/
24. Atluri, P., Stetson, R.L., Hung, G., Gaffey, A.C., Szeto, W.Y., Acker, M.A., Hargrove, W.C.: Minimally invasive mitral valve surgery is associated with equivalent cost and shorter hospital stay when compared with traditional sternotomy. J. Thorac. Cardiovasc. Surg. **151**(2), 385–388 (2016)

μSmartScope: Towards a Fully Automated 3D-Printed Smartphone Microscope with Motorized Stage

Luís Rosado[1]([⊠]), Paulo T. Silva[1], José Faria[1], João Oliveira[1],
Maria João M. Vasconcelos[1], Dirk Elias[1], José M. Correia da Costa[2],
and Jaime S. Cardoso[3]

[1] Fraunhofer Portugal AICOS, Rua Alfredo Allen 455/461,
4200-135 Porto, Portugal
luis.rosado@fraunhofer.pt
[2] Instituto Nacional de Saúde Dr. Ricardo Jorge, Rua Alexandre Herculano 321,
4000-055 Porto, Portugal
[3] INESCTEC and University of Porto, Rua Dr. Roberto Frias,
4200-465 Porto, Portugal

Abstract. Microscopic examination is the reference diagnostic method for several neglected tropical diseases. However, its quality and availability in rural endemic areas is often limited by the lack of trained personnel and adequate equipment. These drawbacks are closely related with the increasing interest in the development of computer-aided diagnosis systems, particularly distributed solutions that provide access to complex diagnosis in rural areas. In this work we present our most recent advances towards the development of a fully automated 3D-printed smartphone microscope with a motorized stage, termed μSmartScope. The developed prototype allows autonomous acquisition of a pre-defined number of images at 1000x magnification, by using a motorized automated stage fully powered and controlled by a smartphone, without the need of manual focus. In order to validate the prototype as a reliable alternative to conventional microscopy, we evaluated the μSmartScope performance in terms of: resolution; field of view; illumination; motorized stage performance (mechanical movement precision/resolution and power consumption); and automated focus. These results showed similar performances when compared with conventional microscopy, plus the advantage of being low-cost and easy to use, even for non-experts in microscopy. To extract these results, smears infected with blood parasites responsible for the most relevant neglected tropical diseases were used. The acquired images showed that it was possible to detect those agents through images acquired via the μSmartScope, which clearly illustrate the huge potential of this device, specially in developing countries with limited access to healthcare services.

Keywords: Microscopy · Mobile devices
Motorized microscope stage · Developing countries · Mobile health

© Springer International Publishing AG, part of Springer Nature 2018
N. Peixoto et al. (Eds.): BIOSTEC 2017, CCIS 881, pp. 19–44, 2018.
https://doi.org/10.1007/978-3-319-94806-5_2

1   Introduction

Neglected tropical diseases (NTDs) are a group of parasitic infectious diseases that affect over 1.5 billion of the world's poorest population, including 875 million children [1]. The gold standard for detection of several NTDs is microscopic examination, particularly via the visualization of different types of human biological products, like blood smears (e.g Malaria, Lymphatic filariasis, African Trypanosomiasis), stool smears (e.g. intestinal helminths), and urine smears (e.g. Schistosomiasis) [2]. Unfortunately, reliable identification of these parasitic infections requires not only proper microscopic equipment, but also high-standard expertise for subsequent microscopic analysis. These requirements represents the most common practical difficulties experienced in rural health facilities, being closely related with the increasing interest of mobile health (mHealth) and computer-aided diagnosis solutions for those particular scenarios.

The mobile phone is currently Africa's most important digital technology. In the year 2000 few Africans had a mobile phone, but today about three-quarters do [3]. So it becomes natural that mHealth is starting to play an important role when it comes to health in Africa, particularly through the usage of solutions that allow skipping over centralized laboratories [4]. For instance, the usage of advanced computer vision approaches coupled to the increasing processing capabilities of mobile devices is already showing promising results in the area of malaria diagnosis [5,6]. Moreover, considering the paramount importance of microscopic examination for NTDs detection, the development of new portable microscopic devices is an area that can greatly improve the chances of the successful deployment of innovative solutions for NTDs diagnosis in underserved areas [7]. To achieve that purpose, the constant advances and increasing possibilities coming from additive manufacturing should certainly be taken into account, since 3D-printing currently allows faster and cheaper prototyping.

In this paper we report our most recent advances towards the development of a fully automated 3D-printed smartphone microscope with a motorized stage, termed μSmartScope [8]. The usage of this prototype can be resumed as follow: the process starts by placing the smartphone in the μSmartScope along with the smear, and have a set of magnified images acquired autonomously by the smartphone camera sensor. This collection of images is then analyzed, either automatically through computer vision approaches, or manually by a specialist on a remote location. It is worth mentioning that we took into account several particularities of the African reality during the design of this device, like the high customs taxes and import duties currently in practice in many African countries; this motivated us to favor solutions easily replicable in developing countries. Several other additional requirements were equally considered, like automating the device as much as possible, discarding the need of considerable expertise and train of the technician in terms of maneuvering the microscope, or supplying the energy needed for the illumination and/or any type of automation through the mobile device battery, thus discarding the need of an additional power source.

This paper is structured as follow: Sect. 1 corresponds to Introduction and presents the motivation and objectives of this work; Sect. 2 summarizes the related work found on the literature; Sect. 3 gives overview of the μSmartScope, with focus for the Optics and Illumination modules; Sect. 4 details the Motorized Automated stage module; Sect. 5 describes the Automated Focus procedure; In Sect. 6 the Results and Discussion are presented; and finally the Conclusions and Future Work are drawn in Sect. 7.

2   Related Work

Some research has been made in the last years to develop cell-phone based systems that provide low-cost alternatives to conventional microscopy. The microscopy designs of the proposed systems can be separated in three different areas: lensless, on-lens and attachment-based approaches.

The lensless approaches are based on the principles of holographic microscopy, i.e. the microscopic images are reconstructed from the holograms captured by the cell-phone. This approach has the advantage of not requiring any lenses or optical component as well as obtaining images with large field-of-view (FOV). However, acceptable resolutions are only obtained for small magnifications (∼40x magnification, NA = 0.65 objective) and processing power is needed to reconstruct the image [9,10].

On-lens approaches usually employ a refractive element directly attached to the smartphone camera at the focus, or a ball lens mounted in front of the camera lens [11,12]. Despite being a low-cost alternative, the ball lens produces a spherical focal plane, which creates aberrations and reduces drastically the usable FOV. Moreover, magnification and radius of the ball lens are inversely linked, so in order to achieve 1000x magnification we need a ball lens with radius of 0.15 mm [12], which can turn the mounting and alignment process with the camera lens really challenging.

The attachment-based approaches covers the majority of the solutions already reported on the literature, which requires coupling additional hardware to the cell-phone, such as commercial lenses or illumination modules [10,13,14]. This approach usually takes advantage of complex optical elements that allow achieving suitable resolutions at high magnifications (e.g. ∼1000x), which increases the overall cost of the system, but is currently a requirement for the microscopic examination of several neglected diseases. With high magnifications also emerges the limitation of having a small FOV, thus requiring the development of mechanisms to move the smears in order to cover a large area of the specimen. Moreover, it was verified that the majority of reported works are designed for a unique cell-phone model, which can greatly compromise the adoption of the proposed solution.

In this work, we present a 3D-printed microscope that can easily be attached to a wide range of mobile devices models. To the best of our knowledge, this is the first proposed smartphone-based alternative to conventional microscopy that allows autonomous acquisition of a pre-defined number of images at 1000x magnification with suitable resolution, by using a motorized automated stage, fully powered and controlled by a smartphone, without the need of human interaction.

3   μSmartScope Overview

Considering that developing a cheap and easily replicable alternative to conventional microscopes was one of the main goals of this work, the μSmartScope was prototyped using Fused Filament Fabrication (FFF) technology. The FFF is a 3D printing technology for rapid prototyping, which works by laying down consecutive layers of material in very precise positions, in our case Polylactic Acid (PLA) termoplastic. Layer by layer, a desired model is built from a digital file. Despite the great advantages of this technology, 3D printing has limitations like any other fabrication process, such as being sensitive to environmental variables like temperature, humidity or dust. Thus, we took those variables into consideration during the design and printing process, for instance by accounting

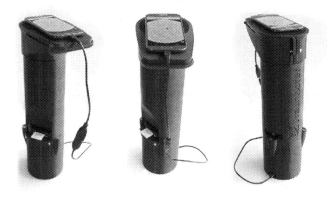

Fig. 1. The μSmartScope prototype, with smartphone attached and microscopic slide inserted.

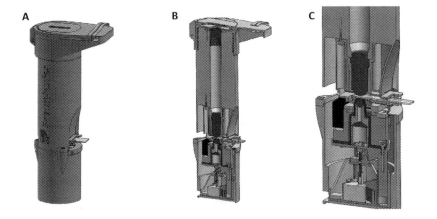

Fig. 2. μSmartScope render models: (A) External view with microscope slide inserted (at yellow); (B) Cut view with optical and electrical components highlighted; (C) Detail of the cut view. (Color figure online)

the expected dimensional contraction during the cooling process or checking the absence of any superficial humidity/dust on the filament, which showed to have a significant impact in the quality and dimensional accuracy of the printed pieces.

As previously reported [8], the μSmartScope can be divided in 3 major modules (see Figs. 1 and 2): (i) Optics; (ii) Illumination; and (iii) Motorized Automated Stage (termed μStage). By analyzing the results previously reported, it becomes clear that the μStage module was the bottleneck of the system. The previous mechanical design had a significant unpredictable behavior due to small irregularities of the 3D printed parts, and it was significantly slower than human technicians in autonomously focusing microscopic fields. Thus, a major refactor was made to the μStage module, which consequently had a pronounced impact on the overall performance of the μSmartScope. Due to these pronounced modifications, we opted to dedicate a separate section on this work to μStage module (see Sect. 4). On the other hand, the Optics and Illumination modules suffered only minor improvements when compared to the previously reported version [8], so we following summarized these two modules under this section.

3.1 Optics Module

The selected commercial lenses used to construct the μSmartScope were supplied by Bresser, a vendor that showed a good price-quality relation for the required optics (see Fig. 3). Particularly, we used the Planachromat 100x oil-immersion objective (Bresser #5941500) and the Wide Angle 10x Eyepiece (Bresser #5941700).

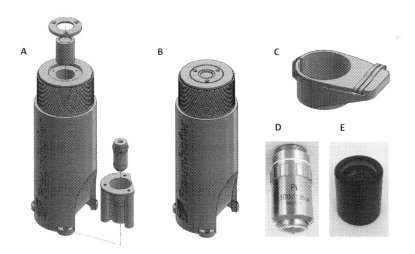

Fig. 3. Optics module: (A) Exploded view; (B) Assembled view; (C) Smartphone holder; (D) Planachromat 100x oil-immersion objective lens; (E) Wide angle 10x eyepiece lens.

3.2   Illumination Module

To allow a uniform illumination of a microsocpic slide, using just a LED is usually not enough because most of the light is lost to parts of the specimen that are not being analyzed. To counter that, a light condenser is normally used in conventional microscopes. The condenser is a lens (or multiple lenses) that concentrates the light from the illumination source and focus it in the part of the specimen that is being analyzed by the amplification device. This device, in turn, magnifies the light beam, allowing an uniform illumination. Since all support materials for the optical components of the μSmartScope are 3D-printed, the minimum resolution of the 3D-printer was taken into consideration during the design of the illumination module.

Several topologies of condensers can be used with their pros and cons. One of the cheapest options with acceptable performance is the Abbe condenser, which uses a plano-convex lens to pre-concentrate the light into a smaller ball or half-ball lens that, in turn, provides the final concentration of light. This arrangement guarantees a good result by using cheaper individual lenses instead of an expensive, custom made, one. To design our condenser we selected a

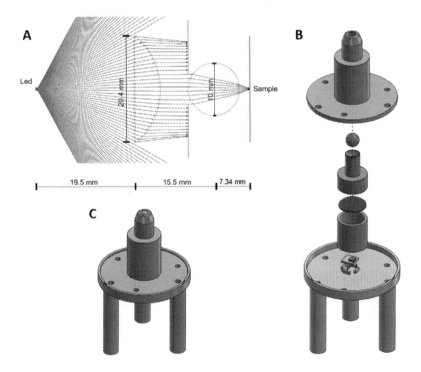

Fig. 4. Illumination module: (A) Schematic of the developed light condenser generated with OpticalRayTracer® optics design software; (B) Exploded view of the light condenser with lenses (at blue) and LED light (at yellow); (C) Assembled view of the light condenser. (Color figure online)

20.4 × 25 mm plano-convex lens (Edmund Optics #43483) and a 10 mm N-BK7 Ball Lens (Edmund Optics #32748). In order to calculate the Back-Focal Length (BFL), i.e. distance on the optical axis between last active optical surface and the specimen plane, we used the following equation [12]:

$$BFL = \frac{1}{2} \cdot \frac{r \cdot (2 - n)}{(n - 1)},$$ (1)

where $r = 5$ mm is the radius of the ball lens and $n = 1.517$ is the Index of Refraction of the N-BK7 optical material. This gives a $BFL = 2.34$ mm, as shown in Fig. 4.

Despite the distances defined on Fig. 4 being strictly respected, during the design we also had to ensure that the center of the ball lens was both carefully aligned with the center of the plano-convex lens and with the center of the objective lens.

4   μStage Module

The microscopic examination of blood smears usually requires the visual analysis of different microscopic fields (i.e. positions) of the specimen. The minimum number of required microscopic fields directly depends on the target disease and used optical magnification, i.e. depends on the size of the target structures. For instance, the World Health Organization (WHO) recomends the analysis of 100 different microscopic fields of a blood sample to perform a malaria microscopy test [15]. It should be noted that this process is manually performed by trained staff and can be extenuating, requiring that the operator takes regular breaks in order to ensure maximum attention.

The approach proposed on this work aims to improve this process by performing the microscopic slide movement autonomously and on-demand using a smartphone. The μStage was developed for that specific purpose (see Fig. 5), which consists on a motorized stage designed to be as cheap as possible, being powered through the USB-OTG connection of the smartphone. In order ensure its flexibility, most of the μStage structure is modular and can be adapted without major refactors of the entire module. It is worth noting that during the design of the μStage we tried to minimize the usage of mechanical components and give priority to 3D-print as many parts as possible, in order to reduce costs and ensure an easy replication of the prototype.

Regarding the μStage mechanical structure, it can be divided in two main functional submodules (see Fig. 6): (i) the **XY-plane Submodule**, responsible to move the stage on the XY plane (i.e. to obtain different microscopic fields); and (ii) the **Z-axis Submodule**, responsible to move the stage in the Z axis (i.e. find the focus point of the specimen in a fixed position on the XY plane).

4.1   XY-Plane Submodule

Composed by 2 parts that slide perpendicularly between each other on the XY plane (see Fig. 6(A)). This submodule moves the μStage to different XY

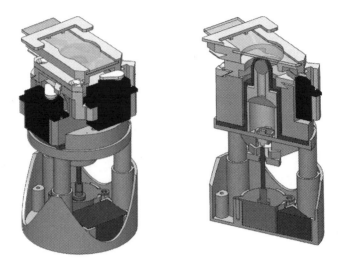

Fig. 5. μStage module: External view (on the left) and cut view (on the right), with detail of servo motors (at black), step motor (at yellow), electronics (at green) and optics (at blue). (Color figure online)

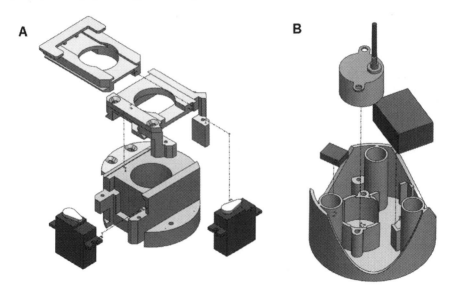

Fig. 6. μStage functional submodules: (A) Exploded view of the XY-plane submodule, with servo motors (at black); (B) Exploded view of the Z-axis submodule, with step motor (at yellow) and electronics (at green). (Color figure online)

positions, in order to obtain distinct microscopic fields of the specimen. Two servo motors are used to provide the movement, together with small elastic bands that ensure the movement in both ways. It should be noted that this arrangement is not linear, since the servo movement is provided in a 90° arc. Nevertheless, it allows the acquisition of different microscopic fields, particularly by moving one of the servos while the other remains static. Taking into account that repositioning to a specific microscopic field location with high precision is usually not required in microscopic blood smear analysis, this module is not required to perform high precision and resolution displacements. Covering a high number of distinct microscopic fields from different XY positions is by far much more important, in order to obtain a reliable overview of the specimen.

4.2 Z-Axis Submodule

Composed by 3 tubular structures that slide against their negatives in the base part (see Fig. 6(B)). This submodule allows the vertical movement of the μStage, in order to find the Z-axis position that corresponds to the focus point of the specimen. A simple stepper motor is used to provide the vertical movement, being the rotary movement of the stepper engine translated to linear motion through a threaded rod and a nut fixed in this part. Moreover, the base part of this submodule is also used to fix the electronic board, the Z-axis actuator and the μUSB connector.

The correct calibration and parameterization of the 3D-printer is evidently important for all μSmartScope printed components, but particularly crucial for this submodule. Obtaining the required gap between each tubular structure and the corresponding negative is mandatory to achieve precise Z-axis displacements. Being the μStage the bottleneck of the previously reported version, two major mechanical changes were made in order to improve the performance of the Z-axis submodule in terms of precision and stability:

- **M2 Threaded Rod:** The previous version of the μStage used a M3 threaded rod with a coarse thread. After extensive testing, we concluded that a higher resolution in the Z-axis movement was required in order to reach the ideal Z position where the specimen is completely focused. For that purpose, we switched to a M2 threaded rod with coarse thread, which theoretically improves the resolution from 0.5 mm to 0.4 mm per revolution. The usage of a M3 rod with fine pitch was discarded due to its low availability and prohibitive cost. It is worth noting that the usage of the M2 thread brings the disadvantage of a lower shaft diameter, so we ensured through calculations that the μStage would not fail under the expected load stress.
- **Buckling Cover:** A good mechanical design practice known to improve the stability of sliding mechanisms was incorporated, which consists on ensuring that each tubular stem should have more than the double of its diameter inside of the outer stem at its maximum Z position [16]. Consequently, the tubular structures that slide against their negative in the base part were redesigned accordingly.

4.3   Electronics

The power board was designed to power the 3 actuators (one stepper and two servos) and the illumination LED, using exclusively the power from a USB connection with 5 V and 500 mA. It should be noted that most of the currently available smartphone models have USB-OTG interface in order to allow the connection of USB peripherals. To be fully compatible with the μSmartScope, the used smartphone model needs to support this power standard, otherwise it will not be capable of powering the μStage. An image of the developed PCB can be observed in Fig. 7, and the electronic system is composed by:

- **Stepper Motor:** The used stepper motor is a 28BYJ-48 5 V, which is the cheapest stepper motor found in common electronic stores. This was a major point in choosing the motor, since the replication of the μSmartScope should be easy and cheap in any part of the world. It is controlled by a DRV8836 from Texas Instruments with current limited to 200 mA, and capable of 512 steps per full rotation. Since we are using a standard M2 threaded rod, we have a theoretical resolution of around 0.78 μm. Furthermore, a simple push-button switch is placed in the Z axis to provide a way to locate the position when the device is turned on.
- **Two Servo Motors:** The used servo motors are the Hitec HS-55 5 V, which is the cheapest micro servo motor found in common electronic stores. Controlled directly by PWM output and limited to 200 mA, their rotation is directly used to generate the linear movement. The servo head has a size of 13 mm meaning that this is our maximum displacement. Using the 90° travel with 2.5° per step, we have 36 steps available while we only need 10 per axis;
- **Illumination:** Since the illumination depends of the specimen under analysis, the control board provides an output based in a power Mosfet capable of providing 150 mA at 5 V. This power can be controlled by changing the PWM duty cycle of the output.
- **Control**: An ATMega32u4 is used to control all the logic of the system, which contains native USB communications and plenty of GPIO ports and PWM support. The native USB connection is seen as a serial port in the smartphone

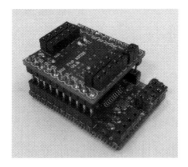

Fig. 7. Prototype PCB to control the μStage [8].

using the *USB serial for Android* library [17]. Moreover, an API for Android was developed to allow interaction with the stage. This API was made to be as simple as possible to integrate in any app, providing every function needed to fully control the stage (i.e. stepping in X, Y and Z axes, as well as control the LED light).

5 Automated Focus

The traditional focusing method in microscopy is usually achieved by manually adjusting the vertical position of the microscope stage, with the objective of obtaining a focused microscopic field. However, for screening processes that requires the analysis of a huge amount of microscopic fields per specimen, this process clearly becomes a cumbersome task. As an illustrative example, for the analysis of malaria-infected blood smears, it is recommended the analysis of 100 distinct microscopic fields for a single specimen. The specialist is even advised to rest regularly, so human errors can be avoided and high performance rates ensured. To tackle this problem, our solution takes advantage of the developed motorized automated stage (see Sect. 4) and real time feedback retrieved from the smartphone camera sensor. But in order to obtain a fully automated solution, we soon realized that we had to develop an automated focus approach that ensures autonomous acquisition of focused microscopic fields.

Automated focus is a long standing topic in the literature, and several focus algorithms have been proposed [18,19]. However, the search for the proper algorithm still remains an open topic, since it can highly depends on the visual characteristics of the specimen and characteristics of the camera sensor. Generally, an autofocus system includes three main components: (i) **Focus Region Selection**; (ii) **Focus Measurement**; and (iii) **Focus Point Search Logic**. In this section we present a detailed description of those components in our approach, with the final goal of obtaining focused microscopic images from malaria-infected thin and thick blood smears without human interaction. As a side note, we opted to use these two types of specimen preparation because they represent quite well two different extreme scenarios in microscopy analysis: the thin usually presents dense concentration of visible structures in each microscopic field (see Fig. 8(A)), while the thick smear presents a low number of visible structures (see Fig. 8(B)).

5.1 Focus Region Selection

Due to lens constrains, it is not possible to obtain maximal focus in the whole area of the microscopic field. Therefore, a square region in the center of the preview image was defined, which generally is the place where distortion interference is lower (see Fig. 8). This square region will be used by the focus algorithm to extract the metrics and make decisions accordingly.

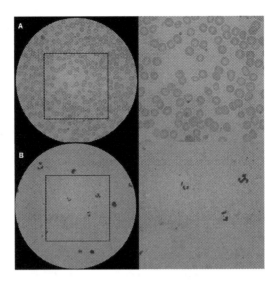

Fig. 8. Focused image obtained using the μSmartScope, and respective central square resulting from focus region selection: (A) Thin blood smear; (B) Thick blood smear.

5.2   Focus Measurement

Taking into consideration several works on the literature targeting the automatic focus for microscopic devices using image processing, in this work we tested and compared a wide range of focus metrics already proposed that were considered highly relevant for automatic focusing. In detail, we tested: derivative-based as the Brenner gradient and the Tenenbaum gradient; statistics based, like the normalized variance; histogram-based, as entropy; and intuitive algorithms, like thresholded content [20,21].

After this comparative analysis, the Tenenbaum gradient [22] standard deviation ($TENG^{STD}$) and sum ($TENG^{SUM}$) were considered the most discriminative focus metrics, i.e. the metrics that allows better differentiation of the ideal focus point. The Tenenbaum gradient is obtained by convolving the previously selected central square of the image with Sobel operators, and by summing the square of gradient vector components:

$$TENG = (G_x(i,j)^2 + G_y(i,j)^2), \qquad (2)$$

where G_x and G_y are the horizontal and vertical gradients computed by convolving the focus region image with the Sobel operators.

Despite the remarkable discriminative power of $TENG^{STD}$ and $TENG^{SUM}$ metrics, in this work we started by testing the previous proposed automated focus approach [8] not only on a wide range of smartphone models, but also on different thin and thick blood smears. After extensive testing, we concluded that improvements to the previously proposed approach were required, mainly because the order of magnitude of the $TENG^{STD}$ and $TENG^{SUM}$ metrics presented a significant variation for different smartphone-specimen combinations. We concluded that this pronounced variation was being cause by two main factor: (i) images of the same specimen captured with different smartphone models may present different image characteristics (e.g. high variation in image contrast and/or color representation) due to the different camera sensor specifications; and (ii) microscopy specimen preparation greatly depends on good-quality reagents and proper human skills, which can lead to huge intensity variations of the stained components.

Despite this shifting behavior, we noticed however that the relative variation of both metrics was considerably more homogeneous when compared with the respective absolute values. So instead of using directly the $TENG^{STD}$ and $TENG^{SUM}$ metrics values, we used the following slope gradients:

$$SLOPE_{ij}^{STD} = \frac{(TENG_i^{STD} - TENG_j^{STD})}{i - j}, \tag{3}$$

$$SLOPE_{ij}^{SUM} = \frac{(TENG_i^{SUM} - TENG_j^{SUM})}{i - j}, \tag{4}$$

where i and j are two different Z-axis positions, with $i, j = \{0, 1, \ldots, Z^{MAX}\}$, being Z^{MAX} the highest Z-axis position reachable by the μStage.

5.3 Focus Point Search Logic

The focus point search logic aims to identify the Z-axis position where the specimen is ideally focused. In order to simplify the explanation and abstract the vertical displacement of the μStage from SI units, a scale from 0 to 7000 was create to represent the possible Z-axis coordinates. In fact, each unit on this scale represents the minimum step allowed by the stepper motor, so taking into account that the stepper motor allows 512 steps per revolution, we can state that the μStage is surely over the specimen focus point after $\sim$13,67 revolutions. The proposed approach can be divided in two main phases, the Rough phase and the Precise phase, according to the following steps:

1. The algorithm starts in the Rough phase, where the goal is to detect a pronounced increase of the focus metrics $SLOPE_{ij}^{STD}$ and $SLOPE_{ij}^{SUM}$, which corresponds to the beginning of the visualization of the microscopic structures. At the beginning of the Rough phase, the μStage is on the bottom Z-axis position ($Z^{Pos} = 0$), which from now on will be called the reset position (Z^{Reset}).
2. While the μStage is on Z^{Reset}, the user inserts the microscopic slide and gives an order through the mobile application to start the image acquisition process. The μStage starts autonomously ascending in the Z-axis to a specific Z position ($Z^{Pos} = 5000$), which from now on will be called the initial position ($Z^{Initial}$). The μStage is surely below the focus point at $Z^{Initial}$, so no focus metrics are computed until this position is reached.

3. When the $Z^{Initial}$ is reached, the μStage starts ascending on specific intervals ($Z_{Step}^{Interval} = 2$). For each $Z_{Step}^{Interval}$, the image preview obtained with the smartphone camera sensor is used to compute the $SLOPE_{ij}^{STD}$ and $SLOPE_{ij}^{SUM}$ focus metrics. It should be noted that in the Rough phase we use a frame rate of 20 frames per second (fps).

4. The transition from the Rough phase to the Precise phase occurs when the following condition is verified: $SLOPE_{ij}^{STD} > 20$ and $SLOPE_{ij}^{SUM} > 20$.

5. When the Precise phase is reached, the μStage keeps ascending with the same $Z_{Step}^{Interval}$, but we decrease the frame rate to 4 fps. This adjustment is directly related with the vibration caused by each mechanical step, which consequently causes motion blur on the image preview. By guaranteeing more time between the mechanical movement and the analysis of the preview image, we ensure that the vibration dissipates and the computation of the focus metrics is not affected by that artifact.

6. During the Precise phase, the $TENG^{STD}$ is computed on the preview image for each $Z_{Step}^{Interval}$. If the $TENG^{STD}$ of the current Z position has the highest value found on the Precise phase, this position is considered the best candidate to focus point. When that happens, an image is captured with 5 Megapixels and saved on the smartphone memory. In the event of an higher $TENG^{STD}$ value for a posterior Z position, a new image is captured and the best candidate to focus point is updated.

7. The focus point search logic ends with successful state when a candidate to focus point was found and: (i) the $TENG^{STD}$ presents always lower value in the following 20 $Z_{Step}^{Interval}$ positions; or (ii) the $TENG^{STD}$ has a value lower than half of the best candidate $TENG^{STD}$ in any of the following $Z_{Step}^{Interval}$ positions;

8. The focus point search logic ends with fail state if the maximum Z-axis position ($Z^{Pos} = 7000$) is reached without a single candidate to focus point. In the event of fail state, a reset procedure takes place: (i) the μStage descends to the Z^{Reset} position; (ii) the μStage moves to a different position in the XY plane; and (iii) the focus point search logic described above is restarted. After extensive testing, we noticed that the most common cause for the occurrence of a fail state is usually the low number of microscopic structures in that specific XY position.

The behavior of the proposed focus point search logic is illustrated on Fig. 9, where is depicted the variation of the $SLOPE_{ij}^{STD}$ and $SLOPE_{ij}^{SUM}$ while the μStage is ascending in the vertical axis.

6   Results and Discussion

In this section we start by presenting the obtained results in terms of resolution, field of view and illumination of the images acquired using the μSmartScope. Moreover, we also evaluated the μStage performance regarding the precision and resolution of the mechanical movement, as well as the power consumption.

We finish this section with a detailed analysis of the proposed automated focus approach, covering the usage of a wide range of smartphone models and different thin and thick blood smears.

6.1 Resolution

The magnified images of the smears obtained with the μSmartScope must have an appropriate resolution over a sufficiently large area, so a conclusive decision about the presence of a specific infectious agent can be made. The 1951 USAF resolution test chart is a resolution test pattern conforming to MIL-STD-150A standard, set by US Air Force in 1951. It is still widely accepted to test the

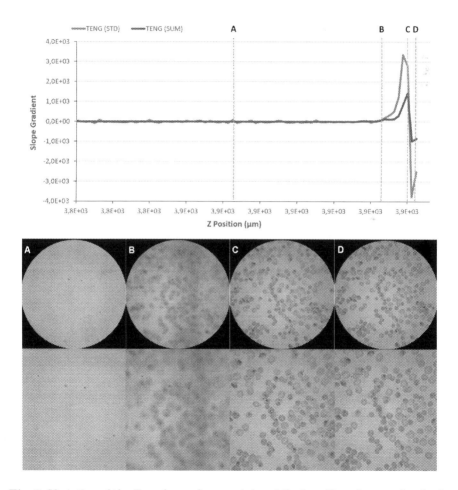

Fig. 9. Variation of the Tenenbaum focus metrics while the μStage is ascending in the vertical axis. Illustrative examples of preview images obtained by the smartphone camera at different Z positions are presented: (A) During the Rough phase; (B) Entering the Precise phase; (C) Focus point; (D) Stopping condition after focus point detected.

resolving power of optical imaging systems such as microscopes, cameras and image scanners. One example is the READY OPTICS USAF 1951 Microscope Resolution Target, which is a target embedded in a standard microscope slide, suitable for oiled objectives and oiled condensers. In terms of resolution, the target allows to check a minimum spacing between lines of 0.197 nm.

Microscopic images of the READY OPTICS USAF 1951 Microscope Resolution Target with 1000x magnification were acquired the μSmartScope and with the Bresser Microscope-5102000-Erudit DLX (see Fig. 10). Both systems use similar objectives and eyepieces, so the main goal is to evaluate image resolution of the μSmartScope.

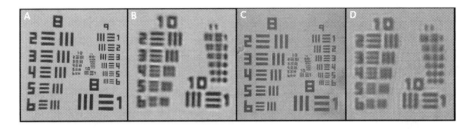

Fig. 10. Images of READY OPTICS USAF 1951 microscope resolution target: (A) Acquired using Bresser Microscope-5102000-Erudit DL; (B) Detail of Group 10 using the Microscope; (C) Acquired using the μSmartScope; (D) Detail of Group 10 using the μSmartScope [8].

To determine the resolution of the μSmartScope and compare it to the resolution of the Bresser commercial microscope, the images acquired with the separate systems were converted to grayscale and the analysis focused on Group 10, which was the smallest resolvable group. In order to determine the smallest resolvable Element of Group 10 in both horizontal and vertical orientations, the images were firstly converted to grayscale and a line for each of the 6 bars of that Element were drawn. Each line starts and ends in a background pixel, and intersects perpendicularly the respective bar. All pixel values of each line were used to calculate the Michelson contrast, which was assigned to the respective bar. In both directions of each Element, the bar with minimum Michelson contrast was selected for analysis purposes (see Fig. 11).

It was defined that an Element is considered resolvable on a particular direction if the minimum Michelson contrast was ≥ 0.1. Thus, Element 3 was defined as the minimum resolvable Element for the μSmartScope, which gives a minimum resolution of 0.388 μm on both directions. For the Bresser commercial microscope, Element 4 was selected as the minimum, which corresponds to a resolution of 0.345 μm for both directions. Although the μSmartScope presents a slightly lower resolution, it is clear on Fig. 11 that both directions have a more homogenous behavior in terms of resolution, while in the Bresser microscope there is an evident discrepancy between the resolving power on different

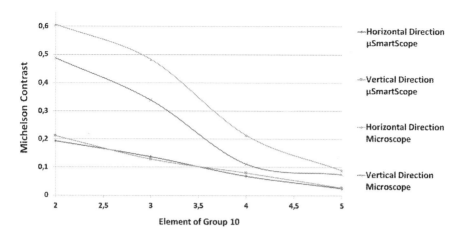

Fig. 11. Minimum Michelson contrast for USAF Resolution Target Elements of Group 10 [8].

directions. The lower values of Michelson contrast for the μSmartScope might be caused by the limitation in terms of the maximum power rate of the smartphone, since both the illumination and motorized automated stage must be powered by USB-OTG. Thus the power that feeds the LED is limited, which diminishes the intensity of the LED and consequently the image contrast.

6.2 Field of View

Resolution and field of view are inversely linked in standard laboratory microscopes. In order to obtain microscopic fields with both high magnification and resolution, the usage of objectives with higher numerical aperture is required, which results in smaller Field of Views (FOV) [10]. To determine the FOV of the μSmartScope, images of the READY OPTICS USAF 1951 Microscope Resolution Target were acquired and used to estimate the microns to pixels (μm/pixel) relationship. The exact distances between bars of a specific Element is given by the specifications of the resolution target, particularly Element 2 and 3 of Group 8 corresponds to 1.740 μm and 1.550 μm, respectively. By measuring the number of pixels between bars of this 2 Elements on the acquired image, a relationship of 0.085 μm/pixel was obtained for Element 2 and 0.084 μm/pixel for Element 3. So we considered the average value, i.e. a relationship of 0.0845 μm/pixel. Furthermore, the number of pixels for the vertical and horizontal axis that passes through the center of the visible optical circle of the acquired image were determined. These values were then combined with the previously calculated μm/pixel relationship, in order to estimate the FOV of the visible optical circle, which resulted in a FOV of 214.38 μm and 206.87 μm for the vertical and horizontal axis, respectively.

6.3 Illumination

In order to evaluate the uniformity of the illumination of the LED coupled to the proposed condenser, an image was acquired with a blank microscope slide (see Fig. 12(A)). A diagonal line scan starting on the top right corner of the image was defined, in order to evaluate the variation of the pixels intensity along this line. Particularly, a total of 200 pixel boxes were considered along the scan line, being each box equally spaced and with a size of 10×10 pixels. The mean and standard deviation of the pixels intensity was computed for each box, as depicted in Fig. 12(B) and (C). This results demonstrate that the proposed illumination set up ensures substantially uniform illumination with low noise, being the small intensity variations probably caused by dust particles on the lenses or components floating in the immersion oil.

6.4 μStage Performance

The μStage performance was evaluated in terms of precision and resolution of the mechanical movement, particularly in terms of the horizontal (XY plane) and vertical (Z axis) directions independently. Moreover, an analysis of the power consumption of the μStage is also presented.

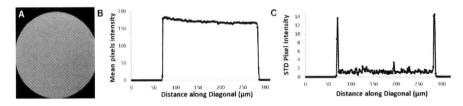

Fig. 12. μSmartScope illumination uniformity analysis: (A) Original image; (B) Mean pixel intensity of the 10×10 pixel boxes on the diagonal direction; (C) Standard deviation of the 10×10 pixel boxes on the diagonal direction [8].

Precision and Resolution. Before analyzing the mechanical movement of the μStage, it should be taken into account the design option of minimizing the usage of mechanical components and give priority to 3D-printed parts, in order to reduce costs and ensure an easy replication of the prototype. Despite the referred advantages, we were aware that using moving parts fully 3D printed might lead to a potential losses in the movement precision, for instance caused by plastic imperfections and/or particles in the sliding portions. Thus, the goal of this section is to measure and assess if the precision and resolution in the mechanical movement offered by the μStage is comparable with conventional microscopy analysis. In Fig. 13 we present the results for the mechanical movement of the μStage in the XY plane and Z axis. Particularly, for each direction we performed 100 steps and the respective displacement was measured using a digital caliper (Mitutoyo Absolute) with resolution of $0.01 \, \text{mm} \pm 0.02 \, \text{mm}$.

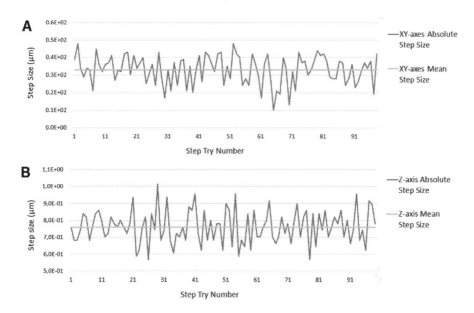

Fig. 13. Measured step size values after 100 repetitions: (A) XY plane; (B) Z axis.

For the displacement in the XY plane, a clear variation of the step size is depict in Fig. 13(A). This behavior is probably caused by two main factors: (i) the non-linear movement of the servo; and (ii) imperfections on the sliding parts that are a consequence of the 3D printing process. Nevertheless, we obtained an average displacement of 330 μm with a standard deviation of 81 μm, a result that attests the suitability of the μStage XY-plane movement for microscopy analysis purposes. As referred before, repositioning to a specific XY position with high precision is usually not required in conventional microscopy analysis, being much more important the coverage of a high number of different XY positions. Please note that the obtained XY μStage displacement is marginally higher than the FOV determined in Sect. 6.2, which means that we are obtaining a new microscopic field every time we take a XY step.

Regarding the displacement in the Z axis, it should be taken into account that our caliper is not able to measure such small steps. To estimate the average step size, one full revolution of the motor was considered (which corresponds to 512 steps), and the respective displacement was measured 100 times. This distance was then divided by the number of steps, in order to estimate the travel of a single step. As we can see in Fig. 13(B), the steps are less dispersed, but some variability is still verified. Each step corresponds to an average of 0.763 ± 0.098 μm, which gives an indication that our steps in the Z axis are within the theoretical values. By comparing these results with the previously reported performance of 0.98 ± 0.18 μm [8], it becomes clear the major impact of the mechanical improvements performed in this work.

Table 1. Power consumption test results [8].

Smartphone	Average current (mA)	Average power consumption (W)	Autonomy (min)
Samsung Galaxy S5	208.64	1.043	164
LG Nexus 5	201.34	1.006	149

Table 2. Average seconds per image for different smartphone models and thin blood smears, calculated over 100 automated focus attempts for each combination.

Thin blood smears	Seconds per image (average time over 100 automated focus attempts)				
	Asus Zenfone 2	HTC One M8	Motorola Moto G5	LG Nexus 5	Samsung Galaxy S6
Slide #1	11.30	8.50	8.39	9.04	7.46
Slide #2	10.76	7.39	8.11	7.37	6.58
Slide #3	10.45	7.25	8.12	7.77	6.99
Slide #4	11.85	7.15	7.95	8.14	7.16
Slide #5	9.21	7.74	7.99	8.11	6.86

Table 3. Average seconds per image for different smartphone models and thick blood smears, calculated over 100 automated focus attempts for each combination.

Thick blood smears	Seconds per image (average time over 100 automated focus attempts)				
	Asus Zenfone 2	HTC One M8	Motorola Moto G5	LG Nexus 5	Samsung Galaxy S6
Slide #1	17.09	18.19	8.76	16.54	23.93
Slide #2	16.49	12.60	13.56	11.49	8.80
Slide #3	13.85	15.24	8.81	10.15	6.64
Slide #4	13.24	9.77	14.64	11.68	8.21

Power Consumption. In order to ensure that we never go over the maximum power rate of the smartphone, the whole system power consumption is always under 400 mA at 5 V. This is achieved by allowing only one actuator moving at any given time. In Table 1, the power consumption of the system can be observed together with the autonomy for two different smartphone models. The profile tested was as close as possible to the real one, i.e. the smartphone was continuously acquiring focused microscopic fields at different XY positions, with the screen turned off and in flight mode until it shut down due to low battery.

It is worth noting that we are currently using the smartphone battery to simultaneously power the actuators of the μStage, the LED light, acquire data continuously with the camera sensor and process each acquired frame for the

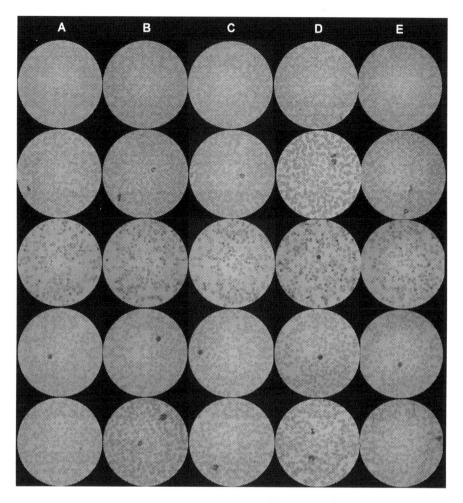

Fig. 14. Illustrative examples of focused images autonomously acquired with the μSmartScope and different smartphone models for 5 different malaria-infected thin blood smears: (A) Asus Zenfone 2; (B) HTC One M8; (C) Motorola Moto G5; (D) LG Nexus 5; (E) Samsung Galaxy 6.

automatic focus of the smear. Considering the current battery capacity of smartphones, this obviously represents a huge burden in terms of power consumption, and it is clear that the current autonomy of the system is low for a day of continuous use. As an alternative, we envision the usage of a power bank coupled to a OTG splitter cable, which we aim to include in the next version of the μSmartScope system.

40   L. Rosado et al.

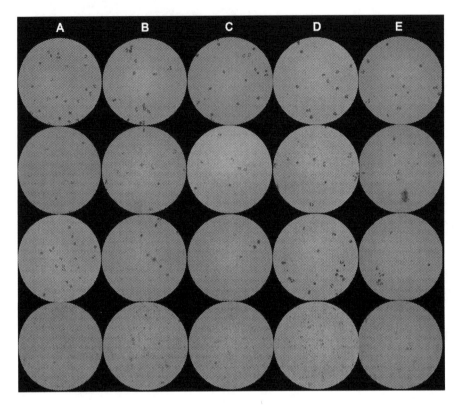

Fig. 15. Illustrative examples of focused images autonomously acquired with the
μSmartScope and different smartphone models for 4 different malaria-infected thick
blood smears: (A) Asus Zenfone 2; (B) HTC One M8; (C) Motorola Moto G5; (D) LG
Nexus 5; (E) Samsung Galaxy 6.

6.5   Automated Focus

In order to evaluate the proposed automated focus approach, we used 9 different
blood smears and 5 different smartphone models, which gave a total of 45 different smartphone-specimen combinations. The automated focus test procedure
consisted on the acquisition of 100 images for each smartphone-specimen combination, i.e. 4500 focused images were acquired without any human interaction.
Two different types of specimens were used: 5 thin blood smears and 4 thick
blood smears. As mentioned before, we opted to use these two different types of
specimen preparations because they represent quite well two different extreme
scenarios we might encounter: the thin blood smears usually presents dense concentration of visible structures in each microscopic field, while the thick blood
smears have a low number of visible structures. The average image acquisition
time per smartphone-specimen combination is depict on Tables 2 and 3.

These results corresponds to an average of 8.31 ± 1.41 sec/image and
12.98 ± 4.20 sec/image, for thin and thick blood smears, respectively. Taken into

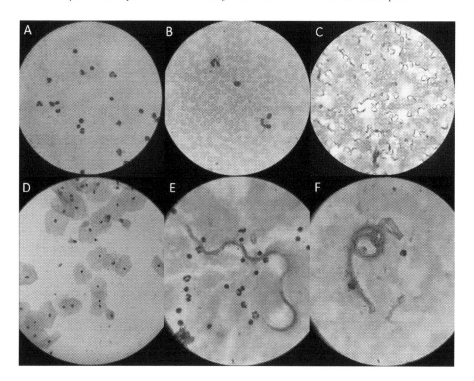

Fig. 16. Images of different smears acquired with the μSmartScope: (A) Thick blood smear infected with malaria parasites (*P.falciparum* species); (B) Thin blood smear infected with malaria parasites (*P. ovale* and *P.malariae* species); (C) Thin blood smear infected with Chagas parasites (*Trypanosome cruzi* species); (D) Liquid-based Pap smear with high grade squamous lesions; (E) Thick blood smear infected with Lymphatic Filariasis parasites (*Brugia malayi* species); (F) Thick blood smear infected with Lymphatic Filariasis parasites (*Wuchereria bancrofti* species). Images (A), (B) and (C) were acquires with a LG Nexus 5, while images (D), (E) and (F) with a Samsung Galaxy S5. All images were acquired with magnification of 1000x, except image (D) which has magnification of 400x [8].

account that on a previous work we reported a performance of 80 s per image [8], this major performance boost clearly illustrates the benefits of the mechanical and software improvements proposed on this work. Particularly, by testing the μSmartScope on such a wide range of smartphone-specimen combinations, we validated that our results were not biased towards a specific specimen type (e.g. amount microscopic structures or staining condition) or specific camera sensor characteristics (e.g. resolution, exposure or white-balancing mode). This good adaptability to different smartphone-specimen combinations conditions is illustrated on Figs. 14 and 15.

6.6   Applicability Examples

The μSmartScope was used to acquire microscopic images of reference blood smears with different parasites, which are responsible for the most relevant NTDs that can be detected through microscopic examination (see Fig. 16). Particularly, the following smears were used: thick blood smear infected with malaria parasites (*P.falciparum* species); thin blood smear infected with malaria parasites (*P.ovale* and *P.malariae* species); thin blood smear infected with Chagas parasites (*Trypanosome cruzi* species); and thick blood smear infected with Lymphatic Filariasis parasites (*Brugia malayi* and *Wuchereria bancrofti* species).

Furthermore, to highlight the versatility of the developed system, a liquid-based Pap smear with high grade squamous lesions was also tested, which is associated with precancerous changes and high risk of cervical cancer. For the analysis of this smear, a magnification of 400x is required, so we had to adapt the optical set up of the μSmartScope, which consisted in the simple procedure of changing the Bresser Planachromat 100x oil-immersion objective for the Bresser Planachromat 40x (Bresser #5941540).

To finalize, considering the acquired images and the feedback received by the specialists that helped us collect the smears, we can state that very promising results were obtained. For all the tested smears, the detection of the considered blood parasites and the precancerous cells on the cervix was considered possible through images acquired via the μSmartScope.

7   Conclusions and Future Work

In this paper we report our most recent advances towards the development of a fully automated 3D-printed smartphone microscope with a motorized stage (μSmartScope). This prototype is the first proposed smartphone-based alternative to conventional microscopy that allows autonomous acquisition of a pre-defined number of images at 1000x magnification with suitable resolution, by using a motorized automated stage fully powered and controlled by a smartphone, without any human interaction.

All the components of the proposed device are described and properly evaluated. In terms of the optical module, a minimum resolution of $0.388\,\mu m$ was determined, with a FOV of $214.38\,\mu m$ and $206.87\,\mu m$ for the vertical and horizontal axis that passes through the center of the visible optical circle, respectively. Regarding the illumination module, the LED light coupled to the proposed condenser demonstrated to achieve an uniform illumination suitable for bright-field microscopy. The developed motorized automated stage (μStage) achieved an average resolution of $330 \pm 81\,\mu m$ for the XY plane steps and an average resolution of $0.763 \pm 0.098\,\mu m$ for the Z-axis steps, results that validates its effective usage for microscopy analysis. Moreover, the proposed automated focus approach was evaluated on 9 different blood smears and 5 different smartphone models, achieving an average performance time of $8.31 \pm 1.41\,sec/image$ and $12.98 \pm 4.20\,sec/image$, for thin and thick blood smears, respectively.

Several smears infected by different blood parasites responsible for the most relevant neglected tropical diseases were used to test the device. The acquired images showed that it was possible to detect those agents through images acquired via the µSmartScope, which clearly illustrate the huge potential of this device, specially in developing countries with limited access to healthcare services. As future work, we want to test the performance and assess the practical usefulness of the µSmartScope on field trials. Particularly, the µSmartScope will represent a component of a mobile-based framework for malaria parasites detection currently being developed. Thus, we aim to integrate this prototype into the referred framework, with the ultimate goal of creating a system that: (i) provides an effective pre-diagnosis of malaria in medically-undeserved areas; (ii) is low cost and mobile based; (iii) is easy to use, even for non-experts in microscopy.

Acknowledgements. We would like to acknowledge the financial support from North Portugal Regional Operational Programme (NORTE 2020), Portugal 2020 and the European Regional Development Fund (ERDF) from European Union through the project 'Deus ex Machina: Symbiotic Technology for Societal Efficiency Gains', NORTE-01-0145-FEDER-000026.

References

1. The END Fund: NTD Overview. http://www.end.org/whatwedo/ntdoverview. Accessed 11 Sept 2017
2. Utzinger, J., Becker, S.L., Knopp, S., Blum, J., Neumayr, A.L., Keiser, J., Hatz, C.F.: Neglected tropical diseases: diagnosis, clinical management, treatment and control. Swiss Med. Weekly **142** (2012)
3. Zachary, G.: Technology alone won't improve health in Africa [Spectral lines]. IEEE Spectr. **52**(1), 7 (2015)
4. Dolgin, E.: Portable pathology for Africa. IEEE Spectr. **52**(1), 37–39 (2015)
5. Rosado, L., da Costa, J.M.C., Elias, D., Cardoso, J.S.: Automated detection of malaria parasites on thick blood smears via mobile devices. Procedia Comput. Sci. **90**, 138–144 (2016)
6. Rosado, L., da Costa, J.M.C., Elias, D., Cardoso, J.S.: Mobile-based analysis of malaria-infected thin blood smears: automated species and life cycle stage determination. Sensors **17**, 2167 (2017)
7. Rosado, L., da Costa, J.M.C., Elias, D., Cardoso, J.S.: A review of automatic malaria parasites detection and segmentation in microscopic images. **14**(1), 11–22 (2016). http://www.eurekaselect.com
8. Rosado, L., Oliveira, J., Vasconcelos, M.J.M., da Costa, J.M.C., Elias, D., Cardoso, J.S.: µSmartScope: 3D-printed smartphone microscope with motorized automated stage. In: Proceedings of the 10th International Joint Conference on Biomedical Engineering Systems and Technologies - Volume 1: BIODEVICES, (BIOSTEC 2017), pp. 38–48. INSTICC, SciTePress (2017)
9. Tseng, D., Mudanyali, O., Oztoprak, C., Isikman, S.O., Sencan, I., Yaglidere, O., Ozcan, A.: Lensfree microscopy on a cellphone. Lab Chip **10**(14), 1787–1792 (2010)
10. Pirnstill, C.W., Coté, G.L.: Malaria diagnosis using a mobile phone polarized microscope. Sci. Rep. **5**, 13368 (2015)

11. Arpa, A., Wetzstein, G., Lanman, D., Raskar, R.: Single lens off-chip cellphone microscopy, pp. 23–28. IEEE, June 2012
12. Cybulski, J.S., Clements, J., Prakash, M.: Foldscope: origami-based paper microscope. PLoS ONE **9**(6), e98781 (2014)
13. Smith, Z.J., Chu, K., Espenson, A.R., Rahimzadeh, M., Gryshuk, A., Molinaro, M., Dwyre, D.M., Lane, S., Matthews, D., Wachsmann-Hogiu, S.: Cell-phone-based platform for biomedical device development and education applications. PLoS ONE **6**(3), e17150 (2011)
14. Switz, N.A., D'Ambrosio, M.V., Fletcher, D.A.: Low-cost mobile phone microscopy with a reversed mobile phone camera lens. PLoS ONE **9**(5), e95330 (2014)
15. WHO: Basic malaria microscopy. Number Part 1. World Health Organization (1991)
16. Budynas, R.G., Nisbett, K.J.: Shigley's Mechanical Engineering Design, 10th edn. McGraw-Hill Education, New York (2014)
17. Wakerly, M.: USB Serial for Android (2012)
18. Krotkov, E.: Focusing. Int. J. Comput. Vis. **1**(3), 223–237 (1988)
19. Shih, L.: Autofocus survey: a comparison of algorithms. In: Electronic Imaging 2007, International Society for Optics and Photonics, p. 65020B (2007)
20. Sun, Y., Duthaler, S., Nelson, B.J.: Autofocusing algorithm selection in computer microscopy. In: 2005 IEEE/RSJ International Conference on Intelligent Robots and Systems, pp. 70–76. IEEE (2005)
21. Liu, X., Wang, W., Sun, Y.: Dynamic evaluation of autofocusing for automated microscopic analysis of blood smear and pap smear. J. Microsc. **227**(1), 15–23 (2007)
22. Tenenbaum, J.M.: Accommodation in computer vision. Ph.D. dissertation. Technical report, DTIC Document (1970)

A Portable Chemical Detection System with Anti-body Biosensor for Impedance Based Monitoring of T2-mycotoxin Bioterrorism Agents

V. I. Ogurtsov[(✉)] and K. Twomey

Tyndall National Institute, Lee Maltings, University College Cork, Cork, Ireland
vladimir.ogurtsov@tyndall.ie

Abstract. The work describes the development of a portable and autonomous biosensing label free platform for detection of biotoxin substances. The biosensor is realized as an on-chip package-free micro electrochemical cell consisting of a counter electrode (CE), a reference electrode (RE) and a working electrode (WE) patterned on a single silicon chip. To improve sensor sensitivity, the WE was implemented as a microelectrode array of 40 micron diameter gold disks with 400 micron centre-to-centre distance, which underwent corresponding surface modification for antibody immobilisation. The interfacial biosensor changes produced by T2-mycotoxin antigen-antibody reaction were sensed by means of Electrochemical Impedance Spectroscopy in a frequency range from 10 Hz to 100 kHz. The signal processing algorithm for mycotoxin quantification was based on analysis of biosensor impedance spectra and its equivalent electrical circuit. It is implemented in corresponding software at microcontroller and single-board computer level in such a manner that the results can be produced at point-of-need or in the decision center without user intervention. The instrumentation represented a mix signal measurement system which consisted of analog and digital parts. The analog part constituted a low noise, highly-sensitive hardware which implemented impedance measurements on the basis of a quadrature signal processing of the biosensor in response to a harmonic stimulation signal. The key unit of the digital part of the device was an Atmel microcontroller with inbuilt 12-bit ADC and external 16-bit DAC, which are responsible for device configuration, stimulation signal generation, biosensor signal digitalization, its initial signal processing and communication with the single-board computer. A calibration of the platform in the range of 0–250 ppm of T2 toxin concentrations confirmed that the system can provide successful detection of the toxin at the levels above 25 ppm.

Keywords: Label-free biosensor · T2-mycotoxin · Immunosensor
Surface modification · Electrochemical Impedance Spectroscopy
Portable instrumentation · Equivalent circuit · Signal processing

© Springer International Publishing AG, part of Springer Nature 2018
N. Peixoto et al. (Eds.): BIOSTEC 2017, CCIS 881, pp. 45–73, 2018.
https://doi.org/10.1007/978-3-319-94806-5_3

1 Introduction

The development of miniaturized, portable biosensing systems for the rapid, reliable and low cost determination of contaminating bio agents in the environment (atmosphere, water, food etc.) has received considerable attention in recent years particularly with the advancements in biotechnology. In the last decade with the growing threat of bioterrorism, the demand on development of systems that can rapidly and accurately detect bio agents, that can threaten human life or health, is significantly increased. There exist a few options for the detection of bioterrorism agents [1]:

1. Generic detectors that provide an on/off alert
2. Biosensors for rapid screening and presumptive identification [2, 3] and
3. Identification systems for definitive confirmation.

Of the three technologies, biosensors can play an important role in detection of Chemical, Biological, Radiological, Nuclear, and Explosive (CBRNE) materials because they can provide a sensitive monitoring tool whilst also being amenable to miniaturization and forming part of a portable system. Beside security, biosensing systems are increasingly used in a range of other different applications including environmental, clinical, food and agriculture [4–15]. The conventional approaches are mainly lab-based and cannot be easily deployed at point-of-need. Modern microfabricated biosensors, on the other hand, offer the advantages of a cost-effective and rapid sample analysis, and specific and sensitive measurements over the traditional methods, which tend to be a multi-step (e.g. ELISA), or to involve sophisticated and expensive equipment (e.g. HPLC). The ability to apply semiconductor processing technologies, more commonly used in the IC industry, in the sensor chip fabrication [8, 10] enables large batch production and subsequent availability of cheap and disposable devices.

The International Union of Pure and Applied Chemistry (IUPAC) defines a biosensor as follows "A biosensor is a self-contained integrated device which is capable of providing specific quantitative or semi-quantitative analytical information using a biological recognition element (biochemical receptor) that is in direct spatial contact with a transducer element" [11, 12]. Thus, according to this classification a biosensor is essentially composed of two elements:

1. A bioreceptor that is an immobilized sensitive biological element (e.g. enzyme, DNA, antibody) recognizing the analyte (e.g. enzyme substrate, complimentary DNA, antigen).
2. A transducer that converts (bio) chemical signal resulting from the interaction of the analyte with the bioreceptor into its electrical equivalent. The intensity of the signal generated is either directly or indirectly proportional to the analyte concentration.

Essentially, the selectivity or specificity of the biosensor depends on the biorecognition element, which is capable of "sensing" the presence of an analyte [13, 14]. There are currently three generations of biosensors in existence. The term generation was originally created to describe the stages of integration in biosensors. Biosensors with mediated response mainly generated by membrane-bound or membrane entrapped biocomponents (first generation), were followed by virtually reagentless biosensors where biocomponents are fixed directly to the sensor surface and either the reaction of coimmobolised cosubstrates (bound to the electrode, polymer or enzyme itself) or the direct heterogeneous electron transfer between the prosthetic group and the electrode is exploited (second generation). While the immobilisation of the receptors directly on an electronic circuit leads to systems with integrated signal generation, transduction and processing (third generation) having the potential of considerable miniaturisation [15]. The devices investigated in this study should be considered as the third generation under this classification and this highlights the progress sensing systems since their relatively recent development.

Antibody-based biosensors or immunosensor are found on an antigen-antibody interaction where antibody (Ab), Y-shaped proteins, bind with a target, an invading antigen (Ag), through a high affinity binding reaction. The specificity of the reaction is due to a chemical constitution of antibody which is specific to the target antigen that defines similarity of the antigen-antibody reaction to a lock (antibody) and key (antigen) operation. This conditions such advantages of immunosensors as high versatility, selectivity, stability and sensitivity. At the same time, the strong antigen-antibody binding makes it very difficult to break these bonds, thus, a typical immunosensor is a disposable one-shot sensor that cannot be used after the target detection [16–20].

Immunosensors utilizing antibody-based recognition elements, have been developed on a wide range of transduction platforms. The transducer element translates the selective recognition of the analyte into a quantifiable signal and thus, has major influence on sensitivity [21]. Since 1959 when an antibodies based biosensor for the first time was used with radiolabeled assay for detection of insulin in the body fluids [22] immunosensors have revolutionized impact on detection of a whole lot of different target analytes such as disease markers, food and environmental contaminants, biological warfare agents and illicit drugs. Nowadays, transduction approaches used with immunosensors include electrochemical, piezoelectric and optical systems [15, 23] where the mostly used methods are based on optical and electrochemical methodology. However, the classical optical transduction mechanism has suffered from poor sensitivity when coupled with radioimmunoassay, the short half-life of radioactive agents, concerns of health hazards, and disposal problems. As well the optical methods usually require a complicated sample preparation that increases risk of sample contamination, rises cost and time of analysis and makes them difficult for implementation in a portable device capable of working in field conditions outside of specialized labs. Electrochemical detection overcomes the most of these problems and provides means for fast, simple, reliable and economical realization of portable autonomous immunosensing systems capable of working at point-of-need without end-user intervention [19, 24]. The advantage of electrochemical biosensors is also that they can monitor bimolecular interactions in real time. In this process the biorecognition components are immobolised on a solid surface (usually the sensor chip), and the component to be detected is present in the solution phase [25].

A typical electrochemical biosensor usually represents an electrode or an array of microdiscs/bands with corresponding bio functionalization acting as the working electrode within a three-electrode electrochemical cell containing also a reference electrode (i.e. Ag/AgCl) and an auxiliary/counter electrode (which varies) [26]. The working electrode provides the sensing capability, the reference and the counter electrodes facilitate the measurements. A design option for the electrochemical biosensor is a bio specific membrane that selectively interacts with the analyte. A physical transducer coupled to the membrane detects this biointeraction and generates the resulting electrical signal. The bio specific membrane can be made up of a material that undergoes electron exchange reactions with the analyte so a direct electrical output signal consisting of a potential or a current can be detected and interpreted [27].

Typical microfabricated biosensors incorporate a gold electrode, or other materials e.g. platinum, Si_3N_4, active layer upon which different surface chemistries are applied to form a complete device that is specific and sensitive to a target of interest [28, 29]. Within the branch of electrochemical sensors, there are amperometeric, potentiometric, impedimetric and field-effect transistor (FET) biosensors [19, 23, 30, 31]. With the amperometric type biosensors, the sensor current is monitored with time; for the potentiometric – the voltage is monitored. Both of these types offer relatively straight forward measurements and a rapid analysis. The impedimetric is more complex and more sensitive technique. Its classical implementation is based on the measurement of an AC current that forms in the response on the application to the sensor a sinusoidal voltage over a set of frequencies. The advantage of impedemetric biosensor is that they can directly sense the changes in interface between the bio functionalized electrode and the sample solution due to the biorecognition reaction through monitoring of the sensor impedance variations. For that they do not need any additional labelling that is very often required in case of optical biosensor [22]. This circumstance along with relative simplicity of electrochemical instrumentation defines the ease and cheapness of impedemetric biosensors operation (no additional expensing labelling or sample preparation) that with such their advantages as high sensitivity and the ability to miniaturise the associated measurement instrumentation explains a growing interest in label-free impedimetric biosensors for different application [4, 32]. A further advance in electrochemical biosensors can be obtained by using of micro-sized electrodes, which improve the mass transport (and hence the sensor sensitivity) owing to the occurrence of radial diffusion over planar diffusion from macro-size electrodes resulting in an increase in the signal-to-noise ratio and reduction in the iR drop [33].

The presented study describes the development of such portable biosensing platform with immunosensor on the base of microfabricated microelectrode array capable of biotoxin detection. The performance of the platform was validated by detection of T2-toxin. It is a trichothecene mycotoxin, which is toxic to humans and animals. It is naturally occurring mould byproduct of Fusarium spp. fungus that can be found in grains such as barley, wheat and oats. It is well-known that some mycotoxins can be used as chemical warfare agents [34, 35]. Inside of this group, trichothecenes can act immediately upon contact, and exposure to a few milligrams of T-2 is potentially lethal. The symptoms exhibited by purported victims included internal hemorrhaging, blistering of the skin, and other clinical responses that are caused by exposure to trichothecenes.

Detection methods for T-2 toxin can be classified into two types: screening methods like ELISA and analytical methods like GC and HPLC [36, 37]. Since low ppb concentrations are usually required to be detected, very sensitive analytical methods are hence needed. Advantages of screening methods like ELISA are that these methods generally do not require a clean-up other than dilution of the extract and/or filtration before analysis. ELISA type screening methods rely on antibodies to detect the T-2 toxin. The specific antibodies (monoclonal or polyclonal) distinguishes the 3D structure of T-2 toxin. Usually an incubation period of about 1-2 h is required to complete this bio recognition procedure. The T-2 toxin present in the sample being tested competes with a labelled toxin for a limited number of antibody binding sites. The more toxin in the sample solution, the lower the binding of the labelled toxin and the lower the signal generated by the assay. The presence of the T-2 toxin is indicated by a specific color change. However, there are disadvantages to this particular mechanism of detection. These two main disadvantages are high matrix dependence and overestimation of the T-2 toxin concentration, which can occur if structurally related mycotoxins or constituents present in the matrix interfere with the competitive antibody-binding site mechanism required for the detection of T-2 toxin by ELISA [38]. Hence, this could lead to false results. However, there are advantages of screening methods like ELISA. They are high sample throughput and ease of operation. Thus, detection limits of 0.1 ng/g obtained with this methodology have been reported [37]. Other recent screening methods include Molecularly Imprinted Polymers (MIPs) [38] and Dipstick and Lateral Flow tests, where detection limits of 4 and 50 ng/kg were stated [39].

The presented study describes the development of a portable autonomous impedimetric biosensing system with a label-free electrochemical immunosensor for T2-toxin detection for using at point of need. The immunosensor is based on a bio functionalized microelectrode array [24, 40] which works as a part of a microfabricated electrochemical cell realized as a single silicon packageless chip. The developed biosensing system played role of a biohazard detection unit in a portable HANHOLD platform developed for detection of CBRN threads for operating at point of need. The platform was created during fulfilment an FP7 collaborative project called Handhold (Handheld Olfactory Detector) [41] and included also an optical sensing module for detection of chemical thread (explosive) and a radioactivity detector. All modules were operating under integrated control from a single board PC that has possibility of wirelessly transmitting the platform data to an outside decision center. The platform was creating by the analogy of a sniffer dog that is used at airport custom control. While the dog will remain a central part of the detection process at border crossing and airports, sensor technology and low power computer based embedded system are improving to the extent that the time is now right to develop substantially improved mobile detection devices that can successfully complement the role played now mostly by dogs. Moreover, these detection devices can be networked together to provide enhanced alert facilities and also to enable easier management and field deployment of the platforms themselves.

2   Experimental

2.1   Description of the Bio Sensing System

The aim of the presented work was to develop a modular sensor platform which is reconfigurable and which can be deployed for a stand-off detection mimicking the operational characteristics of a sniffer dog. Unlike the situation with dog retraining, this platform can be retargeted simply by removing one set of sensors and adding others, the software load reacting dynamically to the reconfiguration. Figure 1 illustrates the different technologies that play a role in the development of the Handhold biosensing system.

These technologies include microfabrication and surface chemistry that will be used for biosensor preparation, mix signal electronic design – for instrumentation hardware development, signal processing algorithm and corresponding software – for implementation of the autonomous system operation without end-user interference and integration – for completion of the system and providing its operability in the Handhold CBRN threads detection platform.

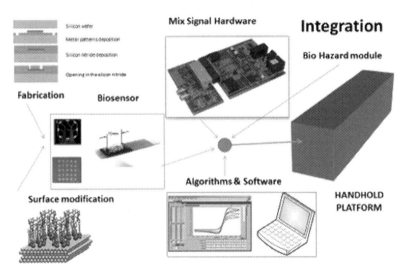

Fig. 1. The Handhold biosensing system.

2.2   Biosensor

As shown in Fig. 1 the biosensor consists of two main parts. They are a transducer (working electrode in the three-electrode micro electrochemical system) and a bio recognition layer that adds the bio specificity to the electrochemical sensor. For improving biosensor sensitivity a microelectrode array structure was selected for working electrode implementation. The development of the sensor transducer was started from simulation of different electrode designs including single disc, disc array, single band and band array. The simulation was performed in Multiphysics Engineering Simulation Software Comsol. The aim of this part of the work was to analyse the diffusion transport mechanism that occurs between the interface of the electrode and the sample solution and to determine the optimum transducer layouts according to its electrochemical performance. In this simulation, the model was created where each microelectrode was positioned at a set distance below the sensor surface. This was to represent the physical fabrication process where an etch layer opens up areas of exposure in the top passivation layer to allow electrode contact with the environment. This technological process allows very fine electrode patterning but supposes that each electrode is located below the chip surface at the depth of few hundred of nm which is the range of possible thicknesses of the silicon nitride layer deposited on the metal. The hexagonal array configuration providing the most compact electrode placement [33] was considered with this simulation. For the disc array model, the diffusion zone approach was applied [42, 43], as schematically shown in Fig. 2.

The species concentration on the electrode surface was defined from the Nernst equation Eq. (1)

$$\frac{C_A}{C_B} = \exp\left(\frac{nF}{RT}\left(E - E'\right)\right) \tag{1}$$

where C_A and C_B are concentrations of the electro active species involved into the electrochemical reaction, n is a number of electrons participated in electron exchange, R is the universal gas constant, F is the Faraday constant, E' is the formal potential. The electrode current was determined from integration of the diffusion flux over the electrode area, Eq. (2):

$$i = 2\pi nFD \int_0^{r_a} \left.\frac{\partial C(r,x,t)}{\partial x}\right|_{x=x_s} r dr \tag{2}$$

where D is diffusion coefficient of electro active species. Some results attained for the different electrode designs from this simulation are discussed below.

Examples of the calculated concentration profiles (occurring due to the diffusion mechanism taking place) at the different disc electrode structures and dimensions are shown in the diagrams presented in Fig. 3 in 10 s span after applying to the electrode a voltage that changes, according to Nernst equation Eq. (1), the concentration of the electro active species on the electrode surface to zero level.

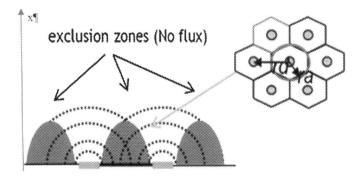

Fig. 2. Array model with the diffusion zone approach implemented.

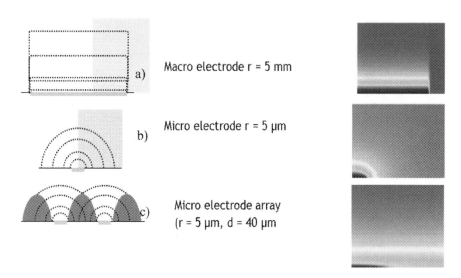

Fig. 3. Concentration profiles for macro, micro and micro electrode array after 10 s. (Color figure online)

As one can note, for a macro electrode, a planar type of diffusion occurs near the electrode (Fig. 3a). Diffusion zones can be seen in the changing color from blue to bright red. The dark red color situated at a distance from the electrode relates to the bulk concentration, where no or minimal diffusion is occurring. A reduction in electrode size from macro to micro changes the diffusion type from planar to radial. It can be seen by an example of a microelectrode of radius 5 μm that spans out a semicircular concentration wave from the electrode (Fig. 3b). This type of diffusion results in a high current density that leads to increase of signal to noise ratio, hence it is desirable to have. However, because of a small area of the microelectrode its total current is reduced in absolute value that can be difficult to measure in practice due to existence of electrochemical and electronic noises. To overcome this problem an array of microelectrodes can be used to increase the total signal. Care needs to be taken to ensure that there is no diffusion zones overlap between the neighboring electrodes. A general rule-of-thumb is to separate the electrodes in array by the length of more or equal to a specific center-to-center distance $d_c = 20r$ [44]. An example of overlapping diffusion zones is shown in Fig. 3c for a microdisc array of radius 5 μm and center-to-center distance of 40 μm (8 disc radii). As can be seen here, at a short distance from the array the concentration profiles transfer to the plain profile as in case of a macro electrode (Fig. 3a). This circumstance reduces the transducer signal. In order to avoid this situation, the center-to-center spacing in the transducer in the biosensor chip prototype for this disk radius was increased to 100 μm.

Dependence of the transducer current and current density from the time for the micro electrode array of different designs can be seen in Figs. 4 and 5. The current density of the whole electrode array is shown in the left plots and current of the whole electrode array is presented in the right plots of these figures. The transient process for a

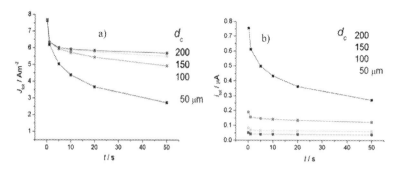

Fig. 4. Transient current density (a) and total current (b) for a microdisk electrodes array with $r_a = 5$ μm and different values of d_c and N_{el} as indicated in Table 1. (Color figure online)

time period of 50 s calculated for an array of microdisc electrodes of radius (r_e) of 5 μm and 1 μm with varying number of electrodes per array (N_{el}), center-to-center spacing (d_c), distance between electrode row (d_r) and the total electrode array area (S_A) as given in Table 1.

The results of the simulations show that for the largest center-to-center separation (blue curve) there is no or only slight interaction of the diffusion zones over the time span of 50 s and the current reaches a steady-state. The effect of diffusion zones overlap is two-fold. First, the current density is becoming smaller with decreasing center-to-center spacing values. Second, with decreasing d_c, the transients deviate from the steady state behavior. A complete overlap of the diffusion zones results in purely planar diffusion and the current starts to decrease at $t^{-1/2}$, as observed for macro electrodes and can be seen for the microdisc array of 5 μm radius and 50 μm center-to-center spacing in Fig. 4 and for the microdisc array of 1 μm radius and 10 μm center-to-center spacing Fig. 5.

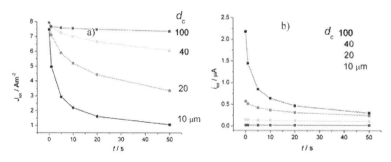

Fig. 5. Transient current density (a) and total current (b) for a microdisk electrodes array with $r_a = 1$ μm and different values of d_c and N_{el} as indicated in in Table 1.

As was mentioned above, due to the technological peculiarities after fabrication the microelectrode of radius r_e is located at the bottom of the pore in the isolation layer of thickness d_p deposited on the top of the metal. Thus, in the reality the microelectrode

Table 1. The electrode arrays geometrical parameters.

r_a, μm	d_c, μm	d_r, μm	N_{el}	S_A, m²
5	200	170	85	6.676E−9
5	150	130	137	1.076E−8
5	100	86	314	2.466E−8
5	50	43	1260	9.896E−8
1	100	86.6	264	2.606E−9
1	40	34.6	1863	1.838E−8
1	20	17.3	7314	7.218E−8
1	10	8.7	29508	2.912E−7

represents a recessed electrode with aspect ratio $\gamma = d_p/r_e$ and performance of the microelectrode depends on this ratio. The simulation results for a single inlaid electrode and a recessed electrode with pore walls perpendicular to the electrode surface are shown in Figs. 6 and 7. Figure 6a demonstrates transient currents for an inlaid disk electrode (black curve) and for a recessed electrode with $\gamma = 0.2$ ($r_a = 5$ μm, $d_p = 1$ μm) (red curve) normalized to steady-state current of the inlaid electrode. Figure 6b shows dependence of the normalized steady-state current of the recess electrode as a function of the pore aspect ratio. Figure 7 presents the concentration profiles for the recess electrode at different times after application of the stimulation voltage: at 0.01 s - Fig. 7a, at 0.1 s - Fig. 7b, at 1 s - Fig. 7c and at 10 s - Fig. 7d. As can be seen from comparison of the inlaid and recess electrodes behavior the existence of the electrode recess leads to decrease of the steady-state current that can be quite significant for the large aspect ratio. From the concentration profiles follows that at start time (high frequencies) until concentration wave is inside of the pore the diffusion processes in a recess electrode are similar to macroelectrode behavior with a planar type of diffusion (Fig. 3a).

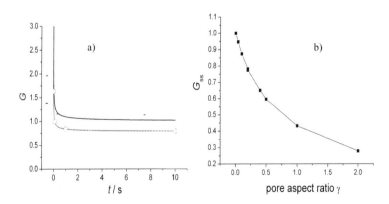

Fig. 6. Normalised transient current for an inlaid disk electrode (black curve) and for a recessed electrode with $\gamma = 0.2$ ($r_a = 5$ μm, $d_p = 1$ μm) (red curve) (a); the normalized steady-state current as a function of the pore aspect ratio (b). (Color figure online)

The results on the electrode topology optimization formed the basis of the design of the biosensor chip prototype. The biosensor was realized as an on-chip packageless three electrode microelectrochemical cell, which includes a counter electrode (CE), an reference electrode (RE) and a working electrode (WE) patterned on a single silicon chip as shown in Fig. 8. The WE was located at the end of the chip to provide its separation from RE and CE. Such an arrangement was implemented in order to facilitate the bio functionalization chemistry and prevent both RE and CE from interference with this process. The chip size was 10.16×37.70 mm. To provide connectivity to the instruments the chip is equipped with 4 rectangular contact gold pads of 2.50×5.00 mm dimensions with a standard 2.54 mm pitch. The CE was made from platinum of 5.25×5.00 mm dimensions. The RE was a circular Ag/AgCl electrode of 1.00 mm diameter. The WE represents an array of microdisk or microband electrodes of different parameters as shown in the Table 2. The best results for the biosensor were obtained with the microdisc array with 40 μm diameter recessed gold disks, arranged in a hexagonal configuration with 400 μm center-to-center spacing which subsequently underwent surface modification as will be described below.

The on-chip micro electrochemical cell was fabricated at the Central Fabrication Facility at Tyndall National Institute. For fabrication of the chip was used a standard photolithography and lift-off techniques with different masks associated with the cell electrodes as schematically shown in Fig. 9 and previously discussed in [10, 24, 45]. In brief this process can be described as follows. Firstly, a silicon oxide layer of 1 μm thickness was thermally grown on the silicon substrate of N-Type, <111>-orientation and alignments marks were patterned on it. The selection of the substrate type is related to its high resistivity. Then the 20 nm thick titanium and 150 nm thick gold layers were patterned on the wafers to prepare for electrodes, connecting tracks and pads. The titanium layer acts as an adhesion layer, which improved the quality of the gold layer

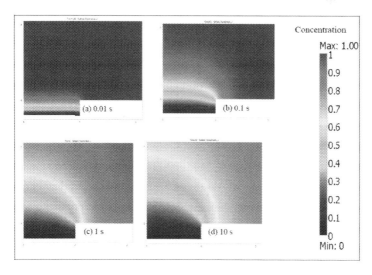

Fig. 7. Concentration distributions around the electrode for the recessed configuration electrode at the indicated times in s.

Table 2. Parameters of working electrode arrays.

Geometry	Disc diameter/ band width, μm	Band length, μm	Center-to-center separation, μm	Number of electrodes	Surface area, m^2
Disc	1	-	10	32592	2.56e-8
	5	-	50	1326	2.60e-8
	5	-	50	663	1.30e-8
	10	-	100	323	2.54e-8
	10	-	100	163	1.28e-8
	20	-	200	85	2.67e-8
	40	-	400	23	2.89e-8
Band	1	50	20	81	4.05e-9
	5	250	100	17	2.12e-8
	10	500	100	17	8.50e-8
	10	500	100	34	1.70e-7
	10	500	100	9	4.50e-8
	20	1000	400	5	1.00e-7
	40	2000	800	3	2.40e-7

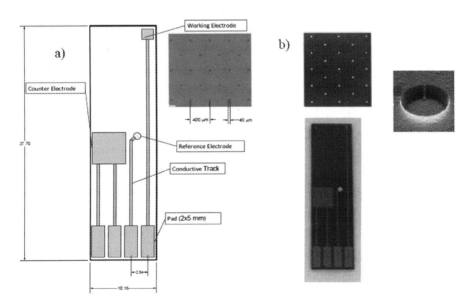

Fig. 8. Biosensor chip layout (a) and photos of fabricated chip, working electrode array and a single recessed microdisk (b).

deposit. Another 20 nm thick titanium adhesion layer was used before the deposition of the 150 nm thick Pt and of 250 nm thick Ag metals on the gold connection areas for the counter and reference electrodes where to promote the adhesion of Ag the Ti layer

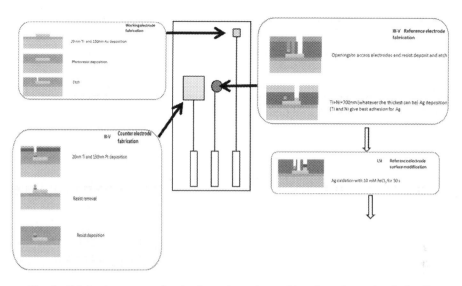

Fig. 9. Fabrication process for the three electrode on-chip micro electrochemical cell.

was supplemented by 20 nm of Ni. Then, 500 nm of silicon nitride was deposited on the whole wafer by plasma-enhanced chemical vapor deposition. The role of the silicon nitride is to insulate the connecting tracks from the solution. Openings for the electrodes and the connecting pads were obtained by plasma etching. Silver–silver chloride reference electrodes were prepared with help of chemical oxidation by immersion of the wafer in a 10 mM FeCl3 solution for 50 s. The metal was then lifted and a resist layer was spin coated on top of the wafer to protect the electrodes during the dicing of the wafer into individual chips.

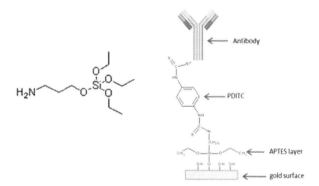

Fig. 10. Scheme of the electrode biofunctionalisation.

The required sensor specificity to the defined biotarget was introduced through application of a bio functionalization procedure which attached an antibody to the surface of a working electrode. Three surface modification techniques were investigated including carboxymethyl dextran (CM-dextran) [46], and two silanisation based methods mainly (3-Glycidyloxypropyl) trimethoxysilane (GOPTS) with poly (ethylene glycol) (PEG) linker (GOPTS – PEG) [47] and (3-Aminopropyl)tri-ethoxysilane (APTES) with 1,4-Phenylene diisothiocyanate (PDITC) linker (APTES - PDITC) [48].

The best results from the biosensor stability, reproducibility and sensitivity per-spectives were obtained with APTES – PDITC methodology. This surface modification procedure is straight-forward and requires for its realization less time than two others that should be also referred to its merits. Here PDITC is a homobifunctional cross-linker containing two amine reactive isothiocyanate groups on a phenyl ring. Reaction with the amine group on silanised surface forms a thiourea linkage leaving the second isothiocyanate group free to couple with amine groups on the antibody (Fig. 10). This allows PDITC layer plays role of effective antibody cross-linker on APTES modified surface [49].

This procedure consisted of the following steps: Pretreatment, Silanisation, Acti-vation and Biofunctionalisation that can be briefly described as follows [24, 40].

Pretreatment: The fabricated gold on silicon electrode chips are stayed in oxygen plasma cleaner for 10 min. Then, they are placed in Hydrogen chloride – methanol (HCl:MeOH, 1:1, v/v) solution for 15 min. After they are sonicated in acetone and isopropyl alcohol for 5 min each and finally are carefully rinsed in DI water and dry under a stream of nitrogen.

Silanisation: The treated chips are immersed in 3% APTES in MeOH:DI water (19:1) solution for 30 min at room temperature. Then the chips are rinsed with MeOH and DI water before left to be cure in the oven (dust free) for 15 min at 120 °C.

Activation: Following the curing step, the silanised WE are immediately drown in 18 mL of DMF solution containing 2 mL of 10% pyridine and 0.098 g 1,4-phenylene diisothiocyanate (-PDITC) (produces 25 mM PDITC) for 2 h for PDITC cross-linker attachment. Then the electrodes are carefully washed with DMF and DCE and dry under N2.

Biofunctionalisation: For antibody immobilisation anti-T2 toxin antibody was diluted in 0.1 M sodium borate pH 9.3 and the working electrodes were immersed in 100 μL of diluted antibody solution for 2 h at RT, wrapped in aluminium foil. Then the electrodes were removed, rinsed with DI water and dried with N2. All modification steps involving the chip treatment in the surface modification reactants are performed in such way that only the surface of working electrode (WE) is staying in contact with the solution to prevent contamination of other electrode on the chip.

2.3   Instrumentation

Instrumentation architecture implements impedance spectroscopy technique and rep-resents low noise, highly sensitive measurement unit (analog part) under microcon-troller control (digital part). The hardware provided stimulus signal, the front-end control, conditioning of the biosensor signal, its amplification, filtration, frequency transformation, data acquisition and communication with a control embedded computer. The instrumentation implements the technique, which is known as electro-chemical impedance spectroscopy (EIS) [50, 51]. It uses complex sensor impedance values (real and imaginary impedance components) obtained in a wide frequency range of the stimulation signal for analysis of the biosensor interfacial behaviour. The simplified block-diagram of the circuitry that provides measurement of real and imaginary components of the biosensor impedance Z_S is shown in Fig. 11.

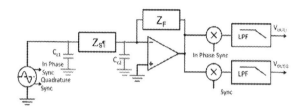

Fig. 11. Simplified block-diagram of impedance measurement circuitry.

It contains a stimulation signal source, which provides in-phase and quadrature AC signals, a transimpedance amplifier with feedback impedance Z_F and two (in-phase and quadrature) detection channels each consisted of a mixer and a low-pass filter. The output of the impedance measurement circuitry includes two DC signals, which contain information on biosensor complex impedance. Assuming that the multipliers have a unitary conversion gain the DC signals can be expressed as follows

$$V_{OUT\_I} = -\frac{V_{STIM}}{2}\frac{|Z_F|}{|Z_S|}\cos(\varphi_S - \varphi_F) \tag{3}$$

$$V_{OUT\_Q} = -\frac{V_{STIM}}{2}\frac{|Z_F|}{|Z_S|}\sin(\varphi_S - \varphi_F) \tag{4}$$

where V_{OUT_I} and V_{OUT_Q} are the output voltages of the two signal paths, V_{STIM} is the amplitude of the stimulation voltage; Z_F is the feedback complex impedance with module $|Z_F|$ and phase φ_F; Z_S is the sensor complex impedance with module $|Z_S|$ and phase φ_S. From the measured output voltages and the known feedback impedance the module and phase of the sensor impedance Z_S can be calculated as defined below

$$|Z_S| = -\frac{V_{STIM}}{2}\frac{|Z_F|}{\sqrt{V_{OUT\_I}^2 + V_{OUT\_Q}^2}} \tag{5}$$

$$\varphi_S = \arctan\left(\frac{V_{OUT\_Q}}{V_{OUT\_I}}\right) - \varphi_F \tag{6}$$

The method of signal extraction, which is used here, is called the lock-in technique. The advantage of this method is the reduction of impact of transimpedance flicker ($1/f$) noise on the measurement. This is because the noise in this technique can be reduced by a final low-pass filter. Thus, if this filter has a narrow bandwidth, only the noise around the measurement frequency will influence the measurements.

The instrumentation architecture implemented in the system is shown in Fig. 12.

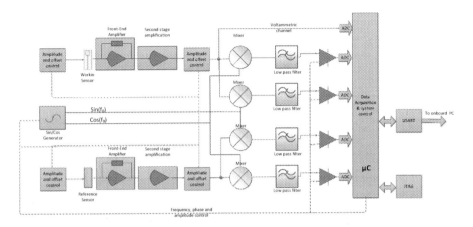

Fig. 12. Instrumentation architecture.

It represents a two channels impedance measurement system with a common signal generator providing in-phase and quadrature AC signals. Each channel includes a current to voltage converter (transimpedance amplifier) and two (in-phase and quadrature) demodulators, each is consisted of a mixer and a low-pass filter, and a level-shift circuit realised on the base of I^2C controlled DAC as shown in Fig. 13. The level-shift circuit is designed to match the sensor double polarity signal with a single polarity microcontroller analog to digital converter (ADC) and to facilitate fine module tuning and calibration. These two detection paths are a sensor channel for the actual measurement and a reference channel to compensate for the background signal.

The sensor connected to the reference channel should be not specific to the target analyte thereby capable of providing information on the sensor background signal resulting from varying parameters such as temperature, pH, nonspecific binding etc. If the background signal is of negligible value, the reference channel can be used as the second sensing channel for another bio target. It is based on the measurement technique

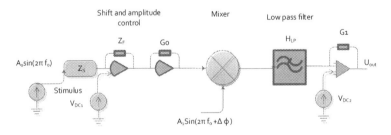

Fig. 13. Block-diagram of the measurement channel.

described above but has some additional features to facilitate its practical implementation. A known AC voltage that is generated by the signal generator is applied across the sensor and the current is converted to a voltage by the transimpedance amplifier. The voltage is amplified and demodulated in the I/Q demodulator yielding real and imaginary impedance components as described above. To increase the dynamic range of the module, 2-bit electronically controlled instrumentation amplifiers are included in the system structure after the transimpedance amplifier.

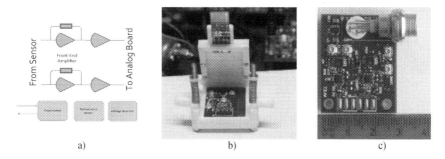

Fig. 14. Block diagram of potentiostat and front-end amplifiers module (a) and photographs of the packaged unit with the sensor chip (b) and the unit PCB (c) (photographs are taken from [24]).

The biosensing system hardware is realized by two modules: Potentiostat and Front-End Amplifiers (PFEA) and Signal Processing and Microcontroller (SPM) units. The PFEA (Fig. 14) is designed as a separate small size unit in order to locate it close to a reservoir where the biosensor tests the sample solution. This shortens the length of the connection wires whose link the biosensor and front-end amplifier, therefore decreases the leakage current and attenuates the noise and electromagnetic interference. The PFEA unit consists of a potentiostat, a temperature sensor and two transimpedance amplifiers providing current to voltage transformation of the sensor and reference (calibration) signals. The potentiostat is realized on three operational amplifiers OPA2211. Two identical transimpedance amplifiers are assembled from OPAMP ADA4647 and instrumentation amplifier AD8253. The unit is implemented on a small four-layer PCB of 25 mm × 35 mm dimensions.

The Signal Processing and Microcontroller (SPM) unit includes mixing and Analog Signal Processing (ASP), microcontroller and peripheral (μC) and Power Supply (PS) blocks. These three blocks forming the main body of the instrumentation are implemented in three separate 4 layer FR4 PCBs of 51 mm × 90 mm dimensions, which are integrated in a stack manner taking 55 mm of height as shown in Fig. 15.

The ASP block consists of Input, Switch, Level-Shifter and four identical Mixer/Low Pass Filter (LPF) lock-in circuits, which form two identical analog processing channels. Four-channel 16-bit digital to analog converters (DAC) incorporated into the SPM circuit is used to adjust DC levels in the SPM unit. The block was assembled from AD630 (Mixer), UAF42 (Low Pass Filter), ADG1419 (Switch), DAC8574 (DAC with buffered voltage output and I^2C compatible two wire serial interface), AD8253 (Instrumental amplifier with 2-bit electronically controlled gain) and LM4140 (1.024 V voltage reference). The μC block is based on a high performance 8-bit ATxmega128A1U microcontroller. It realizes functions of instrumentation control, data acquisition and communication. It also contains the signal generator and four 16-bit DACs. The signal generator is based on AD9854 chip, which is a DDS synthesizer capable of parallel generation of precision sine and cosine signals in a wide frequency range. The SPM unit contains JTAG interface that allows in-circuit system programming and debugging. The PS block supplies stabilized low noise voltages of +8 V, −8 V, +3.3 V and −3.3 V to power the signal generators, microcontroller, ASP and PFEA system units. The PS block can be powered from a voltage source in the range of +5 V−+12 V.

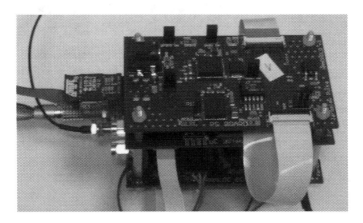

Fig. 15. Photograph of signal processing and Micro-controller unit (the photograph is taken from [24]).

2.4 Signal Processing and Corresponding Software

The associated instrumentation software consists of two highly interrelated parts written for a host computer and an ATxmega128A1U Atmel microcontroller. The software supports communication between the instrumentation and the computer, provides control of the hardware settings and its operation, implements biosensor impedance measurements, their signal processing and the target concentration determination. The computer software is realised with option of a user-friendly multi-tab GUI software that will be described below. Here each tab associated with the program window contains means for solutions of assigned tasks. There are three tabs/windows, namely 'Protocol', 'System configuration', and 'EIS'.

The tab/window **'Protocol'** shown in Fig. 16 is intended for careful design of frequency sweep protocol at each frequency point by applying values of frequency and a repetition number with possibility of adjustment all electronically controlled hardware parameters associated with the impedance measurements. As well all cells in the table including the frequency value can be edited to provide an individual trimming of the measurement mode at the selected frequency. Two command buttons in the upper right corner allow for populating the table with default values (the upper large button) or with parameters, which are set in the SpinEdit controls (the lower small button) for a fast filling of table with the sweep parameter and hardware settings. Sweep parameters include the start *Fmin* and finish *Fmax* frequencies and a number of frequencies per decade, which are used to calculate frequency values distributed between *Fmin* and *Fmax*. Hardware settings duplicate the tuning parameters from the Hardware Config-uration panel that will be discussed below. Accurate adjustment of the sweep param-eters at each table raw (frequency) is available with the help of the SpinEdit control that can be activated in each cell. Frequency is tuned between the neighboring values in the table; hardware settings are limited by the corresponding hardware specification. The created Protocol table can be saved in the Excel file and conversely downloaded from the file.

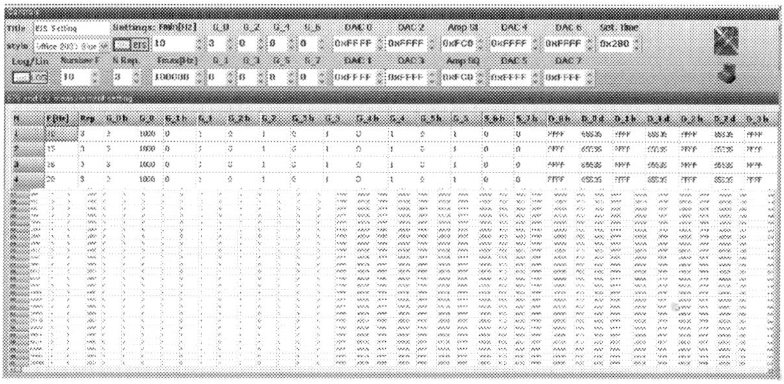

Fig. 16. Screen short of Protocol tab/window.

The tab/window '**System configuration**' shown in Fig. 17 supports communica-tion control including received and transmitted data stream visualization, detection and control of communication and stream errors, data extraction from communication stream, instrumentation and measurement settings control and configuration and system operability testing. Tools for operability testing include Self-Test command, which starts Self-test measurement procedure followed by reporting about the measurement results in the 'Test parameters' plot and in the 'Test parameters' table in 'Hardware Configuration' panel. The program monitors these parameters before each impedance spectrum measurements that allows for easy identification of the hardware and the biosensor operability problem.

The tab/window '**EIS**' is the main instrumentation software part designed to pro-vide all raw impedance measurements and corresponding signal processing and to present the obtained results in different forms as shown in Fig. 18. These include raw sensor impedance measurements presented by Nyquist (Imaginary impedance part vs. Real impedance part - 'Zim vs Zre') and Bode (Imaginary impedance part vs.

Frequency - 'Zim vs F', Real impedance part vs. Frequency - 'Zre vs F' and Phase vs. Frequency - 'Phase vs F') plots as well as the processed Nyquist spectra obtained after Kernel smoothing and subtraction of the reference background spectrum from the measured spectra with analytical signal extraction (see the plot 'Zim vs Zre processed' where the analytical signals extracted are highlighted by red points on the corresponding processed impedance spectra) and calculated analyte concentration in respect to the biosensor calibration (plot 'Anal. Signal vs. Concentration') in both graphical and table forms.

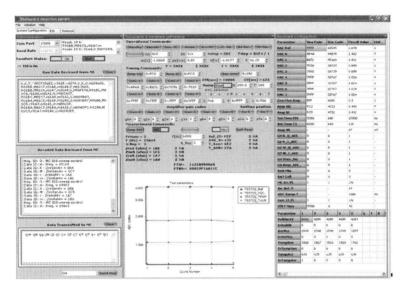

Fig. 17. Screen short of System configuration tab/window (the image is taken from [24]).

The measurements of imaginary Zim, real Zre, phase Ph values of the sensor impedance is based on the Eqs. (3)–(6) and the corresponding module calibration. For determination of the target concentration the special algorithm was developed. It is based on analysis of equivalent circuit of the electrochemical biosensor followed by experimental validation of the approach. The most used model for analysis of impedimetric biosensors is the modified Randles equivalent circuit [52] shown in Fig. 19. It includes resistor Rs that represents the resistance of the sample solution, in which the biosensor is immersed, and the resistance of the working electrode itself and the contacting track connecting the electrode with a corresponding pad presented an external electrical contact of the biosensor; capacitor C_D that arises from the series combination of several capacitive elements, such as analyte binding (C_{An}) to a sensing layer (C_{Se}) on an background electrode (C_{Bg}) capacitances; charge transfer resistor Rct that comprises the series connection of resistors incorporating the analyte binding (R_{An}) to a sensing layer (R_{Se}) on an electrode (R_{Bg}) and diffusion impedance Z_D whose frequency behaviour depends on the electrode system structure, shape and size of its elements [53]. The C_{An} capacitance is most sensitive to binding of large species, such

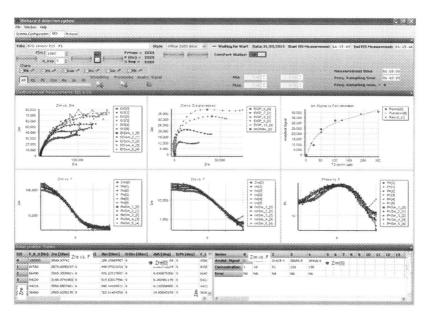

Fig. 18. Screen short of EIS tab/window (the image is taken from [24]). (Color figure online)

as proteins or cells. One difficulty with capacitive based sensors is that their sensitivity depends on obtaining the proper thickness of the sensing layer [54]. The charge transfer resistor Rct can also be quite sensitive to analyte binding, particularly in case of large species, such as proteins or cells, which significantly impede electron transfer.

It was found that for any (macroelectrode, microdisk or microband array) implementation of the biosensor transducer and any mechanism of manifestation of biorecognition reaction through changes in charge transfer resistence or sensor capacitance, the best results can be obtained through application of a differential measurement scheme, realized by subtracting the reference spectrum from the measured impedance spectrum. In this case the measured spectrum is the biosensor impedance spectrum after reaction with the target analyte and the reference spectrum is the biosensor impedance spectrum before reacting with the target analyte or an impedance spectrum obtained from the reference sensor if the last presents in the system. After subtraction, the maximum value of the imaginary part of the differential impedance spectrum can be taken as an analytical signal in the biosensor calibration step and also determination of the target analyte concentration. Using this quantity as an analytical signal instead of such equivalent circuit parameters as C_D or R_{ct} makes the signal processing algorithm straightforward, thus it does not require high calculation power from the control computer for its implementation. Additionally, this impedance spectrum value is located in the middle of the frequency sweep. It reduces requirements on the desired sweep range and therefore simplifies the hardware realization that is also very important for the portable devices. Overall, the application of a differential measurement scheme allows an increase in sensitivity and a reduction in the background signal. At the same time this approach suffers from noise. The injurious effects

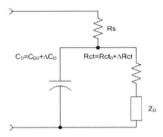

Fig. 19. The modified Randles equivalent circuit for biosensor analysis.

of noise can be reduced by both signals undergoing smoothing before their subtraction. Different smoothing approaches including median, adaptive and Gaussian kernel smoothing algorithms were tested to find the procedure that fits application specification in the best way. It was found that Gaussian kernel smoothing method provides required noise suppression and meets application requirement on simplicity and low power of calculation. Since the window based smoothing methods start working effectively only after the smoothing window is fully filled with samples the suggested approach does not work in the beginning and at the end of the impedance frequency sweep. This disadvantage is not critical in our case as the extracted parameter selected as the analytical signal is located in the middle of the frequency sweep and this limitation does not it affect.

2.5   Method and Chemicals

All electrochemical experiments were performed in a Faraday cage, and each measurement used for obtaining sensor calibration was carried out three times. EIS measurements were performed with the described system over a frequency range from 10 Hz to 100 kHz at an applied potential of DC bias of 0.2 V and an AC amplitude of 10 mV. The frequency range was defined by hardware specification and application objective to determine analyte concentration. The appropriate bias potential was determined from cyclic voltammetry over a range 0 V to 0.6 V at a scan rate of 100 mV/s. All chemicals used in this work including T2-toxin and corresponding antibodies were purchased from Sigma Aldrich Ireland Ltd. and used as received.

3   Results and Discussion

The developed portable immunosensing impedimetric system and suggested approach for the analytical signal extraction was validated with experimental data obtained with T2-toxin in the concentration range of 0–250 ppb. The transducer topology that produced the best sensing result for immunosensor prototype with APTES-PDITC bio-funtionalisation chemistry described above and applied to the 40 μm microdisk array with parameters as indicated in Table 2. Experimental raw and smoothed and differential impedance spectra (in the Nyquist form) obtained with the developed biosensing system for different T-2 toxin concentrations (0, 25 ppb, 50 ppb, 100 ppb, 250 ppb)

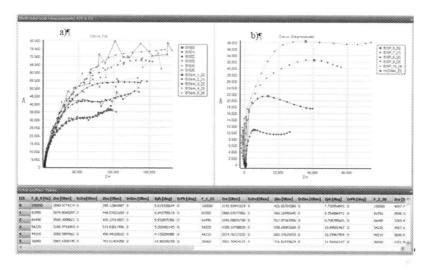

Fig. 20. Experimental raw and smoothed (a) and processed differential impedance spectra with extracted analytical signals (red points) (b) obtained with the developed biosensing system for different T-2 toxin concentrations (0, 25 ppb, 50 ppb, 100 ppb, 250 ppb). (Color figure online)

can be seen in screenshot presented in Fig. 20. In order to provide better spectra distinguishability the measurements were made without repetitions thus zero measurement errors are shown in the corresponding table below the plots. Due to a relatively high low boundary of the frequency sweep (10 Hz) the obtained impedance spectra accounted only for high and middle frequency parts of a depressed semicircle response of a microdisc electrode array associated with semi-infinite radial spherical diffusion. When concentration of T2-toxin increases, real and imaginary impedance parts both also increase that reflects a growth of a layer with targeted species captured by antibodies due the antibody-antigen binding reaction. If toxin concentration exceeds the certain level, this impedance increase is saturated due to a depletion of the free antibodies capable of biorecognition reaction. The raw impedance spectra were subjected to noise impact and application of Kernel's smoothing algorithm allowed for

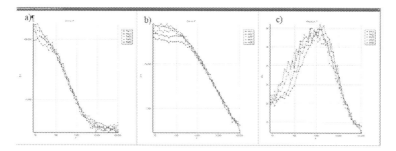

Fig. 21. Experimental smoothed Bode plots for real (a), imaginary (b) and phase (c) of the immunosensor obtained with the developed biosensing system for different T-2 toxin concentrations (0, 25 ppb, 50 ppb, 100 ppb, 250 ppb).

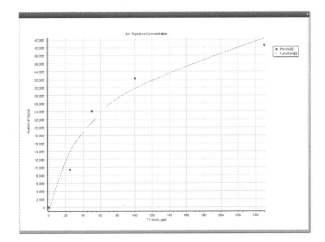

Fig. 22. Calibration curve of the immunosensor obtained with the developed biosensing system with five T-2 toxin concentrations (0, 25 ppb, 50 ppb, 100 ppb, 250 ppb). (Color figure online)

effective noise suppression. As was mentioned above the Kernel's smoothing cannot not work in the beginning and the end of the frequency sweeping that explains the signal oscillation in the plot with the smoothed differential spectra at high frequencies (area of the small impedances in Fig. 20b). At the same time since for the analytical signal are taken the maximal value of the imaginary part of the impedance located fare away from this zone this attribute of the smoothing method does not affect its measurement.

As follows from the smoothed Bode plots presented in Fig. 21 the most significant difference between the spectra corresponding to the different toxin concentrations is located in a low frequency range below 250 Hz. Here, the imaginary impedance values are more than 2 times less than their real counterparts (80000 vs. 180000); they are also more sensitive to variation of T2 toxin concentration. If frequency increases, both impedance components decrease but the imaginary impedance stays relatively constant at the frequencies below 250 Hz where the influence of the toxin concentration on the biosensor impedance is most noticeable. This frequency behavior of the imaginary impedance of the biosensor leads to the fact that frequency dependence of the impedance phase represents unimodal smooth function with maximal values in the range of 56–62° around the frequency of 1 kHz. The dependence of imaginary impedance against toxin concentration becomes more apparent from the differential impedance spectra obtained by subtraction of the spectrum at zero concentration, which is used as the reference background spectrum, from the impedance spectra corresponding to nonzero toxin concentrations as demonstrated in Fig. 20b.

The maximum values of the imaginary impedances on the differential impedance spectra marked by red points in this figure were used as the analytical signals to build a calibration curve of the developed label-free impedimetric immunosensor. This curve together with the analytical signals automatically extracted from the smoothed differential impedance spectra presented by the red squares is shown in Fig. 22.

The calibration curve represents a nonlinear function that reflects the competitive nature of the antibody-antigen binding reaction. The model can be presented by Eq. (7)

$$y = a \ \ln(x+b) + c \tag{7}$$

where y is analytical signal, x is T-2 toxin concentration. Other parameters of the model were determined by fitting the model with obtained experimental data. The following values of these parameters were attained slope $a = 2.667 \cdot 10^4$, $b = 22.449$ and $c = -8.393 \cdot 10^4$. The squared determination coefficient $R^2 = 0.982$ and the total approximation error was $3.929 \cdot 10^3$. As follows from the calibration curve, the developed biosensing portable system can successfully detect biotoxin at the levels below 25 ppm.

4   Conclusions

World-wide increase in bioterrorism activities has led to a corresponding focus on the available tools and techniques that can be deployed in the monitoring of biowarfare agents in the environment. The majority of technologies reside in a lab setting or have been boxed into a benchtop instrument with minimal or no portability possibilities. Portability leads to the potential to deploy at various points-of-need and currently, very few options exist. This paper presented a portable biosensing platform for impedance based detection and quantification of biotoxin substances capable of operation in autonomous mode has been developed. This has been made possible through the incorporation of cutting edge technologies from various disciplines e.g. sensor chip design and fabrication, application of surface chemistry approaches to develop a hybrid sensor chip with biotarget detection capabilities, highly miniaturized instrumentation, and the development of signal processing and data interpretation algorithms. The platform implements a label-free approach, which is based on detection of the biosensor interfacial changes due to a bio recognition reaction. The interfacial changes are sensed by means of Electrochemical Impedance Spectroscopy (EIS) in a frequency range from 10 Hz to 100 kHz. Traditionally, EIS instrumentation has been a relatively large, lab based piece of equipment due to its complexity in the generation of wave-forms over a range of frequencies. corresponding data acquisition of the generated waveforms, and determination of the Nyquist/Bode plots. Advances in chip technology and embedded computing have now lead to increased functionality being possible in highly miniaturized off-the-shelf chips, and it is these advances that are incorporated here. The platform comprises of an electrochemical biosensor, portable low-noise mix signal hardware with embedded microcontroller and associated software incorporating hardware and measurement control together with signal processing algorithms for extraction biotarget concentration from the biosensor response. The biosensor is realized as an on-chip package-free three electrode micro electrochemical cell consisted of a Pt counter electrode, an Ag/AgCl reference electrode and an Au working electrode patterned on a single silicon chip. The WE represents an array of 40 micron diameter gold disks with 400 micron center-to-center distance, which were undergone of surface modification for antibody immobilisation. The surface modification was based on

APTES – PDITC procedure. The instrumentation was realised as a two channel EIS system, which used in-phase and quadrature demodulation of AC signal for extraction of the real and imaginary impedance components. The biosensing system hardware consisted of two modules: Potentiostat and Front-End Amplifiers (PFEA) and Signal Processing and Microcontroller (SPM) units. The corresponding software capable of autonomous operation contains two interrelated parts written for the host computer and the embedded microcontroller. An automated procedure for analytical signal extraction consists of: smoothing of the initial biosensor impedance spectrum by Kernel smoothing procedure; subtraction of a reference background spectrum from the measured impedance spectrum; and extraction from differential impedance spectrum the maximum of the imaginary component, which is used as an analytical signal for biosensor calibration and calculation of the target analyte concentration. The PC software was implemented with the option of user-friendly multi-tab GUI software where each tab is associated with the program window. These are 'System configuration', 'Protocol' and 'EIS' tabs/windows. They provide communication, instrumentation and measurement setting control, and system operability testing; allow for design of impedance measurement protocol for each frequency sweep point; and present results of EIS and analyte concentration quantification in graphical and table forms. The developed biosensing system was validated with the developed on-chip T2 toxin biosensor. Calibration of the system was obtained for five toxin concentrations from 0 ppm to 250 ppm. It showed that the developed portable biosensing system can provide successful detection of the biotoxin at the levels below 25 ppm.

Acknowledgements. Financial support of this work by European Commission projects FP7-SEC-2011.3.4-2 "HANDHOLD: HANDHeld OLfactory Detector" and H2020-NMP-29-2015 "HISENTS: High level Integrated SEnsor for NanoToxicity Screening" is gratefully acknowledged.

References

1. Shriver-Lake, L.C., Ligler, F.S.: The array biosensor for counterterrorism. IEEE Sens. J. **5**(4), 751–756 (2005)
2. Ahmad, A., Moore, E.J.: Comparison of cell-based biosensors with traditional analytical techniques for cytotoxicity monitoring and screening of polycyclic aromatic hydrocarbons in the environment. Anal. Lett. **42**(1), 1–28 (2009)
3. Brennan, D., Lambkin, P., Moore, E.J., Galvin, P.: An integrated optofluidic platform for DNA hybridization and detection. IEEE Sens. J. **8**(5), 536–542 (2008)
4. Bryan, T., Luo, X., Bueno, P.R., Davis, J.J.: An optimised electrochemical biosensor for the label-free detection of C-reactive protein in blood. Biosens. Bioelectron. **39**(1), 94–98 (2013)
5. Zhang, W., Du, Y., Wang, M.L.: Noninvasive glucose monitoring using saliva nano-biosensor. Sens. Bio-Sens. Res. **4**, 23–29 (2015)
6. Wang, X., Lu, X., Chen, J.: Development of biosensor technologies for analysis of environmental contaminants. Trends Environ. Anal. Chem. **2**, 25–32 (2014)
7. Yong, D., Liu, C., Zhu, C., Yu, D., Liu, L., Zhai, J., Dong, S.: Detecting total toxicity in water using a mediated biosensor system with flow injection. Chemosphere **139**, 109–116 (2015)

8. Herzog, G., Moujahid, W., Twomey, K., Lyons, C., Ogurtsov, V.I.: On-chip electrochemical microsystems for measurements of copper and conductivity in artificial seawater. Talanta **116**, 26–32 (2013)

9. Ogurtsov, V.I., Twomey, K., Herzog, G.: Development of an electrochemical sensing system for environmental monitoring of port water quality to integrate on-board an autonomous robotic fish. In: Hashmi, S. (ed.) Comprehensive Materials Processing. Sensor Materials, Technologies and Applications, vol. 13, pp. 317–351. Elsevier Science, Oxford (2014)

10. Said, N.A.M., Twomey, K., Ogurtsov, V.I., Arrigan, D.W.M., Herzog, G.: Fabrication and electrochemical characterization of micro- and nanoelectrode arrays for sensor applications. J. Phys. Conf. Ser. **307**, 012052 (2011)

11. Thevenot, D.R., Toth, K., Durst, R.A., Wilson, G.S.: Electrochemical biosensors: recommended definitions and classification. Pure Appl. Chem. **71**, 2333–2348 (1999)

12. Scheller, F.W., Wollenbergera, U., Warsinkea, A., Lisdata, F.: Research and development in biosensors. Curr. Opin. Biotechnol. **12**, 35–40 (2001)

13. Vo-Dinh, T., Cullum, B.: Biosensors and biochips: advances in biological and medical diagnostics. Fresen. J. Anal. Chem. **366**(6–7), 540–551 (2000)

14. Hock, B., Seifert, M., Kramer, K.: Engineering receptors and antibodies for biosensors. Biosens. Bioelectron. **17**(3), 239–249 (2002)

15. Wollenberger, U.: Third generation biosensors - integrating recognition and transduction in electrochemical sensors. In: Gorton, L. (ed.) Biosensors and Modem Biospecific Analytical Techniques, pp. 65–130. Elsevier, Amsterdam (2005)

16. Koyun, A., Ahlatcıoğlu, E., İpek, Y.K.: Biosensors and their principles. In: Kara, S. (ed.) A Roadmap of Biomedical Engineers and Milestones. INTECH, Rijeka (2012)

17. Sharma, S., Byrne, H., O'Kennedy, R.J.: Antibodies and antibody-derived analytical biosensors. Essays Biochem. **60**(1), 9–18 (2016)

18. Byrne, B., Stack, E., Gilmartin, N., O'Kennedy, R.: Antibody-based sensors: principles, problems and potential for detection of pathogens and associated toxins. Sensors **9**(6), 4407–4445 (2009)

19. Perumal, V., Hashim, U.: Advances in biosensors: principle, architecture and applications. J. Appl. Biomed. **12**(1), 1–15 (2014)

20. Dodeigne, C., Thunus, L., Lejeune, R.: Chemiluminescence as diagnostic tool. A review. Talanta **51**, 415–439 (2000)

21. Jiang, X., Li, D., Xu, X., Ying, Y., Li, Y., Ye, Z., et al.: Immunosensors for detection of pesticide residues. Biosens. Bioelectron. **23**(11), 1577–1587 (2008)

22. Yalow, R.S., Berson, S.A.: Assay of plasma insulin in human subjects by immunological methods. Nature **184**, 1648–1649 (1959)

23. Patel, Pd.: (Bio)sensors for measurement of analytes implicated in food safety. A review. Trends Anal. Chem. **21**(2), 96–115 (2002)

24. Ogurtsov, V.I., Twomey, K., Pulka, J.: A portable sensing system for impedance based detection of biotoxin substances. In: 10th International Joint Conference on Biomedical Engineering Systems and Technologies Proceedings, BIODEVICES, (BIOSTEC 2017), Porto, Portugal, vol. 1, pp. 54–62 (2017)

25. Sadana, A.: Biosensors: Kinetics of Binding and Dissociation Using Fractals, 1st edn. Elsevier, Amsterdam (2003)

26. Zhang, S., Zhao, H., John, R.: Development of a generic microelectrode array biosensing system. Anal. Chimica Acta **421**(2), 175–187 (2000)

27. Willner, I., Katz, E., Willner, B.: Layered functionalized electrodes for electrochemical biosensor applications. In: Yang, V.C., Ngo, T.T. (eds.) Biosensors and Their Applications. Elsevier, Amsterdam (2000)

28. Arrigan, D.W.M.: Electrochemical Strategies in Detection Science. Royal Society of Chemistry, Cambridge (2016)
29. Twomey, K., O'Mara, P., Pulka, J., McGillycuddy, S., et al.: Fabrication and characterisation of a test platform integrating nanoporous structures with biochemical functionality. IEEE Sens. J. **15**(8), 4329–4337 (2015)
30. Kafi, A.K.M., Lee, D.-Y., Park, S.-H., Kwon, Y.-S.: Potential application of hemoglobin as an alternative to peroxidase in a phenol biosensor. Thin Solid Films **516**(9), 2816–2821 (2008)
31. Zhou, Y., Tang, L., Zeng, G., Zhang, C., Xie, X., Liu, Y., Wang, J., Tang, J., Zhang, Y., Deng, Y.: Label free detection of lead using impedimetric sensor based on ordered mesoporous carbon–gold nanoparticles and DNAzyme catalytic beacons. Talanta **146**, 641–647 (2016)
32. Rushworth, J.V., Ahmed, A., Griffiths, H.H., Pollock, N.M., Hooper, N.M., Millner, P.A.: A label-free electrical impedimetric biosensor for the specific detection of Alzheimer's amyloid-beta oligomers. Biosens. Bioelectron. **56**, 83–90 (2014)
33. Arrigan, D.W.M.: Nanoelectrodes, nanoelectrode arrays and their applications. Analyst **129** (12), 1157–1165 (2004)
34. Bennett, J.W., Klich, M.: Mycotoxins. Clin. Microbiol. Rev. **16**(3), 497–516 (2003)
35. Gupta, R.C. (ed.): Handbook of Toxicology of Chemical Warfare Agents, 1st edn. Elsevier, Amsterdam (2009)
36. Ler, S.G., Lee, F.K., Gopalakrishnakone, P.: Trends in detection of warfare agents detection methods for ricin, staphylococcal enterotoxin B and T-2 toxin. J. Chromatogr. A **1133**, 1–12 (2006)
37. Zheng, M.Z., Richard, J.L., Binder, J.: A review of rapid methods for the analysis of mycotoxins. Mycopathologia **161**, 261–273 (2006)
38. Pittet, A.: Keeping the mycotoxins out: experience gathered by an international food company. Nat. Toxins **3**(4), 281–287 (1995)
39. De Saeger, S., Van Peteghem, C.: Dipstick enzyme immunoassay to detect Fusarium T-2 toxin in wheat. Appl. Environ. Microbiol. **62**(6), 1880–1884 (1996)
40. Said, M., Azura, N.: Electrochemical biosensor based on microfabricated electrode arrays for life sciences applications. Ph.D. thesis, University College Cork (2014)
41. http://www.handhold.eu/
42. Britz, D., Strutwolf, J.: Digital Simulation in Electrochemistry, 4th edn. Springer, Cham (2016). https://doi.org/10.1007/978-3-319-30292-8
43. Hermes, M., Scholz, F.: Solid-state electrochemical reactions of electroactive microparticles and nanoparticles in a liquid electrolyte environment. In: Kharton, V.V. (ed.) Solid State Electrochemistry I: Fundamentals, Materials and Their Applications. WILEY-VCH Verlag GmbH & Co. KGaA, Weinheim (2009)
44. Guo, J., Lindner, E.: Cyclic voltammograms at coplanar and shallow recessed microdisc electrode arrays: guidelines for design and experiment. Anal. Chem. **81**(1), 130–138 (2009)
45. Said, N.A.M., Twomey, K., Herzog, G., Ogurtsov V.I.: Fabrication and characterization of microfabricated on-chip microelectrochemical cell for biosensing applications. In: Zaaba, S. K., Zakaria, S.M.M.S., Kamarudin, K., et al. (eds.) Asian Conference on Chemical Sensors 2015, ACCS 2015, vol. 1808, pp. 020032-1–020032-13. AIP, Melville (2017)
46. Masson, J.-F., Battaglia, T.M., Davidson, M.J., Kim, Y.-C., Prakash, A.M.C., Beaudoin, S., Booksh, K.S.: Biocompatible polymers for antibody support on gold surfaces. Talanta **67**(5), 918–925 (2005)
47. Haddada, M.B., Huebner, M., Casale, S., Knopp, D., Niessner, R., Salmain, M., Boujday, S.: Gold nanoparticles assembly on silicon and gold surfaces: mechanism, stability, and efficiency in diclofenac biosensing. J. Phys. Chem. C **120**(51), 29302–29311 (2016)

48. Vashist, S.K., Dixit, C.K., MacCraith, B.D., O'Kennedy, R.: Effect of antibody immobilization strategies on the analytical performance of a surface plasmon resonance-based immunoassay. Analyst **136**(21), 4431–4436 (2011)
49. Raj, J., Herzog, G., Manning, M., Volcke, C., Maccraith, B., Ballantyne, S., Thompson, M., Arrigan, D.: Surface immobilisation of antibody on cyclic olefin copolymer for sandwich immunoassay. Biosens. Bioelectron. **24**, 2654–2658 (2009)
50. Barsoukov, E., Macdonald, J.R. (eds.): Impedance Spectroscopy Theory, Experiment, and Applications, 2nd edn. Wiley, Hoboken (2005)
51. Lasia, A.: Electrochemical impedance spectroscopy and its applications. In: Conway, B.E., Bockris, J., White, R.E. (eds.) Modern Aspects of Electrochemistry, vol. 32, pp. 143–248. Kluwer Academic/Plenum Publishers, New York (1999)
52. Suni, I.I.: Impedance methods for electrochemical sensors using nanomaterials. Trends Anal. Chem. **27**(7), 604–610 (2008)
53. Jacobsen, T., West, K.: Diffusion impedance in planar, cylindrical and spherical symmetry. Elecrochimika Acta **40**(2), 255–262 (1995)
54. Hu, S.Q., Wu, Z.Y., Zhou, Y.M., Cao, Z.X., Shen, G.L., Yu, R.Q.: Capacitive immunosensor for transferrin based on an o-aminobenzenthiol oligomer layer. Anal. Chim. Acta **458**, 297–304 (2002)

Microfluidic Devices Integrating Clinical Alternative Diagnostic Techniques Based on Cell Mechanical Properties

A. S. Moita[(⊠)], D. Vieira, F. Mata, J. Pereira, and A. L. N. Moreira

IN+ - Center for Innovation, Technology and Policy Research,
Instituto Superior Técnico, Universidade de Lisboa,
Av. Rovisco Pais, 1049-001 Lisbon, Portugal
anamoita@tecnico.ist.utl.pt

Abstract. The present paper discusses the development of a microfluidic (lab-on-chip) device to study cells deformability aiming at developing a new diagnostic system for cancer detection. The chip uses electrowetting for droplet transport and cell deformability, on an open configuration. The chip configuration is analyzed towards various steps, from the selection of the materials, to the evaluation of the chip performance. Wetting properties of the selected materials are shown to play a major role. Furthermore, experimental tests confirm the relevance of selecting materials less prone to adsorb the biocomponents, as they tend to locally alter the surface wettability, promoting energy dissipation at the droplet contact line and affecting its manipulation. A rough analysis on droplet evaporation effects suggests that they are not negligible, even at optimum working conditions that minimize the evaporation by mass diffusion (low temperatures and high relative humidity). In this context, exploitation of droplet based microfluidic devices for point-of-care diagnostics in harsh environments should take mass diffusion effects into account.

Keywords: Microfluidic device · Electrowetting · Biofluid droplet dynamics
Wettability · Cancer diagnostics · Cell mechanical properties

1 Introduction

Innovative diagnostic tools are vital for accurate, early and prompt identification of many diseases, which may save peoples' lives. The fast development of microfluidics opened a wide range of possibilities in developing point-of-care microfluidic devices working as diagnostic tools, the so-called lab-on-chips.

Lab-on-chip systems swiftly evolved since their introduction by Manz [1] and are now able to perform several programmed operations and biochemical analysis. One major potential application of these microfluidic devices is in point-of-care diagnostics, as they meet the various requirements identified by the World Health Organization for the development of diagnostic tools for infectious diseases at resource-limited settings, such as affordability, sensitivity, equipment free, robustness and portability [2]. Despite claiming the ability to develop such systems at very low prices (approximately one Euro), researchers working in this field recognize the need for further research, to

© Springer International Publishing AG, part of Springer Nature 2018
N. Peixoto et al. (Eds.): BIOSTEC 2017, CCIS 881, pp. 74–93, 2018.
https://doi.org/10.1007/978-3-319-94806-5_4

devise an effective system, prone to deliver the quick and accurate diagnostics required in developing countries [3]. An important issue is related to the ambient conditions which affect the fluid and therefore the samples transport. This issue, recently approached by Moita *et al.* [4] is discussed in detail in this paper.

A paramount part of lab-on-chips development concerns the successful manipulation and transport operations of the biosamples, which are mainly a matter of momentum, energy and mass transport at liquid-solid interfaces. To cope with this, two main streams were followed, namely the sample transport in microchannel-based continuous microfluidics and the droplet-based digital microfluidics [5]. Although the first has been widely explored in a large number of applications, there are still some limitations associated to these systems, such as the fact that the functionality is not generally reconfigurable after design and fabrication, limiting more flexible applications, the samples are difficult to access, the systems are difficult to clean and maintain, clogging is more likely to occur and numerous auxiliaries such as tubes, valves, pumps, among others, are usually required, thus increasing the complexity of these systems. In addition, the efficiency of the valves and pumps at the micro-scale is still quite low, turning these systems inefficient from the energetic point of view. Conversely, the digital microfluidics based on droplets solves many of these issues, but the accurate control of droplet dynamics is not yet well understood. Most of the droplet based systems use a closed configuration with two plates, working as electrode and counter electrode, respectively. Despite being stable, this configuration keeps some of the problems pointed at the devices using microchannels, such as the clogging, the access to the samples, among others. Alternatively, the open configuration systems have still some problems to overcome. In the EWOD – Electrowettng on dielectric, the electrodes are covered by a thin dielectric layer to avoid the occurrence of hydrolysis [6]. The dielectric material is often hydrophobic to promote the motion of the droplet. As the droplet is deposited on the surface, the liquid-solid-vapour interfacial tensions are in equilibrium, defining the angle formed between the tangent line at the droplet edge and the surface, the so-called equilibrium contact angle [7]. Upon applying an electric potential, the droplet acts as a capacitor and an electric force is generated at the liquid-solid-vapour interface, unbalancing the interfacial tensions and decreasing the contact angle. This mechanism is classically described by the Young-Lippmann equation [7, 8] and despite the basic principles of EOWD are grounded for many decades, as revised for instance by [9], various alternative models (e.g. [10, 11]) strive to explain some unclear phenomena such as the contact angle saturation (i.e. the limiting value of the angle bellow which it remains unchanged, independently of the imposed electric potential), which are not predicted by Young-Lippmann theory.

The EWOD is therefore strongly dependent on the electrochemical properties of the aqueous solutions of the droplets. However, information reported in the literature concerning the transport of biofluids is actually quite sparse. Sirivasan *et al.* [12] report the successful transport of physiological fluids. Also, several authors report the effective electrowetting-induced transport of proteins and DNA [13], but it is not clear which are the most suitable electrochemical properties of the fluids or the most important parameters governing biofluids transport and manipulation. Adsorption of the biocomponents on the dielectric substrate is also a problem that is not completely described yet. For instance, [14, 15] report high adsorption of biocomponents and particularly proteins by substrate materials commonly used as dielectrics in EWOD configurations, e.g. Teflon (PTFE – Polytetrafluoroethylene). The strong affinity of materials such as PTFE for the passive adsorption of proteins has also been recently confirmed by Moita *et al.* [4], who report a local modification of the wettability, which affects droplet motion. Hence, the wetting properties of the dielectric layer with the aqueous solutions in use and the affinity for passive and active adsorption should be inferred at earlier stages of the design and configuration of the microfluidic devices. The dynamic behavior of the biofluids to be manipulated must also be studied *a priori*, to assure the design of an effective device.

Concerning the use of these microfluidic devices, they have been widely explored for DNA manipulation (using electrophoresis working principle) [5] and for bio-chemical analysis of proteins and similar biocomponents (e.g. [13]). Clinical diag-nostics has been less explored, but few authors already report the development of lab-on-chips for the early diagnose of several blood diseases and even cancer [3]. However, they are all based on chemical biomarkers and, exception made to the device developed by Di Carlo's team [3], which can separate circulating tumor cells from the other blood cells, they often still require the previous separation of various components of the sample, following numerous and complex procedures.

Conversely, the device discussed in the present paper will exploit cell mechanical properties to be used for cancer diagnostics. In fact, many cellular functions depend on the mediation and regulation of stress, as well as on the elastic and viscoelastic properties of the cell membrane [16]. Change in cell stiffness is a new characteristic of cancer cells and different types of cancer cells depict similar stiffness [17–19]. Detailed research on cell deformation is therefore proposed in more recent literature to play a vital role towards the early diagnostics of malignancy. Within the various cancer types addressing similar stiffness characteristics, lung cancer, diagnosed by analysis of the cells present in pleural fluid, is a particularly interesting research topic, given the difficulty in distinguishing between healthy and cancer cells based on shape and morphology parameters and even on chemical biomarkers. Also, cytological analysis of pleural fluids is not always reliable and immunofluorescence assays demand for specific sample preparation [20].

2   Experimental Procedure

The experimental procedure described in this section addresses the various steps fol-lowed in the microfabrication of the chips, the protocol defined to characterize the chips performance (mainly focusing on the transport and manipulation section) and diag-nostic procedures to characterize the wettability and infer on the adsorption of the biocomponents.

2.1   Microfabrication of the Chips

The microchips' configurations were modelled in SOLIDWORKS and converted to AutoCAD files to be manufactured at INESC-MN. Here, configurations, mainly composed by arrays of interdigitated electrodes were printed on a 0.6 μm aluminium film by lithography and wet etch on a glass substrate with 102×45 mm^2 and 700 µm width. Finally, a thin film of a dielectric material was deposited on the chip assembly, without covering the contacts. The different configurations tested only vary in the electrodes width, w (between 120 and 1400 µm), being the numerous interdigitated coplanar electrodes displaced with a fixed distance between them, $2a = 60$ µm. The length of the electrodes is 24 mm (Fig. 1a and b).

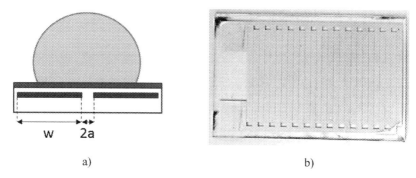

a)   b)

Fig. 1. (a) Definition of the main geometrical parameters for the chip dimensioning. (b) Chip sample.

Since the coplanar electrodes have different polarities, the droplet must cover at least two electrodes. These basic dimensions were taken following the results obtained in the fundamental study previously completed [4]. Then, additional calculations on the chip capacitances and other electrical parameters were performed, following the recommendations of Chen *et al.* [21]. The best performing configurations were then selected empirically, based the analysis of the chips performance, as discussed in the following sections.

2.2 Preparation of the Biofluids and Characterization of Their Physico-Chemical Properties

The experiments are performed using a Green Fluorescent Protein - GFP (produced and purified in house) solution with 1.71×10^{-3} mM concentration and GFP-expressing E. coli suspensions with concentrations of 1×10^9 cells/ml and 2×10^9 cells/ml. The solutions and suspensions are characterized in terms of density, viscosity and surface tension. Density, ρ is measured with a pycnometer for liquids and the dynamic viscosity, μ with an ATS RheoSystems (a division of CANNON® Instruments, Co) under controlled temperature conditions. For the range of accuracy of $\pm 5\%$, the solutions are observed to have density and viscosity values very close to those of water. Hence, all the solutions and suspensions are Newtonian fluids. Surface tension σ_{lv} is measured under controlled temperature conditions (20 ± 3 °C) with the optical tensiometer THETA (Attention), using the pendant drop method. The value taken for the surface tension of each liquid tested is averaged from 15 measurements. The surface tension of

Table 1. Physico-chemical properties of the solutions and suspensions used in the present work [22].

Solution	Density ρ [kg/m^3]	Surface tension σ_{lv} [mN/m]	Dynamic viscosity μ [Ns/m^2]
GFP (1.71×10^{-3} mM)	998	72.2 ± 0.7	1×10^{-3}
GFP-expressing E. coli (1×10^9 cells/ml)	998	73.8 ± 0.04	1×10^{-3}
GFP-expressing E. coli (2×10^9 cells/ml)	998	73.8 ± 0.04	1×10^{-3}

all the solutions used here is very close to that of water, as shown in Table 1, which summarizes the physico-chemical properties of the fluids used in the present work.

2.3   Measurement of the Contact Angles and Dynamic Response of the Biofluid Droplets: Evaluation of the Chips Performance

All experimental assays were performed inside a Perspex chamber with total dimensions of $55 \times 80 \times 90$ mm^3. This chamber has quartz windows to avoid optical distortion, which introduces errors in the image based techniques. The chamber was saturated with the working fluid and the tests were performed under continuous monitoring of temperature and relative humidity of the surrounding air. The measurements were taken with a DHT 22 Humidity & Temperature Sensor, at a sample rate of 0.5 Hz. Relative humidity was measured within 2–5% accuracy, while temperature measurements were taken within ± 0.5 °C accuracy. The temperature was observed to be constant within T = 20 ± 3 °C and relative humidity was kept constant between 75% and 78%. Higher humidity values, up to 99% were then used to evaluate the effect of mass evaporation during the measurements.

The wettability of the dielectric substrates is quantified by the static contact angle θ_e and by hysteresis, determined as the difference between the quasi-static advancing and receding contact angles, measured with the optical tensiometer THETA from Attention. This characterization is performed for all the liquid-substrate pairs considered in the present study. The static angles are measured using the sessile drop method. The size of the images taken with the tensiometer is 640×480 pixels and the spatial resolution of the system for the current optical configuration is 15.6 μm/pixel. The images are post-processed by a drop detection algorithm based on Young-Laplace equation (One Attention software). The accuracy of these algorithms is argued to be of the order of $\pm 0.1°$ [23]. Contact angle hysteresis is assessed at room temperature (20 °C $\pm$ 3 °C), following the procedure described by Kietzig [24]. Briefly, a small water drop is dispensed from a needle and brought into contact with the surface. The volume of the drop is increased and the advancing contact angle is taken as the one just before the interface diameter increases. Afterwards, the drop diameter decreases and the receding contact angle is taken as the one just before the interface diameter decreases. Given the relatively low resolution of these measurements obtained with an optical tensiometer and considering the typical scale of the processes governing the transport of the samples within the droplets (micro-to-nano scale) and the paramount role of wetta-bility, an alternative method is explored to provide more accurate measurements as proposed in Vieira *et al.* [25].

The performance of the chips is evaluated grounded on the dynamic response of the droplets on the chips, which in turn is discussed based on the evaluation of the temporal evolution of the droplet-surface contact diameter. The velocity of the contact line motion is also evaluated. These quantities are determined from high-speed visualization and post-processing. The high-speed images are taken at 2200 fps using a Phantom v4.2 from Vision Research Inc., with 512×512 pixels@2100 fps resolution. For the present optical configuration, the spatial resolution is 25 µm/pixel and the temporal resolution is 0.45 ms. The post-processing is performed using a home-made routine developed in Matlab. Temporal evolution of the contact (spreading and receding) diameters is presented as the average curve of at least 3 events, obtained at similar experimental conditions. Accuracy of the measurements is evaluated to be ± 25 µm for the contact diameter.

Regarding the actuation of the chips, although AC voltage is reported by some authors to lead to better performances of the electrowetting systems, decreasing the contact angle hysteresis and delaying the contact angle saturation [10, 26] these phe-nomena seem to be more related to the wetting characteristics of the surfaces and with the properties of the solutions. Also, to avoid the occurrence of limiting frequencies for which the Lippmann equation is not satisfied [9], DC current was used on the chips provided by a Sorensen DCR600-.75B power supply. The applied voltage was varied from 0 to 245 V. However, since the basic principle for droplet motion in microchips requires switching polarities between neighboring electrodes, within an imposed fre-quency and following a similar approach explored by Fan *et al.* [27], a custom-made frequency controller using an Arduino was applied on the chips using a square wave, to assure the generation of an electrical force in the direction of the desired motion. This wave defines the time during which the electrode is actuated by a certain applied voltage. It has an internal clock with a frequency of 16 MHz. This device can vary the imposed frequency between 50 Hz and 400 Hz, within 50 Hz increments. The negative polarity of the chips was grounded, so, it will have a zero potential, i.e. the overall potential difference applied to the chip corresponds to the voltage applied to the pos-itive polarity of the power supply.

2.4 Characterization of the Dielectric Substrates

To select the most appropriate dielectric substrates to be used, various coatings were tested, namely Teflon (PTFE), Polydimethylsiloxane (PDMS), SU8 resist and Silicon Nitrate (Si_3N_4). The coatings, chosen after extensive literature survey on the most used dielectric materials in EWOD are characterized based on their topography and on their static and dynamic wettability. Surface topography is characterized using a Dektak 3 profile meter (Veeco) with a vertical resolution of 20 nm. Within this resolution all the substrates are smooth. The contact angles are measured using the optical tensiometer THETA from Attention, as described in the previous paragraphs.

2.5   Adsorption Analysis Using Fluorescence Laser Scanning Confocal Microscopy

To infer on the possible adsorption of the biocomponents on the dielectric substrates, simple tests are performed in which droplets of 3.0 ± 0.2 mm of the biofluids (with different concentrations) are deposited on the surfaces. Afterwards, a sequence of tests with and without electrostatic actuation is performed and the "footprints" of the droplets are observed on a Laser Scanning Confocal Microscope (Leica SP8). The images are taken with a 4X magnification (0.10 of numerical aperture), with a pixel size of 5.42 μm × 5.42 μm. The obtained images are then post-processed to determine the mean grey intensity (sum of intensities divided by the number of pixels in the region of interest of the droplet footprint) and the Area Integrated Intensity (sum of intensities of pixels in the region of interest of the droplet footprint normalized by unit of area (μm²). Since the droplet spreads after actuation, the integrated density is weighted with the area. To reduce the noise, the average grey intensity levels of the background image were also subtracted. The final result is the herein so-called Total Corrected Droplet Fluorescence – TCDF, as proposed by Moita *et al.* [4]. Higher values of TCDF can be associated to a larger quantity of protein or cells adsorbed by the substrate.

2.6   Contact Angle Measurements Using 3D Laser Scanning Fluorescence Confocal Microscopy

The 3D Laser Scanning Fluorescence Confocal Microscopy 3D LSFCM is an alternative diagnostic technique, developed as described in [25] which provides static and quasi-static contact angle measurements with high spatial resolution. The measurements were performed with a Laser Scanning Confocal Microscope (Leica TCS SP8), equipped with two lasers of continuous wave length. The maximum light power in the laser output is 350 mW and the excitation wave lengths available are 488 nm and 552 nm.

The measurements proceeded with the laser with 552 nm wavelength, set for the power of 10.50 mW (3.00% of the its maximum power) and gain of the photomultiplier (PMT) of 550 V. These values were set after a sensitivity analysis on the contrast of the image (before the post-processing) and on the Signal to Noise Ratio (SNR). The images are recorded in the format 1024 × 1024 and the scanning frequency is 400 Hz. In addition, the z-step was fixed in 1 μm for all the measurements.

A fluorescent dye - Rhodamine B (Sigma Aldrich) is used, which was chosen taken into account its excitation and emission wavelengths, to be compatible with the wavelengths available in the Laser Scanning Confocal Microscope, but also due to particular characteristics of the experimental conditions, in the present study. For the concentrations used here (0.0007936 mg/ml <Concentration <0.496 mg/ml) the physico-chemical properties of the water-dye solutions are very close to those of water.

While the resolution of the classical tensiometers and goniometers is of the order of tens to hundreds of microns, the pixel size achieved in this technique is, for the worse resolution 5.42 μm, but can be as small as 500 nm. Additional details on this technique can be found in [25].

To validate the 3D LSCFM technique, preliminary results were obtained by measuring the equilibrium contact angles on smooth glass slides. The equilibrium angles θ_{eq} are measured for millimetric and micrometric sizes, from 3 mm down to tens of microns. The measurements obtained are compared with those taken with the optical tensiometer. Various similar slides, from L1 to L4 are used to take into account the heterogeneities associated with material inhomogeneities and even surface defects. Hence, while Fig. 2 compares the equilibrium contact angles θ_e measured with the optical tensiometer with those obtained with the 3D LSFCM technique, for the same plane (XZ), Fig. 3, shows the dispersion of the measurements obtained for each technique, gathering in this case the measures obtained with the 3D LSFCM in 2 different planes (XY and XZ), to infer on possible asymmetries in the droplet shape. These asymmetries, which are not detected with the optical tensiometer are important for the application considered here, as they can distort the droplet and affect its motion in preferential directions.

Overall the results show that both techniques provide similar measurements, although the values obtained from the LSCFM tend to be slightly lower, when compared to those given by the optical tensiometer. This is due to the scale and resolution that are being considered in the LSCFM. The dispersion of the measurements is nevertheless quite similar in both techniques. Furthermore, the measurements in both XZ and YZ planes do not show an evident distortion of the contact line. Vieira *et al.* [25] report, however, significant distortions near the contact line region, when micro-structured surfaces are used. In such cases, the contact angles measured with the tensiometer can be up to 40° higher than those measured with the LSCFM technique, as these distortions affect the material contact angle (measured with the highest resolution) thus parting it from the apparent angle evaluated with the optical tensiometer. These observations of the contact line may also support our previous results (e.g. [4]) which showed that surface topography in these non-stable hydrophobic surfaces promotes energy dissipation at the contact line, thus precluding droplet motion. In line with these

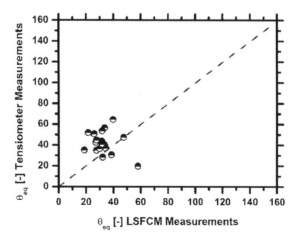

Fig. 2. Comparison between the equilibrium angles measured with the tensiometer and with the LSCFM technique, for a smooth glass surface. Adapted from [22].

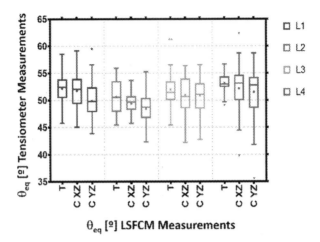

Fig. 3. Dispersion analysis of the static contact angles measured with the tensiometer and with the LSCFM technique, measured for smooth glass surfaces.

results, the safest way to alter wettability, avoiding the aforementioned issues, is towards the chemical modification and/or selection of the appropriate dielectric materials, as discussed in the following sub-section, while keeping the surface as smooth as possible.

3 Device Configuration

The microfluidic device under development has three main working sections, namely, the transport section, the diagnostic section and the selection section. The preferred wetting properties for the materials selected in each of these sections can be quite different. Hence, while in the transport section, droplet motion is governed by electrostatic actuation aided by custom made wetting properties of the dielectric material, so that hydrophobic/superhydrophobic regions are preferred to minimize the adhesive forces, which are proportional to hysteresis and consequently minimize the energy dissipated at the contact line between the droplet and the surface, in the diagnostic section it is desirable to promote adhesion to constrain the sample in the sensor area.

Hence and following the arguments presented in the Introduction, the wettability plays here a paramount role, so its characterization must be as accurate as possible. The materials, namely the dielectric material, which is in contact with the biosolutions, must therefore be chosen with care. For the transport and selection sections, the chosen materials should maximize the hydrophobicity with the fluids in study, minimize the hysteresis (to minimize the energy dissipation at the droplet contact line) and minimize the adsorption, which locally affects the wettability, increasing the adhesion and, consequently the energy dissipation [4]. Opposite trends are desired for the diagnostics section. The various steps followed towards the selection of the materials is discussed in the following sub-section.

3.1 Selection of the Dielectric Substrates Based on Wettability and Adsorption Analysis

As aforementioned, the selection of the dieletric substrates is strongly dependent on their wetting properties. The analysis described in the next paragraphs was performed to select the materials to be used in the transport section. Similar reasoning was then followed for the diagnostic section, considering the specific requirements for this section, as previously discussed.

Hence, Table 2 depicts the equilibrium angles, obtained for each solution tested, on various dielectric coatings which are commonly used in electrowetting chips. Distilled and deionized water is taken as reference fluid. The Table shows that only the SU8 resist and Si3N4 surfaces are hydrophilic, being the others hydrophobic. The highest contact angle of 121° is obtained for the PDMS substrate. Low hysteresis is the complementary characteristic desired in the transport section. However, Fig. 4 shows that the materials depicting the highest contact angles with the working fluids, also depict large hysteresis of the contact angle. To cope with this, the best performing materials were further coated with Glaco®, a commercial coating which is mainly a perfluoroalkyltrichlorosilane combined with perfluoropolyether carboxylic acid and a fluorinated solvent. Its application allowed turning the substrates superhydrophobic to the aqueous solutions in study, portraying high contact angles (>150°) and low hysteresis (<10°), being therefore a good option to consider in the transport section of the microfluidic device. Following this analysis and taking into account the dielectric properties of these materials [28], PDMS and SU8 coated with Glaco® were the dielectric materials selected to coat the electrodes on the transport section.

Table 2. Equilibrium contact angles, obtained for each pair fluid-dielectric substrate considered in the present work [22].

Dielectric coating	Contact angle [°]		
	Water	*E-coli*	GFP
Teflon	112 ± 5	103 ± 6	121 ± 6
Teflon with Glaco	145 ± 1	141 ± 9	153 ± 3
PDMS	121 ± 1	112 ± 1	119.5 ± 0.4
PDMS with Glaco	153 ± 3	153 ± 2	155 ± 3
SU8 *resist*	67.1 ± 0.7	65 ± 2	71.8 ± 0.2
SU8 with Glaco	160 ± 7	162 ± 1	153 ± 4
Si_3N_4	64.1 ± 0.7	59 ± 4	65 ± 2

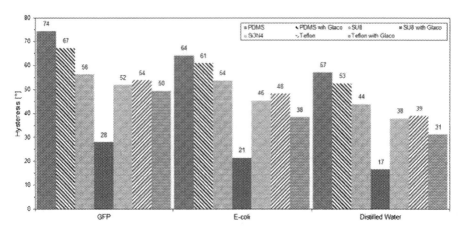

Fig. 4. Contact angle hysteresis evaluated for GFP solution (1.71×10^{-3} mM), GFP-expressing *E-coli* suspension (1×10^9 cells/mL) and distilled water on the tested dielectric substrates [22].

Concerning adsorption, Moita *et al.* [4] report that the GFP was adsorbed by Teflon substrates, leading to a local increase of surface wettability and further contributing to preclude the receding motion, as this wettability increase is irreversible, taking the contact angles to values near saturation. In this context, the following analysis infers on the possible adsorption of the GFP and E-coli cells by the PDMS and SU8 substrates, as depicted in Fig. 5, which shows the TCDF value, as defined in Sect. 2, evaluated for each substrate.

Figure 5a evidences minimum TCDF values for the adsorption of the GFP on PDMS substrates. The alternative material with lower adsorption of the biocomponents tested here was SU8, but the TCDF values obtained are about one order of magnitude higher than those evaluated for PDMS. Even though the adsorption of cells is quite less significant than the adsorption of the protein, Fig. 5b suggests a minor effect of the cell concentration in the solutions in promoting passive adsorption mechanisms, i.e. leading to slightly higher TCDF values. Nevertheless, adsorption of E-coli cells was likewise observed to be minimum on the PDMS substrate. The application of the Glaco® coating is observed to further reduce the adsorption of both proteins and cells, decreasing the TCDF values in about one order of magnitude on the PDMS.

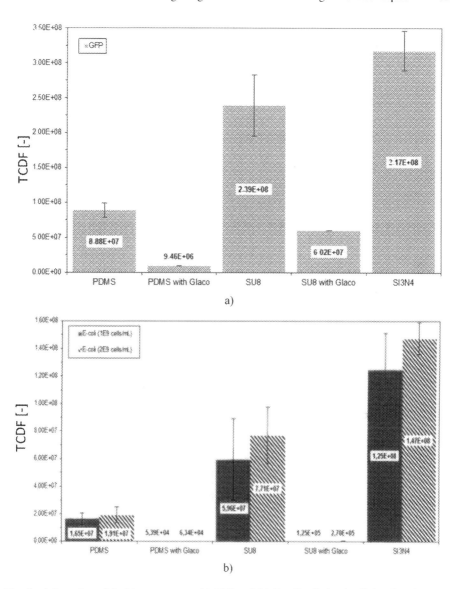

Fig. 5. Adsorption of the biocomponents (a) GFP and (b) E-coli cells by the dielectric substrates quantified by the TCDF.

3.2   Evaluation of the Chips Performance: Analysis of Influencing Parameters

After the selection of the materials, several chip configurations were tested, where the width of the electrodes was systematically varied. The best performing configurations were evaluated based on the dynamic response of the droplets, quantified by the droplet-surface contact diameter and by the velocity of displacement of the contact line.

This analysis determined that the best dynamic response was found for the chips with electrodes width w = 1200 μm and a distance between consecutive electrodes 2a = 60 μm. The detailed study performed is reported in [28].

The wetting properties have an important role in this dynamic response also, together with other parameters such as, for instance, the thickness of the dielectric layer, which is inversely proportional to the change in the contact angle during electrostatic actuation, as predicted by Young-Lippmann equation.

Hence, the spreading diameter of GFP and E-Coli suspension droplets, was evaluated under electrostatic actuation for the test chips coated with PDMS, SU8 resist and both materials further coated with Glaco®. As discussed in the previous sub-section, this coating reduces the adsorption of the proteins and of the cells by the substrates, so the irreversible contact angle decrease associated to the adsorption mechanisms is also minimized. The coating also decreases substantially the contact angle hysteresis. This modification of the wetting properties has a dramatic effect on the droplet transport on the chips, as shown in Fig. 6 which depicts the temporal evolution of the spreading diameter d(t) of a GFP droplet under electrostatic actuation, made non-dimensional with the initial diameter of the deposited droplet, i.e. for 0 V ($d(t)/d_{0V}$). t = 0 ms corresponds to the beginning of the actuation.

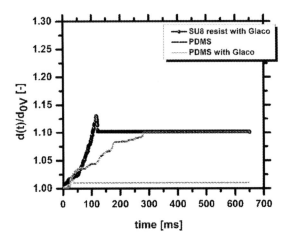

Fig. 6. Electrowetting induced spreading diameter of GFP droplets for different dielectric substrates, between coplanar electrodes for the configuration $w = 1200$ μm, at 230 V and 350 Hz. Initial droplet diameter is 2.8 mm.

The figure shows a significantly larger spreading diameter with the SU8 resist coated with Glaco®, being followed by a pronounced recoiling, allowed by the noteworthy hysteresis reduction. This recoiling will in turn allow the droplet to spread again towards the next electrode, in a continuous motion. The worse response of the droplet to the actuation obtained for PDMS coated with Glaco® is associated to the large final thickness of the substrate, which, according to Young-Lippmann equation, precludes the decrease of the contact angle under actuation. Despite this reduced response, evident recoil is still observed.

However, as one looks at the overall maximum variation of the non-dimensional droplet diameter and of the velocity of the contact line, as a function of different imposed frequencies, the behavior of the droplet on the materials coated with Glaco® is not particularly improved in the sense that the droplet does not depict the largest diameters (Fig. 7a) or the highest velocities (Fig. 7b).

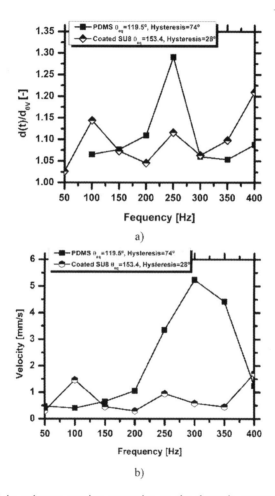

a)

b)

Fig. 7. Effect of the substrate wetting properties on the dynamic response of the droplets, namely on (a) the maximum spreading dimensionless diameter and (b) the maximum spreading velocities of GFP $(1.71 \times 10^{-3}$ mM) and GFP-expressing E-coli suspension $(1 \times 10^{9}$ cells/mL), for droplets moving between coplanar electrodes, for the configuration $w = 1200$ μm, for the configuration $w = 1200$ μm, $2a = 60$ μm. Initial droplet diameter is 2.8 mm.

Once again, this result is attributed to the final thickness of the dielectric substrates, which precludes the actuation. Hence, the final device must be fabricated under strict control of the thickness of the dielectric layers used.

Droplet response is also affected by the nature and physico-chemical properties of the solutions. Figure 8 depicts the dimensional diameter and velocity of droplets of GFP and E-Coli solutions, as a function of the imposed frequency, for the same chip configuration used in the previous analysis.

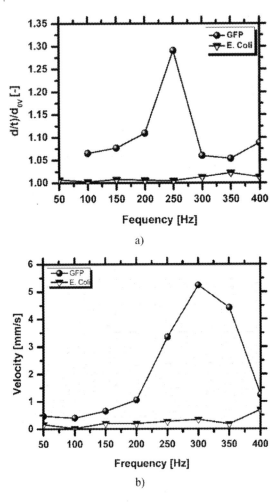

a)

b)

Fig. 8. Effect of the solution composition on the dynamic response of the droplets, namely on (a) the maximum spreading dimensionless diameter [22] and (b) the maximum spreading velocities of GFP (1.71×10^{-3} mM) and GFP-expressing E-coli suspension (1×10^9 cells/mL), for droplets moving between coplanar electrodes, for the configuration $w = 1200$ μm, $2a = 60$ μm. Initial droplet diameter is 2.8 mm.

The figure clearly shows the better response of the droplets of protein solutions, although the surface tension and density only vary slightly between the protein solution and the cell suspensions (Table 1). Hence, this particular behaviour is possibly attributed to local variations in the wettability or in the reorganization of the electrical density of the solution due to cell migration to the contact line region. However, this particular behaviour must be further studied in the near future, by characterizing the flow near the contact line.

3.3   Diagnostics Section

The diagnostic methodology to explore considers the correlation of different ratios of cell stiffness with the degrees of the pathology, being expected to be able to detect cell malignancy at very early stages [18]. Measurements of cell stiffness are usually obtained based on different separate methods (e.g. micro-pipetting, optical tweezers) and require specialized equipment such as Atomic Force Microscope and multiple preparation steps with extremely low output [29]. The work proposed here, on the other hand, addresses the full development of a microfluidic system to measure cell stiffness which does not require such complex equipment. Electrostatic actuation is explored aided by custom made surface wettability to achieve the required deformability ratios.

Cells stiffness is expected to be correlated with the deformation rates of the micro-droplets, which transport the samples. Isolated studies show the application of constitutive models [16] to explain cell stiffness. On the other hand, fluid dynamics research shows that the deformation behavior of even millimetric droplets is highly sensitive to the presence of microparticles or gums [30]. With the joined information, obtained from cell mechanics and flow dynamics, we will test the correlation between cell stiffness and microdroplets deformation. This will allow evaluating the feasibility of our approach.

3.4   Effects of Droplet Evaporation

As pointed in the Introduction, many authors argue for the potential of lab-on-chip devices for point-of-care diagnostics to be exploited for instance in developing countries. The ambient conditions however, can be a problem since to keep the device simple and affordable, there is not much room for the integration of complex systems to control the temperature and the relative humidity. These two parameters however, may strongly promote mass diffusion of the aqueous solutions, thus affecting the viability of the droplet based microfluidic system.

Based on a theoretical analysis, Moita et al. [4] report a non-negligible evaporation of a millimetric sessile droplet (30% of mass) within 1500 s of time intervals, for ambient temperatures of 23 ± 3 °C and a relative humidity of 70%. The evaporation rate of the droplets was also investigated in the present work, evaluating the temporal variation of the height and contact diameter of a sessile droplet, using the LSCFM technique.

To infer on the actual evaporation of the sample droplets, tests were carried out at experimental conditions similar to those reported in Moita *et al.* [4], although for a slightly lower ambient temperature (20 °C $\pm$ 2 °C). Temperature and relative humidity (HR) were monitored using the DHT 22 Humidity & Temperature Sensor. The measurements were performed inside the Perspex chamber, described in Sect. 2.

As discussed in the previous sections, after actuation, the droplet suffers in many cases an irreversible spreading process and the surface becomes locally hydrophilic. In a qualitative approach, under these circumstances, the evaporation of the droplet promotes the decreasing of the contact angle, while the wetting contact area remains approximately constant due to the pinning of the contact line [31].

Looking at our experimental results, in the assay performed at HR = 99.90% two stages can be identified (Fig. 9a): the first, where the liquid-solid contact area remains constant, as the contact angle decreases, in agreement with [31], transiting at t = 58.37 min for the second stage, where both the equilibrium contact angle and the contact area liquid-solid decrease. The height of the droplet decreases continuously over time (Fig. 9b).

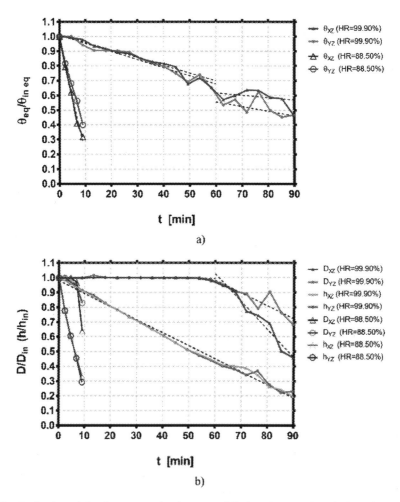

Fig. 9. Evaluation of droplet evaporation by mass diffusion. Temporal evolution of: (a) equilibrium contact angle and (b) droplet height and diameter, for the planes XZ and YZ of the droplet profile. D_{in} and h_{in} stand for the initial diameter and height of the deposited droplet, respectively.

The results further show that the contact angle decreases by about 53% of its absolute initial value. In addition, there is a reduction of the droplet height, evaluated in both planes XY and XZ, of approximately 80% in comparison to its initial height h_{in}. Also, the diameter of the deposited droplet decreases in 54% and 32% in planes XZ and YZ, respectively, compared to the initial values D_{in}.

For HR = 88.50%, the time resolution (2.25 min) is lower relatively to the HR = 99.90% assay (4.49 min) and does not allow identification of the two aforementioned evaporation states. Regarding the contact angle, a linear decrease of 68% and 60% is observed for the XZ and YZ planes, respectively – Fig. 9a.

Furthermore, the diameter of the contact area decreases by 36% (perspective XZ) and 17% (perspective YZ) in comparison to its initial value. In turn, the height decreases linearly throughout the whole period by roughly 67% of its initial height for both planes – Fig. 9b. These trends are qualitatively in agreement with those reported by Sobac and Brutin [32]. Quantitatively, additional experiments must be performed to take more sustained conclusions. For instance, the relative humidity measurements require a more accurate evaluation within the entire chamber, since the evaporative rates are quite high, even for large values of HR, which may be associated to an actual global value of HR lower than that locally measured by the sensor. Despite this limitation, this rough evaluation indicates that the evaporation of the droplets is likely to occur even at controlled ambient conditions, so that a lab-on-chip system to be used in harsh environments (e.g. countries with high temperatures and dry climate) should address the possibility of a local increase of the HR inside the chip, for the time required for the analysis.

4 Conclusions

This paper addresses the development of a microfluidic (lab-on-chip) device integrating alternative diagnostic techniques based on cell stiffness and fluid rheological properties. Namely, the device exploits cell stiffness correlations with different stages of cancer. The samples are transported in microdroplets, manipulated by electrowetting, using an open configuration system.

The chip configuration is analyzed towards various steps and its performance in terms of droplet transport is evaluated based on the measurement of the droplet-surface contact diameter and of the displacement velocity of the contact line, which are observed to be affected by numerous parameters, such as the nature and composition of the biofluids used.

Wetting properties are also shown to play a major role in droplet manipulation.

Following this analysis, a model is now being developed to scale-down the devices, allowing to decrease the size of the droplets and consequently other parameters such as the imposed electric potential.

A rough analysis on droplet evaporation effects suggests that they are not negligible, even at controlled ambient conditions. Hence, lab-on-chip system to be used in harsh environments (e.g. countries with high temperatures and dry climate) should address the possibility of a local increase of the relative humidity inside the chip, for the time required for the analysis.

Acknowledgements. The authors are grateful to Fundação para a Ciência e a Tecnologia (FCT) for partially financing this research through the project UID/EEA/50009/2013, and for supporting D. Vieira with a fellowship. The work was also partially financed by FCT through the project RECI/EMS-SIS/0147/2012, which also funded the fellowships of F. Mata and J. Pereira. A.S. Moita also acknowledges the contribution of FCT for financing her contract through the IF 2015 recruitment program.

Finally, the authors acknowledge the contribution of Prof. Susana Freitas and her team from INESC-MN for the microfabrication of the test chips.

References

1. Manz, A., Widmers, H.M., Graber, N.: Miniaturized total chemical analysis systems: a novel concept for chemical sensing. Sens. Actuators B Chem. **1**(1–6), 244–248 (1990)
2. Yager, P., Edwards, T., Fu, E., Helton, K., Nelson, K., Tam, M.R., Weigl, B.H.: Microfluidic diagnostic technologies for global public health. Nature **442**(7101), 412–418 (2006)
3. Dance, A.: The making of a medical microchip. Nature **545**, 512–514 (2017)
4. Moita, A.S., Laurência, C., Ramos, J.A., Prazeres, D.M.F., Moreira, A.L.N.: Dynamics of droplets of biological fluids on smooth superhydrophobic surfaces under electrostatic actuation. J. Bionic Eng. **13**, 220–234 (2016)
5. Geng, H., Feng, J., Stabryl, L.M., Cho, S.K.: Dielectroetting manipulation for digital microfluidics: creating, transporting, splitting, and merging droplets. Lab Chip **17**, 1060–1068 (2017)
6. Berge, B.: Electrocapillarity and wetting of insulator films by water. Acad. Sci. Ser. II Mec. **317**, 157–163 (1993)
7. Young, T.: An essay on the cohesion of fluids. Phil. Trans. R. Soc. Lond. **95**, 65–87 (1805)
8. Lippmann, G.: Relation entre les phénomènes électriques et capillaires. Ann. Chim. Phys. **5**, 494–549 (1875). (in French)
9. Mugele, F., Baret, J.C.: Electrowetting: from basics to applications. J. Phys. Condens. Matter **17**, R705–R774 (2005)
10. Jones, T.B.: An electromechanical interpretation of electrowetting. J. Micromech. Microeng. **15**, 1184–1187 (2005)
11. Bahadur, V., Garimella, S.V.: An energy-based model for electrowetting-induced droplet actuation. J. Micromech. Microeng. **16**, 1494–1503 (2006)
12. Srinivasan, V., Pamula, V.K., Fair, R.B.: An integrated digital microfluidic lab-on-a-chip for clinical diagnostics on human physiological fluids. Lab Chip **4**, 310–315 (2004)
13. Wheeler, A.R., Moon, H., Kim, C.J., Loo, J.A., Garrell, R.L.: Electrowetting-based microfluidics for analysis of peptides and proteins by matrix-assisted laser desorption/ionization mass spectrometry. Anal. Chem. **76**, 4833–4838 (2004)
14. Rupp, F., Axmann, D., Ziegler, C., Geis-Gerstorfer, J.: Adsorption/desorption phenomena on pure and Teflon® AF-coated titania surfaces studied by dynamic contact angle analysis. J. Biomed. Mater. Res. **62**, 567–578 (2002)
15. Yon, J.Y., Garrell, R.L.: Preventing biomolecular adsorption in electrowetting-based biofluidic chips. Anal. Chem. **75**, 5097–5102 (2003)
16. Suresh, S., Spatz, J., Mills, J.P., Micoulet, A., Dao, M., Lim, C.T., Beil, M., Seufferlein, T.: Connections between single-cell biomechanics and human disease states: gastrointestinal cancer and malaria. Acta Biomater. **1**, 15–30 (2005)
17. Cross, S.E., Jin, Y.-S., Rao, J., Gimzewski, J.K.: Nanomechanical analysis of cells from cancer patients. Nat. Nanotechnol. Lett. **2**, 780–783 (2005)

18. Gosset, G.R., Tse, H.T.K., Lee, S.A., Ying, Y., Lidgren, A.G., Yang, O.O., Rao, J., Clark, A.T., Di Carlo, D.: Hydrodynamic stretching of single cells for large population mechanical phenotyping. PNAS **109**(20), 7630–7635 (2009)
19. Remmerbach, T.W., Wottawah, F., Dietrich, J., Lincoln, B., Wittekind, C., Guck, J.: Oral cancer diagnosis by mechanical phenotyping. Cancer Res. **69**(5), 1728–1732 (2009)
20. Tse, H.T.K., Gosset, D.R., Moon, Y.S., Masaeli, M., Sohsman, M., Ying, Y., Mislick, K., Adams, R.P., Rao, J., Di Carlo, D.: Quantitative diagnosis of malignant pleural effusions by single-cell mechanophenotyping. Sci. Transl. Med. **5**(212), 1–9 (2013)
21. Chen, J.Z., Darhuber, A.A., Troian, S.M., Wagner, S.: Capacitive sensing of droplets for microfluidic devices based on thermocapillary actuation. Lab Chip **4**(5), 473–480 (2004)
22. Vieira, D., Mata, F., Moita, A.S., Moreira, A.L.N.: Microfluidic prototype of a lab-on-chip device for lung cancer diagnostics. In: Proceedings of the 10th International Joint Conference on Biomedical Engineering Systems and Technologies - Volume 1: BIODEVICES, Porto, Portugal, 21–13 February 2017, pp. 63–68 (2017). https://doi.org/10.5220/0006252700630068. ISBN: 978-989-758-216-5
23. Cheng, P., Li, D., Boruvka, L., Rotenberg, Y., Neumann, A.W.: Automation of axisymmetric drop shape analysis for measurements of interfacial tensions and contact angles. Colloids Surf. **43**(2), 151–167 (1990)
24. Kietzig, A.M.: Comments on "an essay on contact angle measurements" – an illustration of the respective influence of droplet deposition and measurement parameters. Plasma Proc. Polym. **8**, 1003–1009 (2008)
25. Vieira, D., Moita, A.S., Moreira, A.L.N.: Non-intrusive wettability characterization on complex surfaces using 3D laser scanning confocal fluorescence microscopy. In: 18th International Symposium on Applications of Laser and Imaging Techniques to Fluid Mechanics, Lisbon (2016)
26. Chen, L., Bonaccurso, E.: Electrowetting - from statics to dynamics. Adv. Colloid Interface Sci. **210**, 2–12 (2014)
27. Fan, S.-K., Yang, H., Wang, T.-T., Hsu, W.: Asymmetric electrowetting–moving droplets by a square wave. Lab Chip **7**(10), 1330–1335 (2007)
28. Mata, F., Moita, A.S., Kumar, R., Cardoso, S., Prazeres, D.M.F., Moreira, A.L.N.: Effect of surface wettability on the spreading and displacement of biofluid drops in electrowetting. In: Proceedings of ILASS – Europe 2016, 27th Annual Conference on Liquid Atomization and Spray Systems, September 2016, Brighton, UK, 4–7 September 2016 (2016). ISBN 978-1-910172-09-4
29. Adamo, A., Sharei, A., Adamo, L., Lee, B., Mao, S., Jensen, K.F.: Microfluidics-based assessment of cell deformability. Anal. Chem. **84**, 6438–6443 (2012)
30. Moita, A.S., Herrmann, D., Moreira, A.L.N.: Fluid dynamic and heat transfer processes between solid surfaces and non-Newtonian liquid droplets. Appl. Therm. Eng. **88**, 33–46 (2015)
31. Picknett, R., Bexon, R.: The evaporation of sessile or pendant drops in still air. J. Colloid Interface Sci. **61**(2), 336–350 (1977)
32. Sobac, B., Brutin, D.: Triple-line behavior and wettability controlled by nanocoated substrates: influence on sessile drop evaporation. Langmuir **27**(24), 14999–15007 (2011)

A Biochip Based Medical Device for Point-of-Care ABO Compatibility: Towards a Smart Transfusion Line

Karine Charrière[1], Alain Rouleau[2], Olivier Gaiffe[2], Pascal Morel[3],
Véronique Bourcier[4], Christian Pieralli[2], Wilfrid Boireau[2],
Lionel Pazart[1], and Bruno Wacogne[1,2(✉)]

[1] INSERM CIC 1431, Besançon University Hospital, 2 place St Jacques,
25030 Besançon cedex, France
[2] FEMTO-ST Institute, Univ. Bourgogne Franche-Comté, CNRS,
15B avenue des Montboucons, 25030 Besançon cedex, France
bruno.wacogne@univ-fcomte.fr
[3] Etablissement Français du Sang Bourgogne/Franche-Comté,
8 rue du Docteur Jean François Xavier Girod, Hauts de Chazal, Temis Santé,
BP 1937, 25020 Besançon cedex, France
[4] Hemovigilance Service, Besançon University Hospital,
1 Bd Alexandre Fleming, 25030 Besançon cedex, France

Abstract. ABO mismatch between donor and patient's blood is still the cause of accidents which are sometimes lethal. The main causes of mis-assignment are human errors and wrong identification of patients or blood product. Only a final compatibility test at the patient's bedside can avoid these errors. In some countries, this test is performed using manual procedures. This does not prevent from human manipulation and interpretation errors. In this paper, we present a prototype able to automatically perform a final ABO compatibility test. It relies on the use of disposable antibodies grafted biochips inserted into a mobile reader/actuator. Red blood cells are selectively captured on biochips grafted with antibodies complementary of antigens present on the cells surface. Detection of captured cells is based on optical absorption techniques. So far, our device achieved blood compatibility test with 99.3% sensitivity and 97.9% specificity.

Keywords: Biosensor · Surface Plasmon Resonance · Human red blood cells
Automated ABO compatibility test · Optical detection · Opto-fluidic prototype

1 Introduction

In all countries before blood transfusion, a concordance verification test between patient's data and red cells to be transfused is performed at the patient's bedside. In most countries, a cross-match test is performed in a biology laboratory before the concordance test. However, it becomes useless when an error occurs after the delivery (the wrong blood bag to the wrong patient, the most frequent case). In very few countries (in France for example), a biologic compatibility test is performed at the patient's bedside.

© Springer International Publishing AG, part of Springer Nature 2018
N. Peixoto et al. (Eds.): BIOSTEC 2017, CCIS 881, pp. 94–105, 2018.
https://doi.org/10.1007/978-3-319-94806-5_5

In countries for which the hemo-vigilance is reliable and where a unique test is performed, the ratio of adverse effects due to ABO incompatibility approaches 1/40000 red cell concentrates (RCC). This was the case in France before 2003 when only ABO compatibility was tested. After this date, the use of both concordance and ABO tests at the patient's bedside reduced the adverse effects to about 1/600000. However, in most countries, only the concordance test is considered.

There is a need for a second test at the patient's bedside in order to reduce the number of ABO errors. There exist ABO test cards, but they rely on delicate manual operation and require a long and specific training. Furthermore, the compatibility card requires a human interpretation of the agglutination test. Therefore, this method is a source of various errors: manipulation, reading and interpretation difficulties. Also, medical staff is exposed to blood when sampling patient's blood. Concerning the interpretation difficulty, iso-group compatibility is relatively straightforward but non iso-group compatibility still leads to interpretation errors or stressful situations.

For these reasons, a point-of-care device able to automatically perform an ultimate compatibility test with minimum manipulation and without human interpretation would be profitable, in particular when considering the increase of blood product distributed during the last decade. For example in France an increase of the RCC delivery of almost 24% has been observed between 2000 and 2011 [1]. In 2016, more than 3 million of RCC where distributed [2].

Several methods have been proposed for blood typing. They are mainly based on gel agglutination [3, 4]. SPR [5–7] and Surface Plasmon Resonance imaging (SPRi) [8–11] techniques can also be used. However, these studies demonstrate the possibility to detect captured cells with commercial laboratory apparatuses. Therefore, a direct translation to the patient's bedside may be difficult because the entire device used should be re-thought for point-of-care use.

Recently, long-range surface plasmon-polaritons to detect red blood cells (RBC) selectively captured by the surface chemistry was demonstrated [12]. However, because packed RBC must be diluted in a buffer of controlled refractive index, translation of the device to clinical use is still challenging. Techniques based on image processing on plate test have been reported [13, 14]. In this case, image processing is used to objectively observe and interpret red cell agglutination obtained manually. Issues concerning blood and antibodies manipulation still exist. Spectroscopic methods have also been reported [15, 16]. However, the use of an optical spectrometer to measure absorption of diluted red cells may be difficult in clinical practice. In fact, although these new devices are able to realize blood typing by objectively reading agglutination, they still require hard translational research work before to be installed in the patient's room.

In this paper, we present a mobile device meant to address the above mentioned issues. The main idea is to replace the four reaction zones of the current manual compatibility card with four IgMs grafted biochips inspired from Surface Plasmon Resonance (SPR) and SPRi biochips. Hemagglutination is therefore replaced by red cell capture. The detection of captured red cells rely on a simple optical absorption technique. Biochips are inserted in a mobile reader/actuator which drives the fluids (blood, red cell concentrate (RCC) and physiological serum), performs the optical reading and final interpretation. This concept is currently protected by two patents [17, 18] and was describing in a previous paper [19].

Research actions to set-up this device include four main steps. The first series of tests consisted in studying the IgMs grafting and red cell capture using SPR and SPRi methods with homemade biochips. This has been previously reported [20, 21]. The second set of experiments consisted in translating the SPR biochip to biochips inserted into cartridges and to detect the capture of red cells in these half-bulk conditions together with the correlation between the number of captured cells and optical reading [19].

The third part of the experiments is the subject of the current publication. It consists in using a large number of whole blood (WB) and RCC samples to test the automated fluid flow control, optical reading and software interpretation of the ABO compatibility result. The goal is to determine sensitivity and specificity of the device together with the blood group concordance between what is expected and what the device reads. We also studied the performance of the device according to the age of RCC. The last part of the work consists in experimenting the use of the venous return to drive patient's blood into the device with reduces risk of exposure to blood for medical staff [18].

2 Materials and Methods

2.1 Biochip Fabrication

The fabrication and testing of biochips using SPR and SPRi techniques has been previously reported [20]. The antibodies used were IgM anti-A or IgM anti-B (DIAGAST, France). The running buffer was saline physiological serum (NaCl 0.9%).

2.2 Description of the Device

The heart of the device consists of two cartridges, one used to test the patient's blood, the other for the RCC (see Fig. 1). Both of them contain two IgMs grafted biochips, one with anti-A, the other with anti-B antibodies. When blood (either WB or RCC) is applied to the biochips, antigen-antibody recognition occurs.

These microfluidic cartridges are placed into an optical clamp which consists of blue LEDs and photodetectors. Each biochip can then be interrogated with its own LED/Detector pair. Red cells trapped onto the biochip absorb light. The detection principle consists in measuring the transmission before red cells are driven onto the chip, when physiological serum fills the circuitry, (reference measurement) and after red cell/surface interaction followed by washing with physiological serum (final measurement).

The optical reading is therefore an absorbance measurement given by:

$$Absorbance = (reference - final)/reference \tag{1}$$

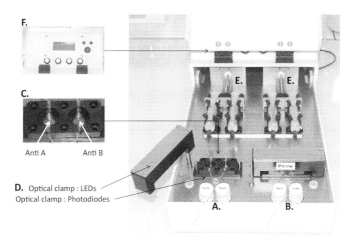

Fig. 1. Views of the device. A.B. There is 1 cartridge for the patient and another one for the red cell concentrates. C. Each cartridge includes 2 biochips grafted with anti-A and anti-B antibodies. D. Optical clamps are used to detect the capture of red cells at the chip's surface. E. Fluids are driven using syringes controlled by the internal micro-processor. F. The human-machine interface allows setting the opto-fluic parameters and displaying compatibility test results.

In what follows, positive chips are defined as chips that have captured red cells, regardless of the blood group. Conversely, negative chips correspond to chip with no capture.

Fluids (blood, RCC and physiological serum) are driven by means of automated syringes controlled via dedicated software. This software also drives the optical measurement, human-machine interface and USB connection to a PC for data recording and processing.

2.3   Surface Analysis

After experiments, cartridges were removed from the laboratory prototype and observed with a macroscope (Leica MSV266; soft-ware Leica Application Suite V3.7.0). The percentage of RBC trapped on surfaces was estimated with ImageJ for each biochip by averaging the percentage of RBC on surface of 5 random macroscopic fields.

2.4   Statistical Analysis

Statistical comparisons were made with the Kruskal–Wallis test followed by Dunn's multiple comparison tests using GraphPad prism 5.

2.5   First Validation of the Use of the Venous Return

Experiments were conducted using an intravenous trainer arm (Adam, Rouilly, AR251). A Baxter Y-type transfuser (RMC 5849) was modified. 2 ways valves were inserted in the patient's end of the transfuser. They are used to drive the red cell concentrate to the patient and to drive patient's blood to the device. They are also used to isolate the patient during the test and to protect the medical staff from contact with the patient's blood. The tested fluids were physiological serum and colored solution to represent blood. Fluidic behavior of the device was assessed visually.

3   Results

3.1   Device's Testing

The device was tested using 148 blood aliquots. This represents 296 biochips and therefore 148 cartridges. Blood comes from both RCC and WB. Samples were provided by the Etablissement Français du Sang in accordance with the ethical rules and with informed consent obtained from donors.

Among these 296 chips, 4 are not taken into account because errors occurred while assembling the cartridges.

Therefore, only 292 biochips were tested. Remember that 2 biochips are required to test 1 sample. For two samples, inversions of the anti-A and anti-B biochips were made. Although the biochips behave correctly and are taken into account for biochip testing, the corresponding samples were not taken into account for compatibility testing. At the end, 142 samples were tested for compatibility.

The repartition of samples in terms of RCC, WB and blood group is given in Table 1.

Table 1.   Number of samples used in this study.

Group	A	B	AB	O
RCC	19	25	14	20
WB	17	13	20	14

3.2   Biochip Efficiency

Here, 292 biochips were tested. The absorbance was measured as a function of positive and negative biochips for both RCC and WB. Positive and negative biochips correspond to the 4 blood groups (see Fig. 2).

There is a strong difference between positive and negative biochips. No statistical variation of the absorbance was observed in negative biochips (0.003 ± 0.001 for RCC neg and 0.007 ± 0.02 for WB neg). Conversely, significant difference is observed in positive biochips between RCC and WB (0.36 ± 0.006 for RCC pos and 0.18 ± 0.008 for WB pos). This result may be related to the large difference of erythrocytes number in samples ($4.3 \times 10^9 \pm 10^8$ RBC/mL for RCC and 10^9 C/mL for WB).

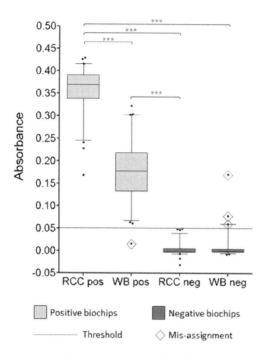

Fig. 2. Absorbance versus positive or negative biochips. Box plot: 5–95 percentiles. Kruskal-Wallis test followed by Dunn's multiple comparison tests. *** p < 0.001. Negative values are due to a slight drift of the electronics. Red diamond shows cases of mis-assignment when the threshold is set to 0.05. (Color figure online)

The best absorbance threshold to discriminate between positive and negative biochip was set to 0.05 (minimization of mis-assignments). In this way, only 4 errors occurred. One biochip represents a false negative. For it, not enough red cells were captured although the biochip should have been positive. Indeed, red cell capture is not homogenous on the surface, maybe due to an antibodies grafting problem. This means that 1 patient of group AB was detected as A. Three other biochips were false positive. For them a strong non-specific retention of red cells was recorded due to washing problem. This means that 1 patient of group O was detected as A and 2 patients B detected as AB.

From these results and differentiating between A and B biochips allows calculating sensitivity and specificity of the device. This is summarized in Table 2. Almost all sensitivities are 100%, except for anti-B biochips (97%) used with WB (false negative described earlier). It is the same for specificities: all biochips are 100% specific, except the anti-A biochips used with WB (3 false positives described previously).

Table 3 presents the same parameters regardless of the blood type and for the entire device. At the end, specificity of the device is 99.3% and specificity is 97.9%. Improving fabrication of the cartridges would probably resolve these mis-assignments and improved sensitivity and specificity.

Table 2. System performance (in terms of biochips).

	RCC		WB	
	Anti-A	Anti-B	Anti-A	Anti-B
Number of Biochips	82	78	68	64
Expected positives	36	39	39	33
Recorded positives	36	39	39	32
Sensitivity	**100%**	**100%**	**100%**	**97%**
Expected negatives	46	39	29	31
Recorded negatives	46	39	26	31
Specificity	**100%**	**100%**	**89.7%**	**100%**

Table 3. System performance (in terms of antibodies and for the entire device).

	RCC + WB		Entire device
	Anti-A	Anti-B	
Number of Biochips	150	146	292
Expected positives	75	72	147
Recorded positives	75	71	146
Sensitivity	**100%**	**98.6%**	**99.3%**
Expected negatives	75	70	145
Recorded negatives	72	70	142
Specificity	**96%**	**100%**	**97.9%**

Biochips performance was also tested as a function of the age of the blood donation. In this case, only RCC were considered because WB is meant to be fresh. For this
test we used 30 positive biochips with 6 to 8 days old donations, 31 negative biochips
with 6 to 8 days old, 29 positive with 43 to 44 days old and 40 negative with 43 to 44
days old. Figure 3 shows the absorbance obtained in terms of positivity/negativity. No
difference was observed between all kinds of positive biochips: 0.35 ± 0.011 for 6 to 8
days old RCC and 0.37 ± 0.01 for 43 to 4 days old RCC. The same is observed
between negative biochips: 0.001 ± 0.002 for 6 to 8 days old RCC and 0.005 ± 0.002
for 43 to 44 days old RCC. It is quite clear that the age of the blood donation does not
impact device performances (see Fig. 3).

For compatibility interpretation, 74 tests were performed. In all cases the software
delivered the right compatibility information, perfectly coherent with what happened at
the biochip surface. Of course, we mentioned cases where mis-assignments occurred.
However, this part of the test concerns the fact that the device delivers the right
information from the result of the optical measurement. For example, with sample
SO11 (WB of group O), a strong non-specific RCC retention has been observed on the
anti-A biochip, with an absorbance of 0.06 corresponding to a percentage of red cells of

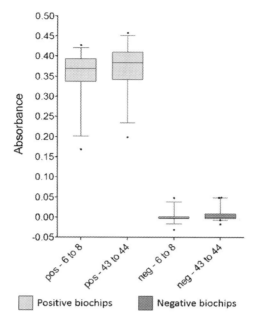

Fig. 3. Absorbance versus the age of the red cell concentrates in terms of positive and negative biochips. Box plot: 5–95 percentiles.

21% on the biochip surface. This "patient" was considered A group. When testing the compatibility with B group RCC, the device concluded that the transfusion should not be allowed. Therefore the optical reading and the interpretation software work properly.

Experiments to test the ability of the device to correctly identify blood groups have been conducted. Among 142 concordance tests performed 4 mis-assignments occurred. The concordance performance is therefore 97% (see Table 4). Mis-assignments reported here correspond to those already mentioned above.

Table 4. Detail of the concordance test (m-a: mis-assignment).

		Groups			
		A	B	AB	O
RCC	N° of tests	19	25	14	20
	Concordance (%)	100	100	100	100
WB	N° of tests	17	13	20	14
	Concordance (%)	100	84.6 (2 m-a)	95 (1 m-a)	94.4 (1 m-a)
		All groups			
RCC + WB	N° of test	142			
	Concordance (%)	97 (4 m-a)			

The next experiment concerned the percentage of red blood cells on the biochips surfaces as a function of the positive or negative nature of the biochips. While the threshold in terms of absorbance was set to 0.05, the threshold in terms of percentage of the surface covered with red blood cells is about 17.5% (see Fig. 4).

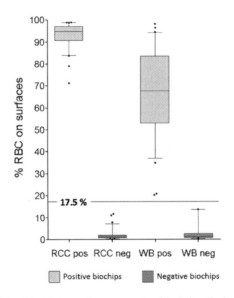

Fig. 4. Percentage of the biochip's surface covered with red cells in terms of positive and negative chips. RCC: red cell concentrate. WB: whole blood. Box plot: 5–95 percentiles.

3.3   Venous Return

The last experiment concerned the validation of the use of the venous return to sample patient's blood. For this, preliminary fluidic tests were performed using an intravenous trainer arm. This is illustrated in Fig. 5 which shows frames of a video filmed during the experiments. Preliminary tests show that a slightly modified conventional transfuser can be used to correctly drive fluids the device (see Fig. 5). As seen in Fig. 5(a), the colored solution to represent blood rises in the catheter when the catheter is placed. When the 3 ways valve is correctly positioned, the patient's blood is correctly driven toward the device (Fig. 5(b)). In Fig. 5(c), the patient's is correctly isolated from the physiological serum used to rinse the tubes. Tubes and device connection are correctly rinsed (Fig. 5(d)).

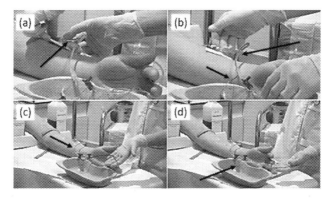

Fig. 5. Frame captures of a video filmed while testing the efficiency of the blood venous return.

4   Discussion

In this paper, we presented a new device able to semi-automatically perform an ultimate ABO compatibility test. It is based on biochips grafted with anti-A and anti-B antibodies. They are inserted into disposable cartridges and placed into a mobile and re-usable reader/actuator. The latter includes embarked software that drives and controls the fluid flows, performs the optical detection of captured red cells and interpret the result in terms of ABO compatibility. 292 biochips were tested. The device exhibits sensitivity and specificity equal to 99.3% and 97.9% respectively. At this stage of the project, different aspects can be discussed.

Concerning the automatic fluid driving, cartridges proved to be efficient in driving the fluids onto the biochip with minimum non-specific interactions. Taking into account the very strong affinity-avidity of the antigen-antibody couple, the test duration do not exceed a few minutes, which is perfectly compatible with clinical constraints.

The optical absorption detection method also proved to be efficient. We demonstrated efficient detection with low hematocrit levels (down to about 10%).

We still need to fully understand why 4 mis-assignments occurred during the tests. However, for the 3 false positives, washing was imperfect, probably due to a slight motor dysfunction. For false negative biochips, IgMs were probably not optimally grafted which may explain the non-uniform red cells capture. Optical reading and software interpretation are not to be blamed. However, just after these 4 false results have been observed, the same samples used with new biochip were re-tested. This time, everything worked correctly and no mis-assignment was observed. In fact, these problems will probably be solved when transferring the device for industrial development according to the quality policy of the involved company.

More generally, the immune-opto-fluidic cartridge we present here proved to be able to detect red cell capture even when only a few red cells are trapped. Therefore, a large number of applications can now be envisaged like anti-D detection for example.

5   Conclusion

To conclude, we believe that the concept described here may help enhancing blood transfusion safety, not only in countries where a double ultimate test is already performed, but especially in countries where only one test is considered. Furthermore, such a device is meant to drastically reduce ABO compatibility accidents in countries where the whole transfusion process (blood donation, conservation, delivery and transfusion) is not yet fully satisfactory.

Acknowledgements. This work was partly supported by the EFS (grant DECO-13-0128), the INSERM-CNRS (patent file CNRS/REF:02682-V), OSEO and the University of Franche-Comté (grant A11050051). This work is developed in the frame of the French RENATECH network and the Biom'@x transversal axis at FEMTO-ST.

References

1. EFS: Rapport d'activité (2011). http://www.dondusang.net/rewrite/article/4900/efs/publicati ons/feuilletez-en-ligne-le-rapport-d-activite-2011-de-l-efs.htm?idRubrique=790
2. ANSM: Bilans/Rapports d'activité - Bilans et rapports d'activité - ANSM : Agence nationale de sécurité du médicament et des produits de santé. http://ansm.sante.fr/Mediatheque/ Publications/Bilans-Rapports-d-activite-Bilans-et-rapports-d-activite#folder_26762
3. Cid, J., Nogués, N., Montero, R., Hurtado, M., Briega, A., Parra, R.: Comparison of three microtube column agglutination systems for antibody screening: DG Gel, DiaMed-ID and ortho BioVue. Transfus. Med. **16**, 131–136 (2006). https://doi.org/10.1111/j.1365-3148. 2006.00655.x
4. Langston, M.M., Procter, J.L., Cipolone, K.M., Stroncek, D.F.: Evaluation of the gel system for ABO grouping and D typing. Transfusion **39**, 300–305 (1999)
5. Malomgre, W., Neumeister, B.: Recent and future trends in blood group typing. Anal. Bioanal. Chem. **393**, 1443–1451 (2009)
6. Quinn, J.G., O'Neill, S., Doyle, A., McAtamney, C., Diamond, D., MacCraith, B.D., O'Kennedy, R.: Development and application of surface plasmon resonance-based biosensors for the detection of cell-ligand interactions. Anal. Biochem. **281**, 135–143 (2000). https://doi.org/10.1006/abio.2000.4564
7. Quinn, J.G., O'Kennedy, R., Smyth, M., Moulds, J., Frame, T.: Detection of blood group antigens utilising immobilised antibodies and surface plasmon resonance. J. Immunol. Methods **206**, 87–96 (1997). https://doi.org/10.1016/S0022-1759(97)00092-6
8. Berthier, A., Elie-Caille, C., Lesniewska, E., Delage-Mourroux, R., Boireau, W.: Label-free sensing and atomic force spectroscopy for the characterization of protein-DNA and protein-protein interactions: application to estrogen receptors. J. Mol. Recognit. **24**, 429–435 (2011). https://doi.org/10.1002/jmr.1106
9. Boozer, C., Kim, G., Cong, S., Guan, H., Londergan, T.: Looking towards label-free biomolecular interaction analysis in a high-throughput format: a review of new surface plasmon resonance technologies. Curr. Opin. Biotechnol. **17**, 400–405 (2006). https://doi. org/10.1016/j.copbio.2006.06.012
10. Campbell, C., Kim, G.: SPR microscopy and its applications to high-throughput analyses of biomolecular binding events and their kinetics. Biomaterials **28**, 2380–2392 (2007). https:// doi.org/10.1016/j.biomaterials.2007.01.047

11. Mansuy-Schlick, V., Delage-Mourroux, R., Jouvenot, M., Boireau, W.: Strategy of macromolecular grafting onto a gold substrate dedicated to protein–protein interaction measurements. Biosens. Bioelectron. **21**, 1830–1837 (2006). https://doi.org/10.1016/j.bios.2005.11.021

12. Krupin, O., Wang, C., Berini, P.: Selective capture of human red blood cells based on blood group using long-range surface plasmon waveguides. Biosens. Bioelectron. **53**, 117–122 (2014). https://doi.org/10.1016/j.bios.2013.09.051

13. Ferraz, A., Carvalho, V., Soares, F.: Development of a human blood type detection automatic system. In: Eurosensors Xxiv Conference, vol. 5, pp. 496–499 (2010)

14. Ferraz, A., Carvalho, V.: A prototype for blood typing based on image processing. In: SENSORDEVICES 2013: The Fourth International Conference on Sensor Device Technologies and Applications, pp. 139–144 (2013)

15. Ramasubramanian, M.K., Alexander, S.P.: An integrated fiberoptic–microfluidic device for agglutination detection and blood typing. Biomed. Microdevices **11**, 217–229 (2009). https://doi.org/10.1007/s10544-008-9227-y

16. Ramasubramanian, M., Anthony, S., Lambert, J.: Simplified spectrophotometric method for the detection of red blood cell agglutination. Appl. Opt. **47**, 4094–4105 (2008)

17. Wacogne, B., Boireau, W., Morel, P., Pazart, L., Pieralli, C.: Device for taking a sample of a body fluid and method for implementing same (2011)

18. Wacogne, B., Boireau, W., Morel, P., Pazart, L., Pieralli, C.: Secure perfusion system (2011)

19. Charrière, K., Rouleau, A., Gaiffe, O., Fertey, J., Morel, P., Bourcier, V., Pieralli, C., Boireau, W., Pazart, L., Wacogne, B.: Biochip technology applied to an automated ABO compatibility test at the patient bedside. Sens. Actuators B Chem. **208**, 67–74 (2015). https://doi.org/10.1016/j.snb.2014.10.123

20. Charrière, K., Guerrini, J.-S., Wacogne, B., Rouleau, A., Elie-Caille, C., Pieralli, C., Pazart, L., Morel, P., Boireau, W.: SmarTTransfuser - a biochip system for the final ABO compatibility test. In: Présenté à International Conference on Biomedical Electronics and Devices (BIODEVICES 2012), Vilamoura, Portugal (2012)

21. Charrière, K., Rouleau, A., Gaiffe, O., Morel, P., Bourcier, V., Pieralli, C., Boireau, W., Pazart, L., Wacogne, B.: An automated medical device for ultimate ABO compatibility test at the patient's bedside - towards the automation of point-of-care transfusion safety. In: Présenté à International Conference on Biomedical Electronics and Devices (BIODEVICES 2015), Lisbon, Portugal (2015)

Novel Pattern Recognition Method for Analysis the Radiation Exposure in Cancer Treatment

Dmitriy Dubovitskiy$^{(\boxtimes)}$ and Valeri Kouznetsov

Oxford Recognition Ltd, 10 Maio Road, Cambridge CB4 2GA, UK
{dda,vk}@oxreco.com
http://www.oxreco.com

Abstract. A novel pattern recognition technique has been deployed in the treatment of cancer tumours to provide improved targeting of ionising radiation and more accurate measurement of the radiation dose. The radiation beams enter the body from different directions to concentrate on the tumour. The centre of the tumour has to be precisely located relatively to patient's skin surface, so the radiation does not affect healthy tissue and produces successful treatment. Existing methods of 3D dose measurement are highly labor-intensive and generally suffer from low accuracy. In this publication, we propose a new method of 3D measurement of the dose in real-time by using skin pattern recognition technology. The textural pattern of the patient's skin is analysed from an image sensor in a specially designed camera using Fractal Geometry and Fuzzy logic. A specially designed net sensor is then placed over the area of skin exposed to the treatment in order to measure the radiation dose. The algorithms discussed below enable the precise focussing of the radiation. The novel object recognition technique provides a mathematical tool to build a volume model of the dose distribution inside the patient's body. This paper provides an overview and specific information on the technology and necessary background for future industrial implementation into health care infrastructure.

Keywords: Cancer treatment · In vivo dosimetry
Radiation sensors · Pattern analysis · Decision making
Object recognition · Image morphology · Image recognition
Pattern recognition · Texture classification · Computational geometry

1 Introduction

For the purposes of the dosimetry of the small areas in radiotherapy, typically uses traditional micro ionisation chambers, semiconductor diode dosimeters and, in the recent years, increasingly uses a very handy MOSFET transistors. The MOSFET transistors provide good accuracy and repeatability of the results with dimensions of a few millimetres, which is sufficient for practical applications in

© Springer International Publishing AG, part of Springer Nature 2018
N. Peixoto et al. (Eds.): BIOSTEC 2017, CCIS 881, pp. 106–118, 2018.
https://doi.org/10.1007/978-3-319-94806-5_6

medical diagnostics. In addition, they are joined harmoniously with the systems of scanning and information processing [1,2]. For 3D doisimetry, Gel Dosimeters proposed in the mid 80-s are widely used. However, this method is rather inconvenient as it is associated with the use of special phantoms (models) made of gel-like material changing its optical properties under the influence of ionising irradiation. At the same time, it allows customising the parameters intensity and the 3D geometry of irradiation. Polymer gel dosimetry remains one of the most promising and widely used tools for 3D dose measuring [3]. There are also methods of extrapolating measurements at individual points or 2D measurements to 3D models.

The most modern methods [4] of measurement suggest usage of linear array diodes with 98 measurement points for scanning of a water phantom. Then the data are linked to the patient CT image and after Monte Carlo method are used to extrapolate dose distributions inside the patient body and to control measurements with point dosimeters (diodes) performed during the process treatment in vivo. Impact of ionising irradiation at different MOS (metal oxide semiconductor) structures have been studied for quite a long time, at least since the mid 70-s due to the start of using of electronics based on MOS technology in space systems [5]. The processes occurring in such structures under the influence of radiation of various types and intensity is very well studied and described in numerous articles addressing radiation hardness of MOS IS [6–9]. For medical applications measuring of the accumulated radiation dose with such structures is still rather new. As an indication of the accumulated dose the effect of degradation of MOS structure is used, particularly the under-gate dielectric (SiO2). Without going deep into the details of physical processes, we mention only the main effect that is used for dosimetry.

Under irradiation, gate dielectric accumulates a positive charge which leads in particular to a shift of the threshold voltage in a MOSFET transistor or to a shift of the volt-farad characteristics of the MOS capacitor. Inducing of a positive voltage on the Gate of a transistor (MOS capacitor) in the process of irradiation, leads to the increase of the amount of accumulated charge. In the case of no voltage applied, it makes possible to irradiate the passive MOS structure, and then to measure the charge that is equivalent to the dose. Other effects occurring in dielectrics during irradiation can be ignored in this case. In the range of doses used in medicine, the charge accumulation is linearly proportional to the dose and only at high doses about 6–8 Gy (depends on the technology) tends to saturation and loses linearity. Moreover, dosimeters based on MOS structures are small in size (around 1 sq. mm) and very simple in production.

The particular focus of this paper is in the use of such sensors for development and imaging technology of a net bandage dosimetry system (Fig. 1), with a MOS capacitor sensor in every node of the grid. Such dosimetry net can be placed (dressed) around any part of the body (or fantom) and will allow controlling the dose of radiation for the incoming and outgoing flow of irradiation and from any direction. This will allow building a 3D model of the absorbed dose inside the patient's body, which is a new and highly demanded product in the market of medical diagnostics tools.

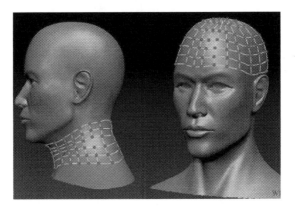

Fig. 1. Net bandage.

The skin pattern recognition system is to deliver the location for net bandage position relatively to body map. The skin patent is mathematically interpreted by Fractal geometry. The self-similarity features of fractals are very suitable for this application. The skin region is translated into the vector of Fractal features. The Fractal features is then identifying the skin map. The first net bandage placement is to select and record the skin regions. The future treatments requires to position the sensor net at the very same skin area.

The automatic decision making system is implemented by Fuzzy logic technology. At the first net sensor bandage application the image recognition system build membership function of Fuzzy logic and memorised skin map. The future net bandage application will be automatically calculated offset to the first position and it is up to future developer to use the offset or to move the sensors net to the exact first position. We will cover the novel mathematical equation in Sect. 3 and begin from dosimetry setup in next section.

2   Structural Scheme of Dosimetry System

The proposed dosimetric network, can be a convenient and inexpensive tool to verify the dose distribution inside the body as well as build three-dimensional models of absorbed dose. The MOSFET was recently highly proven [10–14] as an in vivo dosimeter of the absorbed dose. Here, we have decided to focus on the most simple structures, such as the MOS capacitors, since the phenomenon of charge accumulation in under-gate dielectric of MOSFET (in fact, under-gate MOS capacitor) determines its ability to function as a dosimeter. MOS sensors, in this case, contain a number of advantages. MOS capacitors are extremely simple and inexpensive to manufacture. We can select and vary many parameters of this structure (for example thickness and type of gate-dielectric, the size of the structure) to improve its operation as a dosimeter, due to the fact it's simply a capacitor it is not necessary to take into consideration the parameters required for function as a transistor.

The scheme of the measurement of accumulated charge which corresponds to the absorbed dose requires less number of contacts (only two, and one of them is common for all sensors) that facilitates the creation of matrix or grid with a large number of sensors.

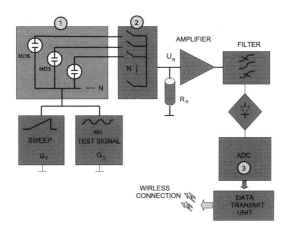

Fig. 2. The measuring system for collecting data from sensors. 1- matrix of sensors, 2-multiplexer, 3-analog to digital converter.

The block diagram of such a system as shown in Fig. 2. The accumulated charge in the oxide (equivalent to dose) proposed to determine by measuring volt-farad characteristics. This method has long been known as the main and classical method for measurement of MOS structures properties [15–17] and have been well tested. A typical view of this characteristic for the silicon substrate n-type is shown in the Fig. 3.

This figure shows the shift of C-V characteristics which occurs as a result of accumulating charge in the gate oxide, the measurement of this shift is our goal in this case. Capacitive Sensors - dosimeters are connected in matrix (1). The date from the sensors is collected consecutively been analog multiplexer (2) switches from one structure to another. The sweep generator G1 provides a slow shift in a range of a few volts on MOS and G2 provides a test signal with a frequency of 1 MHz and amplitude of 10 mV. The alternate voltage amplitude on resistor Rn will be proportional to the capacity of MOS sensor, as demonstrated in the formulas below.

$$Rc = 1/wC, \quad i = Ug_2/Z = Ug_2/\sqrt{Rn^2 + 1/w^2C^2}$$

$$if \quad R_c = 1/wC >> R_n, \quad then \quad i \approx wC(Ug_1)Ug_2$$

$$U_R = iR_n = Ug_2R_nwC(Ug_1) \quad where \quad w = 2\pi f$$

The measurement process for each sensor will take approximately no more than 5–10 ms. This means that the matrix of sensors with dimension of 256 sensors will be scanned in 1.5 to 2.5 s. These data is digitised by ADC (3) and sent to a computer wirelessly, where data can be processed further. The advantages of MOS as an absorbed dose dosimeters is also that they are able keep the charge somewhat stable and readings can be taken for a long period of time after exposure.

When MOS capacitors are exposed to ionizing radiation, the positive charge is captured in the under-gate oxide [18–20]. It leads to a shift of volt-farad characteristics, see Fig. 3. The magnitude of the shift depends on the absorbed dose of ionising radiation and is approximately 200 mV in the absence of gate voltage during irradiation. By applying a positive voltage on the gate, we can increase the sensitivity of the sensors and the shift of the voltage can reach 400–500 mV per Gy.

To confirm the behaviour of MOS structures under radiation by standard medical equipment, the most common samples taken, the gate oxide SiO2 were grown in a dry environment at 1000C, thickness of oxide was 0.6 μm on Si wafer 4.5 Om/cm conductivity of n-type with F(fluorine) doping. Size of crystal was 1 × 1 mm. Irradiation was carried out at Photon clinical linear accelerator 6 MeV (Varian 2100 EX), doses were 0 to 10 Gy, at room temperature. As a control dosimeter, ionisation chamber ROOS was used. Results of the experiment are shown on Fig. 4.

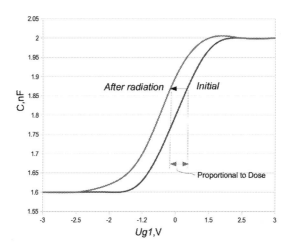

Fig. 3. Volt-Farad characteristic of typical MOS condensator.

For our purposes we are going to use a successfully tested system of pattern recognition [27] and adhere our system of sensors to the skin of the patient. The image recognition system was used for skin cancer diagnostic and has been published in [22–26,28] this redundant system was working well and we expect it to be extremely effective.

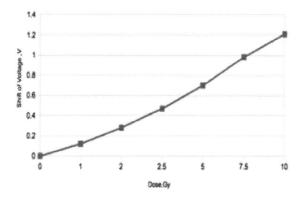

Fig. 4. Characteristic of volt shift for the silicon substrate n-typer.

3   Skin Pattern Positioning System

The current medical practice includes several radiation exposure during the course of treatment with a number of days in between. The position of the net bandage on the patient's skin is very important to allow consistency for the next treatment of the same tumour. In order to address this, data from the CT scan could be used to adjust position for the next treatment. Computation of position is implemented by using Fractal Geometry theory [36] to get the precise pattern of the skin. The precise pattern of the skin is corresponded to the calibration points on the net bandage. The real time computation system [33] will allow a doctor to dynamically move the bandage and see the offset from the last treatment position. When offset approaches zero, the exact same position of the radiation sensors will be reached.

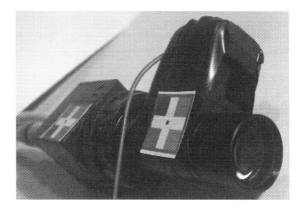

Fig. 5. Dermatological image acquisition camera.

The skin has texture and a particular skin region can be characterised by Fractal features called Fractal parameters [34]. An image of the skin sample is taken by a specially designed dermatological image acquisition camera [38] on Fig. 5.

The correspondent points are calculated from Fractal parameters [35]. If we consider the profile of a typical skin image [37], then the curve does not coincide with a sine-wave signal. To obtain adequate accuracy, it is necessary to magnify the resolution of the image [21], which in turn introduces distortion [29,31]. For increased accuracy on low-resolution data, we consider a convolution function of a form more consistent with the profile of a video signal [30–32]. For a signal I we consider the representation

$$F(k) = \sum_{n=1}^{N} I(n)$$

$$\mathrm{arccos}\left[\cos\left(\frac{2\pi(k-1)(n-1)}{N} - \frac{\pi}{2}\right)\right] - \frac{\pi}{2}$$

$$-i\,\mathrm{arcsin}\left[\cos\left(\frac{2\pi(k-1)(n-1)}{N}\right)\right]$$

and for an image I with resolution $m \times n$,

$$F(p,q) = \sum_{m=1}^{M}\sum_{n=1}^{N} I(m,n) \tag{1}$$

$$\left(\mathrm{arccos}\left[\cos\left(\frac{2\pi(p-1)(m-1)}{M} - \frac{\pi}{2}\right)\right] - \frac{\pi}{2}\right)$$

$$\times \left(\mathrm{arccos}\left[\cos\left(\frac{2\pi(k-1)(n-1)}{N} - \frac{\pi}{2}\right)\right] - \frac{\pi}{2}\right)$$

$$-i\,\mathrm{arcsin}\left[\mathrm{arccos}\left(\frac{2\pi(k-1)(p-1)}{M}\right)\right]$$

$$\times \mathrm{arcsin}\left[\cos\left(\frac{2\pi(k-1)(n-1)}{N}\right)\right] \tag{2}$$

In this work, application of the power spectrum method used to compute the fractal dimensions of a skin surface is based on the above representations for $F(k)$ and $F(p,q)$ respectively. We then consider the power spectrum of an ideal fractal signal given by $P = c|k|^{-\beta}$, where c is a constant and β is the spectral exponent. In two dimensions, the power spectrum is given by $P(k_x, k_y) = c|k|^{-\beta}$, where $|k| = \sqrt{k_x^2 + k_y^2}$. In both cases, application of the least squares method or Orthogonal Linear Regression yields a solution for β and c, the relationship between β and the Fractal Dimension D_F being given by

$$D_F = \frac{3D_T + 2 - \beta}{2}$$

for Topological Dimension D_T. This approach allows us to drop the limits on the recognition of small objects since application of the FFT (for computing the

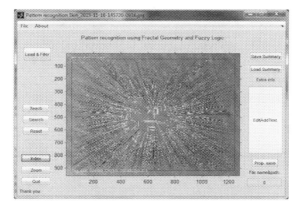

Fig. 6. GUI software.

power spectrum) works well (in terms of computational accuracy) only for large data sets, i.e. array sizes larger than 256 and 256×256. Tests on the accuracy associated with computing the fractal dimension using Eqs. (1) and (2) show an improvement of 5% over computations based on conventional Discrete Fourier Transform.

The setup calculates Fractal features dynamically from the centre of an image. The testing GUI software is presented on Fig. 6:

The original skin image from the camera is presented on Fig. 7.

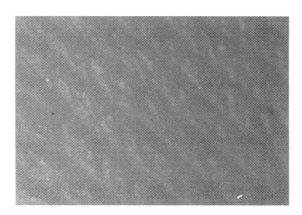

Fig. 7. The original skin image.

The current position of the net bandage and camera is given from optical calibration marks Fig. 8.

The corresponding points of the current Fractal marks and optical position gives us the offset number which guide the doctor to the original position of the sensor net bandage.

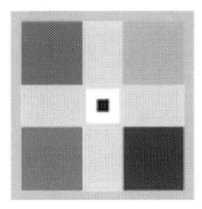

Fig. 8. The optical calibration mark.

In order to map the skin surface, the 'system' has to know its mathematical representation. Here, this representation is based on the features considered in the previous section which are used to create an image of the object in the 'electronic mind'. This includes the textural features for the skin object coupled with the Euclidean and morphological measures defined. In the case of a general application, all objects are represented by a list of parameters for implementation of supervised learning for the first net bandage application in which a fuzzy logic system automatically adjusts the weight coefficients for the input feature set.

The methods developed represent a contribution to pattern recognition based on fractal geometry, fuzzy logic and the implementation of a fully automatic recognition scheme as illustrated in Fig. 9 for the Fractal Dimension D (just one element of the feature vector used in practice). The recognition procedure

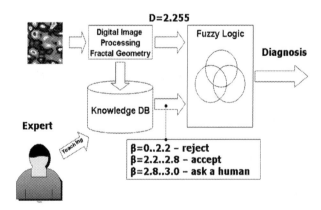

Fig. 9. Basic architecture of the diagnostic system based on the Fractal Dimension D (a single feature) and decision making criteria β.

uses the decision making rules from fuzzy logic theory [39–42] based on all, or a selection, of the features defined above which are combined to produce a feature vector **x**.

3.1 Decision Making

The class probability vector $\mathbf{p} = \{p_j\}$ is estimated from the object feature vector $\mathbf{x} = \{x_i\}$ and membership functions $m_j(\mathbf{x})$ defined in a knowledge database. If $m_j(\mathbf{x})$ is a membership function, then the probability for each jth class and i^{th} feature is given by

$$p_j(\mathbf{x}_i) = \max \left[\frac{\sigma_j}{|\mathbf{x}_i - \mathbf{x}_{j,i}|} \cdot m_j(\mathbf{x}_{j,i}) \right]$$

where σ_j is the distribution density of values $\mathbf{x}_j$ at the point $\mathbf{x}_i$ of the membership function. The next step is to compute the mean class probability given by

$$\langle p \rangle = \frac{1}{j} \sum_j \mathbf{w}_j p_j$$

where $\mathbf{w}_j$ is the weight coefficient matrix. This value is used to select the class associated with

$$p(j) = \min \left[(p_j \cdot \mathbf{w}_j - \langle p \rangle) \geq 0 \right]$$

providing a result for a decision associated with the jth class. The weight coefficient matrix is adjusted during the learning stage of the algorithm.

The decision criterion method considered here represents a weighing-density minimax expression. The estimation of the decision accuracy is achieved by using the density function

$$d_i = |\mathbf{x}_{\sigma_{\max}} - \mathbf{x}_i|^3 + \left[\sigma_{\max}(\mathbf{x}_{\sigma_{\max}}) - p_j(\mathbf{x}_i) \right]^3$$

with an accuracy determined by

$$P = \mathbf{w}_j p_j - \mathbf{w}_j p_j \frac{2}{\pi} \sum_{i=1}^{N} d_i.$$

3.2 Skin Pattern Learning

The Pattern learning procedure is the most important part of the system for operation in automatic recognition mode. The training set of sample objects should cover all ranges of class characteristics with a uniform distribution together with a universal membership function. This rule should be taken into account for all classes participating in the training of the system. An system defines the class and accuracy for each model object where the accuracy is the level of self confidence that the skin object belongs to a given class. During this procedure, the system computes and transfers to a knowledge database, a vector

$\mathbf{x} = \{x_i\}$, which forms the membership function $m_j(\mathbf{x})$. The matrix of weight factors $w_{j,i}$ is formed at this stage accordingly for the ith parameter and j^{th} class using the following expression:

$$w_{i,j} = \left| 1 - \sum_{k=1}^{N} \left(p_{i,j}(\mathbf{x}_{i,j}^k) - \langle p_{i,j}(\mathbf{x}_{i,j}) \rangle \right) p_{i,j}(\mathbf{x}_{i,j}^k) \right|.$$

The result of the weight matching procedure is that all parameters which have been computed but have not made any contribution to the characteristic set of an object are removed from the decision making algorithm by setting $w_{j,i}$ to null.

4 Conclusions

The focus of this paper is the development and validation of a simple, user-friendly system which allows control of the spatial distribution of the accumulated dose of radiation inside a body. The use of modern image recognition techniques allows precise positioning of the sensors net bandage. The calculation of exact accumulation dose and its confirmation by correct measurements is the key to the effective treatment. Simple and reliable monitoring of the 3D dose distribution will allow us to provide treatment in the safest way. The safe way means that the healthy cells will not be subject to unnecessary exposure, which helps to maintain the healthy cells surrounding the tumour. This work represents a new approach to accurate radiation exposure treatments. Implementation in hospitals requires more experiments, calibration and technological input. Feasibility studies, clinical validation and economical evaluation should be the next steps. We hope that this research will contribute to the safer radiation exposure treatment in cancer cure and prolonging the lives of many people.

Acknowledgement. The work reported in this paper is supported by the Oxford Recognition Ltd. The authors are grateful to Richard Spooner, Ann Wallace and Gladys O'Brien for help in the preparation of this paper.

References

1. Soubra, M., Cygler, J., Mackay, G.F.: Evaluation of a dual metal oxide-silicon semiconductor field effect transistor detector as a radiation dosimeter. Med. Phys. **21**(4), 567–572 (1984)
2. Thomson I., Reece M.H.: Semiconductor MOSFET dosimetry. In: Proceedings of Health Physics Society Annual Meeting (1988)
3. De Deene, Y., Jirasek, A.: Uncertainty in 3D gel dosimetry. J. Phys. Conf. Series **573**, 012008 (2015). 8th International Conference on 3D Radiation Dosimetry (IC3DDose)
4. Nithiyanantham, K., Mani, G.K., Subramani, V., Mueller, L., Palaniappan, K.K., Kataria, T.: Analysis of direct clinical consequences of MLC positional errors in volumetric-modulated arc therapy using 3D dosimetry system. J. Appl. Clin. Med. Phys. **16**(5), 296–305 (2015)

5. Ma, T.P., Dressendorfer, P.V.: Ionizing Radiation Effects in MOS Devices and Circuits. Wiley Interscience, New York (1989)
6. Kohler, R.A., Kushner, R.A.: Total dose radiation hardness of MOS devices in hermetic ceramic packages. IEEE Trans. Nucl. Sci. **35**(6), 1492–1496 (1988)
7. Kaschieva, S.: Improving the radiation hardness of MOS structures. Int. J. Electron. **76**(5), 883–886 (1994)
8. Claeys, C.: Simoen, E: Radiation Effects in Advanced Semiconductor Materials and Devices. Springer Science and Business Media, Berlin (2002). https://doi.org/10.1007/978-3-662-04974-7
9. Meurant, G.: New Insulators Devices and Radiation Effects, 1st edn. North Holland, New York (1999). Print book ISBN 9780444818010
10. Kumar, A.S., Sharma, S.D., Paul Ravindran, B.: Characteristics of mobile MOSFET dosimetry system for megavoltage photon beams. J. Med. Phys. **39**(3), 142–149 (2014)
11. Gopidaj, A., Billimagga, R.S., Ramasubramanian, V.: Performance characteristics and commissioning of MOSFET as an in-vivo dosimeter for high energy photon external beam radiation therapy. Rep. Pract. Oncol. Radiother. **13**(3), 114–125 (2008)
12. Choe, B.-Y.: Dosimetric characteristics of standard and micro MOSFET dosimeters as in-vivo dosimeter for clinical electron beam. J. Korean Phys. Soc. **55**, 2566–2570 (2013)
13. Briere, T.M., et al.: In vivo dosimetry using disposable MOSFET dosimeters for total body irradiation. Med. Phys. **32**, 1996 (2005)
14. Scalchi, P., Francescon, P., Rajaguru, P.: Characterisation of a new MOSFET detector configuration for in vivo skin dosimetry. Med. Phys. **32**(6), 1571–1578 (2005)
15. Sze, S.M.: Physics of Semiconductor Devices, 2nd edn. Willey, New York (1981)
16. Nicollian, E.H., Brews, J.R.: MOS (Metal Oxide Semiconductor) Physics and Technology. Wiley, New York (1982)
17. Zemel, J.N.: Nondestructive Evaluation of Semiconductor Materials and Devices. Nato Science Series B. Springer US, New York (1979). ISSN 0258-1221
18. Hughes, H.L., Benedetto, J.M.: Radiation effects and hardening of MOS technology devices and circuits. IEEE Trans. Nucl. Sci. **50**, 500–521 (2003)
19. Oldham, T.R., McLean, F.B.: Total ionizing dose effects in MOS oxides and devices. IEEE Trans. Nucl. Sci. **50**, 483–499 (2003)
20. Adams, J.R., Daves, W.R., Sanders, T.J.: A radiation hardened field oxide. IEEE Trans. Nucl. Sci. **NS–24**(6), 2099–2101 (1977)
21. Davies, E.R.: Machine Vision: Theory, Algorithms, Practicalities. Academic press, London (1997)
22. Dubovitskiy, D.A., Blackledge, J.M.: Surface inspection using a computer vision system that includes fractal analysis. ISAST Trans. Electron. Signal Process. **2**(3), 76–89 (2008)
23. Dubovitskiy, D.A., Blackledge, J.M.: Texture classification using fractal geometry for the diagnosis of skin cancers. In: EG UK Theory and Practice of Computer Graphics 2009, pp. 41–48 (2009)
24. Dubovitskiy, D., Devyatkov, V., Richer, G.: The application of mobile devices for the recognition of malignant melanoma. In: BIODEVICES 2014: Proceedings of the International Conference on Biomedical Electronics and Devices, Angers, France, p. 140, 03–06 March 2014. ISBN 978-989-758-013-0

25. Dubovitskiy, D.A., Blackledge, J.M.: Moletest: a web-based skin cancer screening system. In: The Third International Conference on Resource Intensive Applications and Services, Venice, Italy, vol. 978-1-61208-006-2, pp. 22–29, 22–27 May 2011

26. Dubovitskiy, D.A., Blackledge, J.M.: Object Detection and classification with applications to skin cancer screening. In: International Society for Advanced Science and Technology (ISAST) Intelligent Systems, vol. 1, no. 1, pp. 34–45 (2008). ISSN 1797–1802

27. Dubovitskiy, D.A., Blackledge, J.M.: Targeting cell nuclei for the automation of raman spectroscopy in cytology. In: Targeting Cell Nuclei for the Automation of Raman Spectroscopy in Cytology. British Patent No. GB1217633.5 (2012)

28. Dubovitskiy, D.A., McBride, J.: New 'spider' convex hull algorithm for an unknown polygon in object recognition. In: BIODEVICES 2013: Proceedings of the International Conference on Biomedical Electronics and Devices, p. 311 (2013)

29. Freeman, H.: Machine Vision: Algorithms, Architectures, and Systems. Academic press, London (1988)

30. Grimson, W.E.L.: Object Recognition by Computers: The Role of Geometric Constraints. MIT Press, Cambridge (1990)

31. Louis, J., Galbiati, J.: Machine Vision and Digital Image Processing Fundamentals. State University of New York, New-York (1990)

32. Nalwa, V.S., Binford, T.O.: On detecting edge. IEEE Trans. Pattern Anal. Mach. Intell. 1(PAMI–8), 699–714 (1986)

33. Ripley, B.D.: Pattern Recognition and Neural Networks. Academic Press, Oxford (1996)

34. Clarke, K., Schweizer, D.: Measuring the fractal dimension of natural surfaces using a robust fractal estimator. Cartograph. Geograph. Inf. Syst. **18**, 27–47 (1991)

35. Falconer, K.: Fractal Geometry. Wiley, Hoboken (1990)

36. DeCola, L.: Fractal analysis of a classified landsat scene. Photogram. Eng. Remote Sens. **55**(5), 601–610 (1989)

37. Snyder, W.E., Qi, H.: Machine Vision. Cambridge University Press, Cambridge (2004)

38. Yagi, Y., Gilberson, J.R.: Digital imaging in pathology: the case for standardisation. J. Telemed. Telecare **11**, 109–116 (2005)

39. Zadeh, L.A.: Fuzzy Sets and Their Applications to Cognitive and Decision Processes. Academic Press, New York (1975)

40. Mamdani, E.H.: Advances in linguistic synthesis of fuzzy controllers. J. Man. Mach. **8**, 669–678 (1976)

41. Sanchez, E.: Resolution of composite fuzzy relation equations. Inf. Control **30**, 38–48 (1976)

42. Vadiee, N.: Fuzzy Rule Based Expert System-I. Prentice Hall, Englewood (1993)

Bioimaging

Automatic Segmentation of Neurons from Fluorescent Microscopy Imaging

Silvia Baglietto[1,2(✉)], Ibolya E. Kepiro[3], Gerrit Hilgen[4], Evelyne Sernagor[4], Vittorio Murino[1,5], and Diego Sona[1,6]

[1] Pattern Analysis and Computer Vision, Istituto Italiano di Tecnologia, Genoa, Italy
silvia.baglietto@iit.it
[2] Department of Naval, Electric, Electronic and Telecommunication Engineering, University of Genova, Genoa, Italy
[3] Nanophysics, Istituto Italiano di Tecnologia, Genoa, Italy
[4] Institute of Neuroscience, Newcastle, Newcastle-upon-Tyne, UK
[5] Department of Computer Science, University of Verona, Verona, Italy
[6] NeuroInformatics Laboratory, Fondazione Bruno Kessler, Trento, Italy

Abstract. Automatic detection and segmentation of neurons from microscopy acquisition is essential for statistically characterizing neuron morphology that can be related to their functional role. In this paper, we propose a combined pipeline that starts from the automatic detection of the soma through a new multiscale blob enhancement filtering. Then, a precise segmentation of the detected cell body is obtained by an active contour approach. The resulted segmentation is used as initial seed for the second part of the approach that proposes a dendrite arborization tracing method.

1 Introduction

Thanks to the great advances in microscopy technologies and cellular imaging, we have many tools and techniques allowing to address fundamental questions in neuron studies. We can capture high-resolution images of single cells or neuron population that enable neurobiologists to investigate the neuronal structure and morphological development associated to neurological disorders.

Recent studies [1] claim that the morphology (i.e., size, shape and dendritic arborization) of a neuron is a key discriminant of its functional role. With different morphological features and different functional tasks, distinct neurons have diverse soma shapes and dendrite arborizations. Developmental abnormalities might lead to neuron malfunction and can be early signals for variety of neuropathies and neurological disorders.

To support neuroscientists in this study, fully automated tools for neuron detection and segmentation are required. Different approaches have been proposed [2,3], however still to date, the state of the art is not still satisfactory given the complexity of the problem. For example, the manual interaction that

N. Peixoto et al. (Eds.): BIOSTEC 2017, CCIS 881, pp. 121–133, 2018.
https://doi.org/10.1007/978-3-319-94806-5_7

some tools require [4] is time consuming, expensive and extremely subjective as it depends on the user expertise and diligence.

Moreover the task is quite complex for different reasons. First of all, neuronal samples are highly heterogeneous across different acquisitions. Images can be characterized by high cell density and shape variety and usually there is a low contrast at the neuron boundaries. Indeed, the fluorescence expressed is commonly non-uniform: it might present high intensity variability between soma, its border and the processes, leading to bad morphological segmentation of cell and significant fragmentation in dendrite appearance.

Traditional segmentation approaches that use basic method such as thresholding and morphological operators are not precise enough for the task at hand and lead to wrong segmentations. Learning approaches, nowadays broadly used in object segmentation also thanks to Deep Learning, are not suitable for these images because they require a huge amount of hand-labeled neuron samples for training [5].

Among deformable models, active contour models have demonstrated good performance in segmentation also in correspondence of challenging data [6,7]. Their main issue is the high sensitivity to the initialization, which often requires user setting. To this aim, recent active contour models trying an hybrid approach to automate the initial mask have been introduced [8,9].

Skeletonization is a global technique that extract the binary skeleton from a given neuronal structure [10,11]. The key idea of these methods is an iterative erasure of voxels from the volume of the segmented object preserving the topology of the contained structure. Minimal path based tracing are other global approaches which aim at linking seed points through an optimization problem [12] or through Fast Marching algorithm [13]. Minimum Spanning Tree (MST) tracing deals with the link between detected points into a tree representation [14].

In our work, we present a combined and fully automatic approach in order to detect and segment the whole neuron. The first part [15] starts with soma detection using a multiscale blob enhancement filtering. Then, neuron bodies are segmented by an high performance active contour model. The resulting segmentation is used to initialize the second part of the method, concerning dendrite tree segmentation by hessian-phase based level set model.

The remainder of the paper is organized as follows. In Sect. 2 details on the adopted dataset are provided. We present the combined method in Sect. 3: for the detection and segmentation of cell bodies see Sect. 3.1 and for the dendritic tracing see Sect. 3.2. In Sect. 4 results are presented and conclusions are provided in Sect. 5.

2   Materials

In this work, we use two different datasets: *Mouse Retina* [15] and *Larva Drosophila* [16]. *Mouse Retina* dataset shows populations of Retinal Ganglion Cells (RGCs) which play a central role into the complex and stratified structure of the retina. Retina samples were imaged using Leica SP5 upright confocal

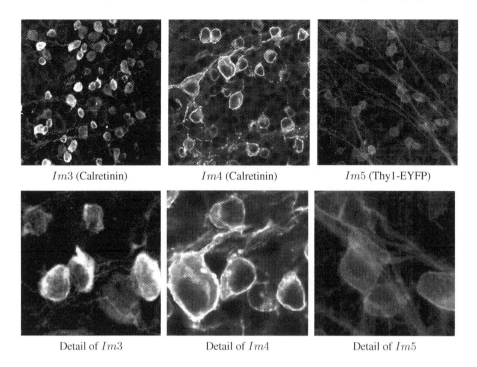

$Im3$ (Calretinin) $Im4$ (Calretinin) $Im5$ (Thy1-EYFP)

Detail of $Im3$ Detail of $Im4$ Detail of $Im5$

Fig. 1. Some images containing Retinal Ganglion Cells (RGCs) used for testing the proposed method [15]. The images show high variability across samples. In the bottom line, there is some magnified crops of the upper images, showing the complexity of images, where the analyzed structures are mixed with background and other structures.

microscope. Images were acquired at (sub)cellular resolution and at high averaging number to reduce the noise level due to the limitation of light penetration in deep layers of the tissue where RGCs are located. A total of 5 images (2048 × 2048 and 1024 × 1024 pixels), showing some hundreds of cells each, were selected from 3 distinct retina samples including: (i) three images obtained from samples with genetic fluorescence expression, (i.e., $Im1$ from PV-EYFP and $Im2$ and $Im5$ images from Thy1-EYFP staining), and (ii) two images from samples with immunofluorescence staining using the Calretinin calcium-binding protein ($Im3$ and $Im4$) (Figs. 1, 2 and 3). The samples were selected to best capture the variability in terms of fluorescence expression, cell and axonal bundle density and background.

Larva Drosophila dataset is acquired on some sensory neurons in wild-type larva *Drosophila* [16] studied over different development phases. This dataset shows single neurons including both cell body and dendritic tree. In our case, we study the $2D$ maximum projection value on xy plane across slices. Figure 2 shows some $2D$ maximum projection of the considered volumes.

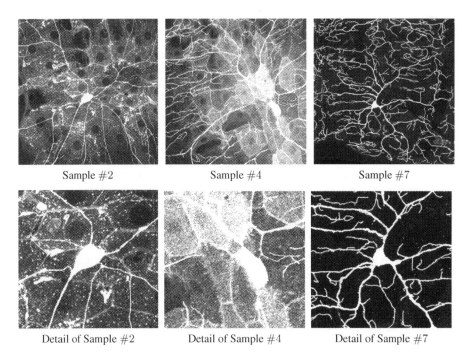

Fig. 2. Some samples from the second dataset imaged single neurons. Images shows, also for this dataset, the heterogeneity across samples and across microscopic acquisitions. In the bottom line there are some details of the correspondent top line images.

3   Method

To automatically study neuron morphology, we need to detect and segment the cell body(i.e. the soma) and trace its dendritic arborization. In this work, we describe the sequence of methods we used to solve the soma detection and segmentation task and the dendrite tracing.

3.1   Soma Detection and Segmentation

The pipeline for cells detection and segmentation is composed of three main steps. As shown in Fig. 3 a Blob-based Filtering (second column) is followed by an Active Contour (third column) and a Watershed Transform (last column).

The Multiscale Blob Enhancement Filtering is used to identify regions where neuronal cells are likely located. After the blob filtering approach, blob-shapes objects are binarized and used as initial ROIs for a Localizing Region-Based Active Contour [17] that traces cell borders. Due to the fuzzy cell boundaries and occlusions, multiple cells can be segmented all together as a unique entity. To cope this issue, we apply a watershed transform.

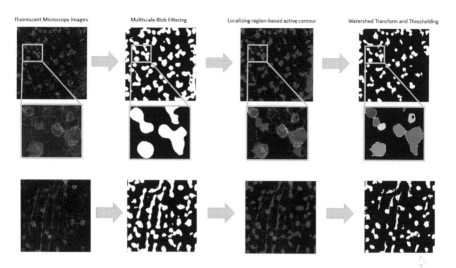

Fig. 3. Pipeline applied to two examples (from the top, $Im1$ (PV-EYFP) and $Im2$ (Thy1-EYFP)) with a crop in the central row, showing the difficulties caused by contiguous cells [15]. In column, starting from the left side: Original Fluorescent Microscopy Images; Results of the multiscale blob filter binarization; Results of the active contour segmentation in blue transparency over the original image for getting the suitable qualitative performance; Results of the watershed transform and of the final threshold. (Color figure online)

Blob-Based Filtering. The Multiscale Blob Enhancement Filtering improves the intensity profile of cell bodies and reduces the contribution of dendritic and axonal structures. The eigenspace of the Hessian matrix $\mathcal{H}$ is analyzed at multiscale to determine the local likelihood that a pixel belongs to a cell, i.e. to a blob profile. The proposed approach is inspired by the work of Frangi et al. [18] that defines a multiscale vessel enhancement filtering. The Frangi filter basically depends on the orientational difference or anisotropic distribution of the second-order derivatives to delineate tubular and filament-like structures.

For $2D$ images, the formulation of Frangi is defined as follows:

$$
\mathcal{V}_s(x_o) = \begin{cases} 0, & \text{if } \lambda_1^{x_o,s} < 0 \\ e^{-\frac{1}{2\beta^2} \cdot \left(\frac{\lambda_2^{x_o,s}}{\lambda_1^{x_o,s}}\right)^2} \cdot \left(1 - e^{-\frac{\Lambda^2}{2\gamma^2}}\right), & \text{otherwise} \end{cases} \tag{1}
$$

where $\lambda_1^{x_o,s}$ and $\lambda_2^{x_o,s}$ are the eigenvalues of the Hessian matrix at point x_o and at scale s, β and γ are two thresholds which controls the sensitivity of the line filter and S is defined as $\Lambda = \|\mathcal{H}\|_F = \sqrt{\sum_{j \leq D} \lambda_j^2}$, where D is the dimension of the image. This measure is used for differing the structures from the background.

Starting from Frangi's idea, we modify the filtering to filter-out line-like patterns in favor of blob-like structures (as [19]).

Instead of a vesselness measure, we define a blobness measure as follows [15]:

$$\mathcal{B}_s(x_o) = \begin{cases} 0, & \text{if } \lambda_1^{x_o,s} < 0 \\ e^{\frac{1}{2\beta^2} \cdot \left(\frac{\lambda_2^{x_o,s}}{\lambda_1^{x_o,s}}\right)^2}, & \text{otherwise} \end{cases} \tag{2}$$

where $\lambda_1^{x_o,s}$ and $\lambda_2^{x_o,s}$ are the eigenvalues of the Hessian matrix at point x_o and at scale s. β is a threshold which controls the sensitivity of the blob filter. In our experiments, both β and the Hessian scale have been selected as the average neuron radius. Equation (2) computes the blobness in the case of bright objects over dark background. In case of dark structures, system conditions should be reversed.

The filter is computed at a multiscale level. The response of the blob filter would be maximum at scale s that is more suited to the diameter of the blob to detect. Our *blob enhancement filtering* is said *multiscale* because we combine the blob measure at different scales to obtain a final blobness estimation defined as:

$$\mathcal{B}(x_o) = \max_{s_{min} \leq s \leq s_{max}} \mathcal{B}_s(x_o) \tag{3}$$

where s_{min} and s_{max} are the minimum and maximum scales where we expect to find structures.

Active Contour. Within active contour models, we exploited Localizing region-based active contour [17], an improved version of traditional ones [6,7]. The advantage of the proposed model is that objects characterized by heterogeneous statistics can be successfully segmented thanks to localized energies, where, instead, the corresponding global AC would fail. This approach allows to remove the assumption that foreground and background regions are distinguishable based on their global statistics. Indeed the improving hypothesis is that interior and exterior areas of objects are locally different. Within this framework, the energies are constructed locally at each point along the curve in order to analyze local regions. The localization radius is chosen following the size range of the objects to be segmented. In our case, for each image, we defined a radius equal to the average soma radius, depending on the image size and on the microscope lens used for the acquisition.

Thanks to this efficient technique, we obtain a segmentation mask which tightly fits real cell bodies.

Watershed Transform and Size Filter. Active contour can fail to separate groups of overlapping or contiguous cells. So, we exploit the simplicity and computational speed of the watershed transform, introduced by Beucher and Lantuéjoul [20], to split cells englomerates into groups of cells.

As a final step, we delete components which are too small or too large for being cell bodies (a given example is in Fig. 3, first line) applying a size filter to remove structures with size outside an acceptable range of soma dimensions. It is possible to fix this range by a statistical analysis of the dimensions removing the tails of the distribution.

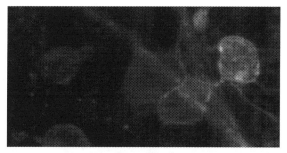

Crop of $Im5$

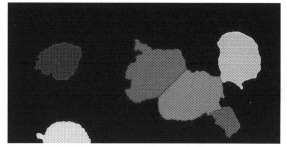

Resulted Crop Segmentation

Fig. 4. Some cells are not easily visible to the human eye just visualizing the retina images, but they are discovered and segmented by our algorithm (for example, in this cropped figure, pink and blue cells were hardly detectable). Adding contrast to the image makes these somata clearer but it increases noise and cell heterogeneity [15]. (Color figure online)

3.2 Dendrite Segmentation

To reconstruct the dendrites, we exploit the soma segmentation as initialization seed to start a level set propagation with local phase and with hessian eigenspace information. The main idea is that local phase is extracted using quadrature filters and this allows to distinguish lines and edges in a image [21,22]. In our case study, a dendrite can appear locally as a line or as an edge pair; then a multiple scale integration is used for capturing information about dendrites of varying width and contrast. Our novel idea is weighting this filter by the Hessian eigenspace that guarantees that only pixel belonging to filamentous structures contributes [18]. In particular we modify Eq. (4) in [21] weighting the evolution term with the first eigenvalue. The new evolving equation becomes:

$$\frac{\partial \Phi}{\partial t} = -|\lambda_1| \; Re(\hat{q}(\sigma)) \; |\nabla \Phi| + \alpha k |\nabla \Phi| \qquad (4)$$

where λ_1 is the first eigenvalue computed in each pixel by the Hessian Matrix, $\hat{q}$ is the normalized phase function, α is a regularizer and k is the mean curvature. With this contribution, the background signal is omitted and λ_1 drives the level set only where the pixels belong to a structure. The result is a "local" filter which can drive a contour towards the dendrite arborization (see Fig. 7).

| 2D projection | Soma detection and segmentation | Neuron final segmentation |

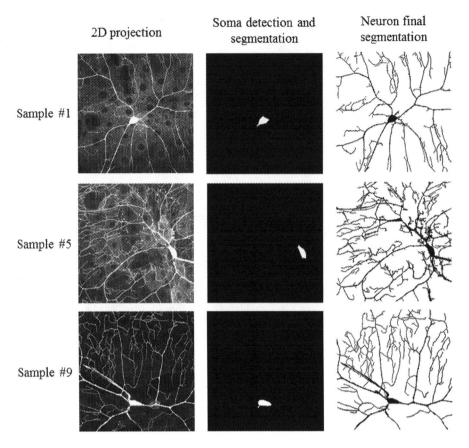

Fig. 5. Some example images from *Larva Drosophila* dataset. In column, from the left side: 2D projection of the original volume; soma detection and segmentation applying the first part of the proposed approach; whole neuron segmentation including dendrites.

4   Results and Discussion

For the evaluation of soma detection and segmentation, we applied our pipeline to two different datasets, *Mouse Retina* [15] and *Larva Drosophila* [16]. For the evaluation of dendrite segmentation, we use *Larva Drosophila* dataset because only this one contains images with the complete dendritic tree labeled for each neuron. As previously described in Sect. 2, the first dataset, *Mouse Retina*, is composed of 5 different retinal images representative of possible variations on the retinal samples, such as brightness, intensity, size and number of cells, presence of axonal structures and processes, strong background signals, etc. These samples show images at the network scale of many dozens of RGCs with higher fluorescence expression into the soma. We generated the ground truth manually segmenting all cells in each image (around 280 cells in total). The second dataset, *Larva Drosophila* contains images made of 11 single neurons representative of spatially inhomogeneous signal-to-noise ratios. Also in this case, we manually segmented all the neurons (both soma and dendrites). For the gold dendritic tracing, we adopted Simple Neurite Tracer [4].

4.1 Soma Detection and Segmentation Results

To give a qualitative evaluation, we report different examples of *Mouse Retina* in Figs. 3 and 4 and of *Larva Drosophila* in Fig. 5 (central column) where it is possible to see that our approach works in different sample conditions.

To quantify the performance of our method, we adopt the Dice Coefficient (DC), a widely used overlapped metric for comparing two segmentation. DC is defined as follows:

$$DC = \frac{2(A \cap B)}{(A + B)},$$

where A is the binary ground truth mask and B is the binary segmentation result. The DC value ranges between 0 (absence of agreement) and 1 (perfect agreement). A DC higher than 0.70 usually corresponds to a satisfactory segmentation [23].

Table 1 shows the quantitative results on our *Mouse Retina* samples. We compute the DC for each of the three steps in the pipeline (Blob-based Filtering, Active Contour and Watershed Transform). Each stage clearly improves the segmentation, reaching satisfactory results for all images. In $Im3$ (Fig. 1), the fluorescence is mainly expressed by the body cells; for this reason, we reach good scores right after the first two steps. The weaker DC values on images $Im2$ and $Im5$ are due to a strong presence of axonal structures which can be hardly removed. As an additional index of performance at the network scale, we also present the percentage of detected cells for each *Mouse Retina* image. Figure 6

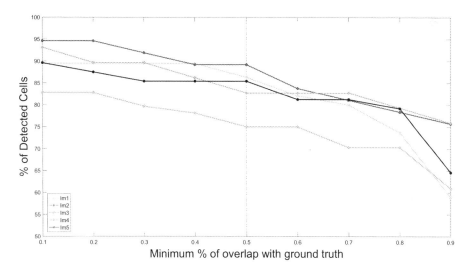

Fig. 6. Variation of the % of detected cells in *Mouse Retina* dataset as a function of the % threshold of overlap between detected cell and the corresponding annotated ground truth [15].

Table 1. Results for soma segmentation on *Mouse Retina* samples [15]. Dice Coefficient is computed for all steps in the pipeline (Blob Filter, Active Contour and Watershed Transform) and it shows improvements after each step. For the final stage of the pipeline, there is also the percentage of detected cells computed assuming as detected a cell with minimum overlap 50% with ground truth fixed at 50%.

Image	# of cells	Blob filter DC	Active contour DC	Final DC	Detected cells
Im1 (PV-EYFP)	95	0.60	0.69	0.81	86.32%
Im2 (Thy1-EYFP)	37	0.43	0.58	0.64	89.19%
Im3 (Calretinin)	64	0.62	0.82	0.83	75.00%
Im4 (Calretinin)	29	0.57	0.71	0.79	82.76%
Im5 (Thy1-EYFP)	48	0.51	0.62	0.70	85.42%

shows the variation of the percentage of detected cells at different thresholds of overlapping between computer-aided segmentation with the ground truth to count a cell as detected. It can be observed that 50% threshold is a good trade off between the certainty of a cell detection and a satisfactory retrieval. So, in Table 1, we consider a cell as detected if it is correctly segmented for more than 50% of its total area, comparing the segmentation mask to the ground truth for each annotated RGC.

Table 2 reports the quantitative evaluation on the *Larva Drosophila* dataset. Worst values are obtained for Sample #4 (see Fig. 2, middle column) and #6, where background noise is strong and leads to confusing borders. In general, however, the values are significantly high with an average reaching 0.88.

Table 2. Soma segmentation results on *Larva Drosophila* dataset. Dice Coefficient has been computed for each segmented soma.

Image	#1	#2	#3	#4	#5	#6	#7	#8	#9	#10	#11	Average
DC	0.89	0.95	0.97	0.74	0.94	0.69	0.93	0.91	0.83	0.89	0.92	0.88

4.2   Dendrite Segmentation Results

A qualitative evaluation of the dendrite segmentation starting from seed soma is shown in Fig. 7 (bottom right) and in Fig. 5. In particular Fig. 7 shows an example of level set initialization, evolution and result; Fig. 5 proposes some

Table 3. Dice Coefficient has been computed comparing our segmentation and Tuff segmentation with manual segmentation done by Simple Neurite Tracer [4].

DC	Volume											
	#1	#2	#3	#4	#5	#6	#7	#8	#9	#10	#11	Average
Our method	0.82	0.71	0.78	0.71	0.80	0.91	0.86	0.86	0.88	0.83	0.85	0.82
Tuff	0.51	0.39	0.40	0.33	0.32	0.77	0.79	0.80	0.71	0.76	0.76	0.56

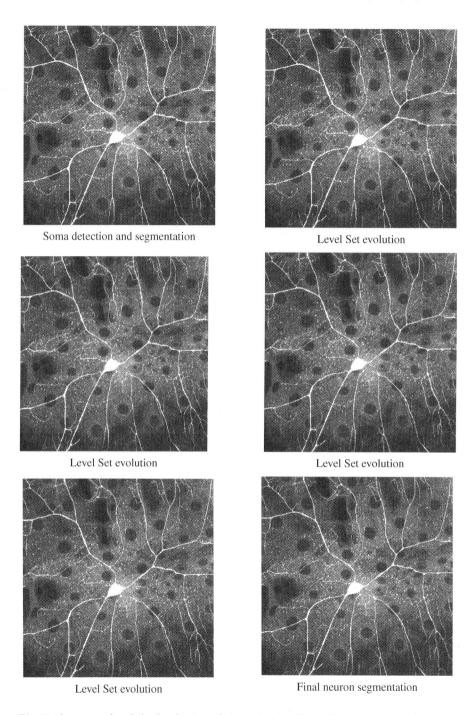

Soma detection and segmentation   Level Set evolution

Level Set evolution   Level Set evolution

Level Set evolution   Final neuron segmentation

Fig. 7. An example of the level set evolution starting from the soma segmentation as seed point in the Sample #1. The level set is shown at different evolution steps.

Larva Drosophila image results after the first part of the segmentation process (middle column) and at the final segmentation (column on the right side).

To quantitatively evaluate our neuron segmentation, we compare our method with a recent state-of-the-art automated approach proposed in [24], Tubularity Flow Field (*Tuff*). *Tuff* is a technique for automatic neuron segmentation that performs directional regional growing guided by the tubularity direction of neurites. We compute the DC on *Larva Drosophila* results for both methods and it can be observed that our method significantly outperform *Tuff* (Table 3).

5   Conclusion

We have presented a new approach for whole neuron segmentation in challenging fluorescent microscopy images. Our method is comprehensive of two main steps: soma detection and dendrite segmentation. In the first stage cell bodies are detected by a new blob filtering approach and segmented by an active contour model and a watershed transform. Then, a novel hessian-phase based level set has been developed allowing to segment the whole neuron morphology. Tests have been performed on large scale and single scale images. We obtained high results for both detection and segmentation of the soma and for the whole neuron reconstruction. Thanks to its generality and automation, this framework could be applied to similar images and it is easily reproducible for the full network reconstruction at the population level. Moreover, we could easily extend the method to $3D$ dimensions since our theoretical model adopted a general dimension formulation. Finally, it also opens new perspectives for the analysis and the characterization of neuronal cells.

Acknowledgements. The research received financial support from the 7th Framework Programme for Research of the European Commision, Grant agreement no. 600847: RENVISION project of the Future and Emerging Technologies (FET) programme.

References

1. Baden, T., Berens, P., Franke, K., Rosón, M.R., Bethge, M., Euler, T.: The functional diversity of retinal ganglion cells in the mouse. Nature **529**(7586), 345–350 (2016)
2. Meijering, E.: Neuron tracing in perspective. Cytom. Part A **77**(7), 693–704 (2010)
3. Basu, S., Aksel, A., Condron, B., Acton, S.T.: Tree2Tree: neuron segmentation for generation of neuronal morphology. In: 2010 IEEE International Symposium on Biomedical Imaging: From Nano to Macro, pp. 548–551. IEEE (2010)
4. Longair, M.H., Baker, D.A., Armstrong, J.D.: Simple neurite tracer: open source software for reconstruction, visualization and analysis of neuronal processes. Bioinformatics **27**(17), 2453–2454 (2011)
5. Zheng, Z., Hong, P.: Incorporate deep-transfer-learning into automatic 3D neuron tracing. In: The First International Conference on Neuroscience and Cognitive Brain Information, BRAININFO 2016 (2016)
6. Chan, T.F., Vese, L., et al.: Active contours without edges. IEEE Trans. Image Process. **10**, 266–277 (2001)

7. Yezzi, A., Tsai, A., Willsky, A.: A fully global approach to image segmentation via coupled curve evolution equations. J. Vis. Commun. Image Represent. **13**(1), 195–216 (2002)
8. Ge, Q., Li, C., Shao, W., Li, H.: A hybrid active contour model with structured feature for image segmentation. Signal Process. **108**, 147–158 (2015)
9. Wu, P., Yi, J., Zhao, G., Huang, Z., Qiu, B., Gao, D.: Active contour-based cell segmentation during freezing and its application in cryopreservation. IEEE Trans. Biomed. Eng. **62**(1), 284–295 (2015)
10. Lee, T.C., Kashyap, R.L., Chu, C.N.: Building skeleton models via 3-D medial surface axis thinning algorithms. CVGIP: Graph. Models Image Process. **56**(6), 462–478 (1994)
11. Palágyi, K., Kuba, A.: A 3D 6-subiteration thinning algorithm for extracting medial lines. Pattern Recognit. Lett. **19**(7), 613–627 (1998)
12. Meijering, E.H., Jacob, M., Sarria, J.C.F., Unser, M.: A novel approach to neurite tracing in fluorescence microscopy images. In: SIP, pp. 491–495 (2003)
13. Benmansour, F., Cohen, L.D.: Tubular structure segmentation based on minimal path method and anisotropic enhancement. Int. J. Comput. Vis. **92**(2), 192–210 (2011)
14. Türetken, E., González, G., Blum, C., Fua, P.: Automated reconstruction of dendritic and axonal trees by global optimization with geometric priors. Neuroinformatics **9**(2–3), 279–302 (2011)
15. Baglietto, S., Kepiro, I.E., Hilgen, G., Sernagor, E., Murino, V., Sona, D.: Segmentation of retinal ganglion cells from fluorescence microscopy imaging. In: BIOSTEC, pp. 17–23 (2017)
16. Gulyanon, S., Sharifai, N., Kim, M.D., Chiba, A., Tsechpenakis, G.: CRF formulation of active contour population for efficient three-dimensional neurite tracing. In: 2016 IEEE 13th International Symposium on Biomedical Imaging, ISBI, pp. 593–597. IEEE (2016)
17. Lankton, S., Tannenbaum, A.: Localizing region-based active contours. IEEE Trans. Image Process. **17**(11), 2029–2039 (2008)
18. Frangi, A.F., Niessen, W.J., Vincken, K.L., Viergever, M.A.: Multiscale vessel enhancement filtering. In: Wells, W.M., Colchester, A., Delp, S. (eds.) MICCAI 1998. LNCS, vol. 1496, pp. 130–137. Springer, Heidelberg (1998). https://doi.org/10.1007/BFb0056195
19. Liu, J., White, J.M., Summers, R.M.: Automated detection of blob structures by Hessian analysis and object scale. In: 2010 17th IEEE International Conference on Image Processing, ICIP, pp. 841–844. IEEE (2010)
20. Beucher, S., Lantuéjoul, C.: Use of watersheds in contour detection. In: International Workshop on Image Processing, Real-Time Edge and Motion Detection (1979)
21. Lathen, G., Jonasson, J., Borga, M.: Phase based level set segmentation of blood vessels. In: 19th International Conference on Pattern Recognition, ICPR 2008, pp. 1–4. IEEE (2008)
22. Läthén, G., Jonasson, J., Borga, M.: Blood vessel segmentation using multi-scale quadrature filtering. Pattern Recognit. Lett. **31**(8), 762–767 (2010)
23. Zijdenbos, A.P., Dawant, B.M., Margolin, R., Palmer, A.C., et al.: Morphometric analysis of white matter lesions in MR images: method and validation. IEEE Trans. Med. Imag. **13**(4), 716–724 (1994)
24. Mukherjee, S., Condron, B., Acton, S.T.: Tubularity flow field—A technique for automatic neuron segmentation. IEEE Trans. Image Process. **24**(1), 374–389 (2015)

Evaluation of Dense Vessel Detection in NCCT Scans

Aneta Lisowska[1,2], Erin Beveridge[1], Alison O'Neil[1(✉)], Vismantas Dilys[1],
Keith Muir[3], and Ian Poole[1]

[1] Toshiba Medical Visualization Systems Europe Ltd.,
2 Anderson Place, Edinburgh, UK
aoneil@tmvse.com
[2] School of Engineering and Physical Sciences, Heriot-Watt University,
Edinburgh, UK
[3] Queen Elizabeth University Hospital, University of Glasgow, Glasgow, UK

Abstract. Automatic detection and measurement of dense vessels may
enhance the clinical workflow for treatment triage in acute ischemic
stroke. In this paper we use a 3D Convolutional Neural Network, which
incorporates anatomical atlas information and bilateral comparison, to
detect dense vessels. We use 112 non-contrast computed tomography
(NCCT) scans for training of the detector and 58 scans for evaluation of
its performance. We compare automatic dense vessel detection to identification of the dense vessels by clinical researchers in NCCT and computed
tomography angiography (CTA). The automatic system is able to detect
dense vessel in NCCT scans, however it shows lower specificity in relation
to CTA than clinical experts.

1 Introduction

Automatic detection of dense vessels in Non-Contrast Computed Tomography
(NCCT) scans of patient with suspected stroke may accelerate treatment triage.
In a thrombolysis-only service, detection of a dense vessel helps to inform the
decision to treat, since the length of the clot observed in thin slice NCCT is
related to the success rate of thrombolysis [1], a treatment aimed to recanalise
occluded arteries. If a thrombectomy service is available, then detection of proximal, large vessel occlusions helps identify a cohort of patients potentially eligible
for this treatment. Subsequent mandatory review of CTA would also benefit from
identification of which vasculature to review rst in the search for a denitive clot.

Detection of clots is complicated by the fact that increased intravascular
density might reect either stasis of blood ow at the clot blood interface, or a
high haematocrit (in which case it is usually symmetrical). In this paper we
aim to evaluate the performance of an automatic dense vessel detector versus
manual identfiication of dense vessel signs in NCCT. Nevertheless, whether a
dense vessel sign represents a true clot can only be determined by looking at the
CT angiography (CTA) scans, therefore we also compare automatic detection
and clinical identification in NCCT with CTA.

© Springer International Publishing AG, part of Springer Nature 2018
N. Peixoto et al. (Eds.): BIOSTEC 2017, CCIS 881, pp. 134–145, 2018.
https://doi.org/10.1007/978-3-319-94806-5_8

2   Dataset

We use data from the South Glasgow Stroke Imaging Database provided by the Institute of Neuroscience and Psychology, University of Glasgow, Southern General Hospital. It includes data from the following studies: ATTEST [2], POSH [3] and WYETH [4]. The database provides information about presence or absence of dense vessel signs in NCCT, and presence or absence of arterial occlusions in the corresponding CTA scans.

For the purposes of this evaluation, we consider only the anterior circulation to the brain which comprises proximal occlusions and more distal dot signs. In order to train the detector, manual segmentations were required. These were generated in 3D Slicer 4.5.0 by a clinical researcher under the supervision of an experienced neuroradiologist. Annotations were collected on the acute NCCT scan with sight of the radiology report which included laterality of symptoms, but blind to additional information such as the CTA, CT perfusion and follow-up scans.

3   Methods

3.1   Data Preprocessing Pipeline

The first steps consist of isotropic resampling to 1 mm voxels and alignment of the NCCT volumes to a reference dataset designated as an atlas. The registration between a given dataset and a reference dataset is performed using landmarks detected by random forest method [5]. A block of interest extending into the sagittal plane is then extracted and folded along the brain midline, similarly to the folding of a butterfly's wings (see Fig. 1). The midline is determined from the aligned atlas. Block intensities are clamped in the range $\{-125, 225\}$ HU.

3.2   Detector

We use a Convolutional Neural Network architecture designed to exploit contralateral features and anatomical atlas information to detect dense vessels [6,7]. The folding of the block results in two 3D CNN intensity channels relating to the target and contralateral sides of the brain. The model weights for these channels are shared, enabling bilateral comparison. Alongside the two intensity input channels, we insert three channels encoding the x, y and z atlas coordinates to the architecture. These are provided at the same input level as the intensity data, rather than later layers in the architecture e.g. pre-classification layer as in [8]. The early incorporation of atlas information results in better detections [7]. For the convolution operations, we use a spatial decomposition of a $5 \times 5 \times 5$ filter resulting in the three layers of orthogonal one-dimensional convolutions: $5 \times 1 \times 1, 1 \times 5 \times 1, 1 \times 1 \times 5$. $N_I = 32$ kernels are used for the data channels and $N_A = 4$ kernels are used for the atlas channels. Channels are then merged and another convolution operation is applied, with $N_M = 32$ kernels. ReLU activation functions are used. The output of the network is fully convolutional.

The model is implemented in Python using the Keras [9] library built on top of Theano [10].

3.3 Detector Training

We used 112 scans from the ATTEST and WYETH studies for training of the detector, 60 of which show dense vessel signs in NCCT. There were 7,319 dense vessel voxels and 26,589,625 normal voxels in the blocks of interest after data augmentation which included only flipping of the datasets.

Training was performed using the Adam optimizer [11] on normalised data samples, with the default parameters of learning rate of 0.001, beta$_1$ = 0.9, beta$_2$ = 0.999 and epsilon = 1e−08. To compensate for the strong class imbalance we experimented with optimising the focal loss function [12].

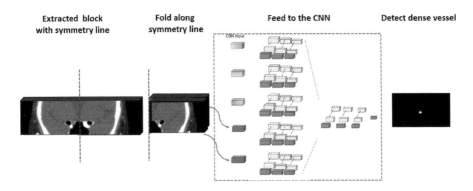

Fig. 1. Steps in the dense vessel detection pipeline. From left to right: (1) Extraction of the block of interest (anterior circulation region) from the novel volume which has been aligned to the atlas. (2) Folding of the block along the anatomical midline. (3) Corresponding bilateral intensity data is input to parallel CNN channels to allow direct comparison of the left and right sides of the brain. The remaining three input channels encode the x, y and z atlas coordinates. (4) CNN outputs probability volumes for the target hemisphere, indicating the voxelwise probability of a dense vessel being present.

Table 1. Description of the connected components detected in the scan shown in Fig. 2. The four detections are ranked from the most to the least confident.

Overlaps with manual segmentation	Size (voxels)	Confidence level
True	164	0.78
True	9	0.33
False	5	0.19
False	1	0.12

3.4   Evaluation Procedure

For the evaluation, we used 58 scans from the POSH study (all patients for which information was available about the presence or absence of dense vessels in NCCT and arterial occlusion in CTA), 25 of which show dense vessel signs in NCCT.

The output probability volumes are thresholded with $t = 0.1$. This threshold is selected such that the geometric mean of precision and recall is maximised on the voxel level predictions for the training data. After thresholding, connected components are identified. If any of the connected components overlap with the manual segmentation, then the the dense vessel sign is considered to be detected i.e. a true positive. If the dense vessel sign is present and a detection is output by the CNN, but the two do not overlap, then this is considered to be a *mislocated* true positive. See Figs. 2 and 3 for examples of a true positive and a mislocated true positive respectively. Table 1 gives details of the connected components detected in one example of a true positive scan. To aid in assessing clinical value, we further report the mean, minimum and maximum number of connected components which require reviewing in a positive scan (either true positive or false positive).

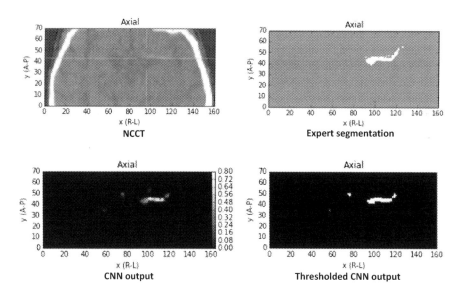

Fig. 2. True positive detection. NCCT is presented at the slice where the largest area of dense vessel is visible. Expert segmentation and CNN outputs are presented as a Maximum Intensity Projection (MIP). The brighter colours of the CNN output suggest stronger confidence and darker weaker confidence. The thresholded output results in 4 connected components with peak confidences of 0.12, 0.19, 0.33 and 0.78 (see Table 1). There is an overlap between at least one of the detected components and the expert segmentation, therefore the detection is treated as a true positive. In this case the number of detections that need reviewing is four; two detected components overlap with manual segmentation and two are false positive detections. (Color figure online)

Since not all arterial occlusions are visible in the NCCT scan (see Fig. 5), we compare the CNN detections and manual segmentations with the thrombus diagnoses according to the database in the CTA scans.

4 Results

Table 2 shows the agreement between the dense vessel identification by the clinical researchers and by the automatic detection system. A good automatic detection system would achieve a level of agreement with a human expert equivalent to the agreement between two human expert annotators. To obtain the inter-rater agreement score we compare the clinical researcher's manual segmentation with the database dense vessel sign annotations. The CNN detection does not reach the level of inter-rater agreement. Table 3 presents more detailed analysis of the automatic detection in comparison to the manual segmentation in NCCT.

Table 3 shows that the CNN detector yielded 17 false positives. Comparing the detection confidence range between the true positives and the false positives suggests that the threshold selected based on the training data is not optimal for the validation datasets (See Fig. 6B). The training data distribution has a

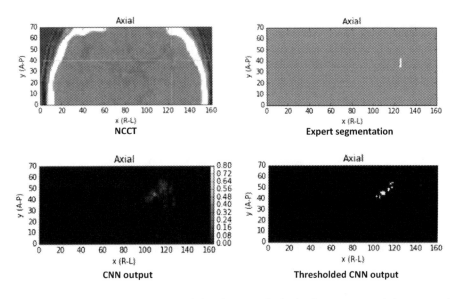

Fig. 3. Mislocated true positive. NCCT slice in which the largest area of dense vessel is visible. The manual segmentation and CNN outputs are presented as a MIP. There are only weakly confident detections. The thresholded output results in 8 connected components with a maximum confidence level between 0.1 for the least confident segment and 0.3 for the most confident segment. There is no overlap between any of the detected components and the manual segmentation, therefore the detection is treated as a false negative detection of dense vessel. We also report that there were 8 detections which needed reviewing.

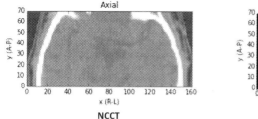

NCCT

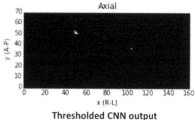

Thresholded CNN output

Fig. 4. False positive. NCCT slice in which the largest area of CNN detected dense vessel is visible. The clinical researcher has not segmented any areas in this scan, therefore this is a false positive detection. The number of components which require review in this scan is 2.

Table 2. Agreement between observers for detection of dense vessel sign in NCCT. The mislocated true positive are counted as missed detections.

	Segmentations	CNN detections
Database annotation	0.84	0.66
Segmentations	X	0.64

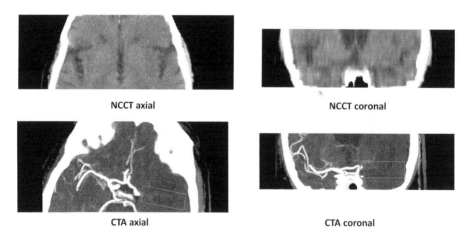

Fig. 5. Large CTA occlusion but dense vessel is not visible in NCCT. Not all occlusions present as dense vessels.

higher percentage of dense vessels (53%) than the validation data (43%), which might affect the choice of threshold. Setting the detection threshold to 0.2 would reduce the number of false positives without affecting the true positives and it would increase the overall agreement with the expert segmentation to 0.7 and with the database score to 0.72. It is worth noting that this would still be lower than the intra-rater agreement.

Table 3. CNN detection vs manual segmentations. See Fig. 6 for complementary boxplots.

	True −ve	True +ve	False +ve	False −ve	Mislocated true +ve
No. cans	16	21	17	1	3
Mean no. detections/scan	0	3.09	3.76	0	3.60
Max no. detections/scan	0	16	12	0	8
Min no. detections/scan	0	1	1	0	1
Top detection confidence	<0.1	0.21–0.82	0.11–0.51	<0.1	0.16–0.30

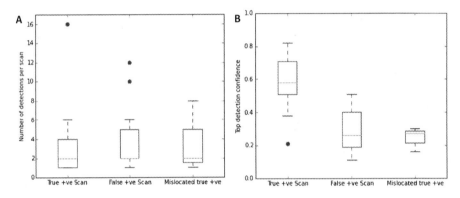

Fig. 6. Box plots of scans with positive detections. (A) Number of connected components idented in the scan for each type of positive (+ve) scan. (B) Confidence level of the most confident connected component for each type of positive scan.

There are 6 datasets which are treated as false positive as dense vessels were not identified in the NCCT scans, however arterial occlusions were identified in the CTA scans. One of these detections turned out to be a true positive when reviewed against CTA i.e. manual identification erroneously missed a dense vessel sign.

There are 4 datasets in which the CNN failed to detect the dense vessel. All of these are dense vessels at the distal segment of the vessel (see Fig. 7). These are usually harder to detect, because they frequently present as dot signs, which may be only a few voxels in size. The larger, easier to identify, distal occlusion cases have been detected (See Fig. 8).

To assess the extent to which the detection of dense vessel signs would help in the review of CTA we compute the agreement between detections in NCCT and CTA (see Table 4). Most of the detected dense vessel cases have been identified in CTA as the clots (arterial occlusion(AO)), however not all clots were visible in NCCT, therefore all detection methods have higher specificity than sensitivity when reviewed against CTA. There is a high proportion of cases that have a dense vessel in our validation set, therefore the sensitivity of detection is higher than reported in larger population studies [13], where the reported sensitivity is 52%

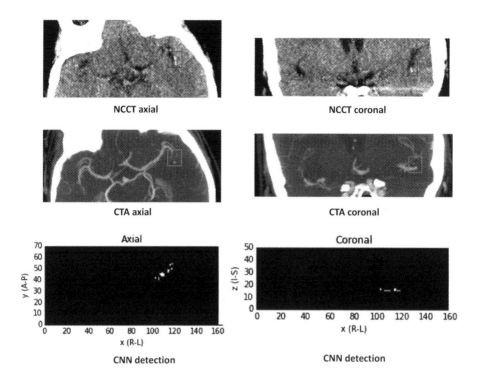

Fig. 7. Missed distal detection. This is a mislocated true positive case i.e. the detections were situated in the wrong part of the scan.

and specificity 95%. The automatic system did not reach detection specificity of the clinical researchers, however the overall detection agreement with CTA remained at the same level as the agreement with human annotations in NCCT.

5 Discussion

When we are considering the automatic detection for use in patient triage for thrombectomy it is important that the CNN detects the dense vessels in patients who have a large vessel occlusion in the internal carotid and in the M1 segment of the middle cerebral artery [14] as these patients would be considered for thrombectomy. In the validation dataset there were 19 patients who presented occlusion in that region and the CNN detected all of them correctly (e.g. see Fig. 9). In one case, a large vessel sign had been erroneously missed during manual segmentation, and the CNN detector picked it up. This illustrates the fact that identification of dense vessel in NCCT is not trivial and some signs can be missed even by a human expert, therefore an automatic detector which acts as a second reader may aid in reviewing the scan.

Any patient considered for thrombectomy would also have CTA to confirm the presence and location of a clot, but this kind of detection could direct the

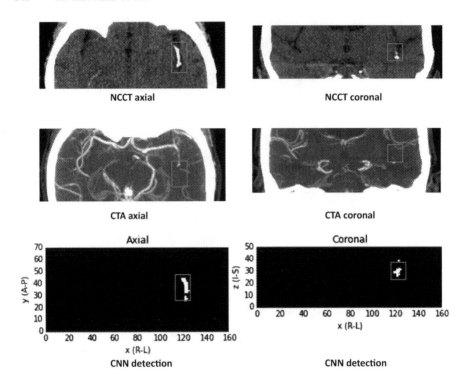

Fig. 8. Large clearly visible distal occlusion.

Table 4. NCCT vs CTA.

		Database dense vessels	Segmentation dense vessels	CNN detections
CTA (AO)	Agreement	0.78	0.79	0.62
	Sensitivity	0.68	0.68	0.59
	Specificity	0.95	1.0	0.67

clinician to the most likely vessel in CTA to speed up the review and treatment decision. In order for an automatic system to be useful, the number of the candidate detections cannot be overwhelming. We report that the median number of detection which required reviewing per positive scan is 2 (See Fig. 6A) and average is between 3 and 4 (See Table 3). The highest number of detections per scan was 16 and in this case it probably would not be clinically useful to run the automatic detector. We do not use morphological operation e.g opening and closing to clean the scans from small detections, which are frequently false positive, because we do not want to remove possible small distal dot signs. Nevertheless we provide the detection confidence rank for each scan (see Table 1) and the clinician may choose to review only the top confident detections. Encouragingly,

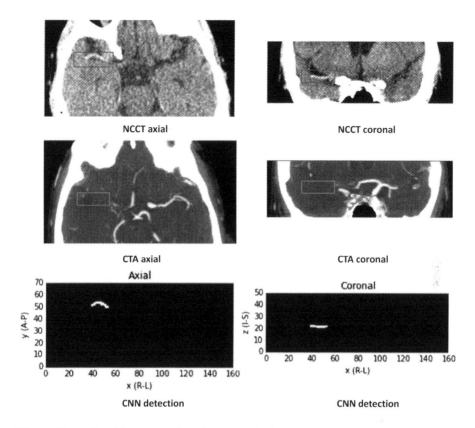

Fig. 9. Example of large vessel occlusion with dense vessel, confirmed by CTA and detected.

in all of the true positive scans, the most confident detection was the true detection.

An interesting possibility would be to train a complementary system on CTA scans, with or without the initial NCCT scan as additional input. In this task, *positive* detection presents as the *absence* of a feature (the vessel) in the scan, and the bilateral comparison inherent in our network might prove to be particularly well suited. Such a network could act as a further second reader to aid the radiologist.

6   Conclusions

In this paper, we have presented an evaluation of a previously reported system [6,7] for the automatic detection of dense vessel signs in NCCT scans. Our system shows promise, detecting all patient cases who present with large vessel occlusions—which is important when selecting patients for thrombectomy.

Whilst there is currently an equal number of false positives, this number might be reduced with better threshold selection.

This system will be beneficial to those patients with arterial occlusion who exhibit the dense vessel sign in NCCT. There is a subset of patients who do not exhibit this sign, and therefore we further propose a future objective of training a system on both NCCT and CTA scans for complete detection of occluded arteries.

References

1. Riedel, C.H., Zimmermann, P., Jensen-Kondering, U., Stingele, R., Deuschl, G., Jansen, O.: The importance of size successful recanalization by intravenous thrombolysis in acute anterior stroke depends on thrombus length. Stroke **42**(6), 1775–1777 (2011)
2. Huang, X., Cheripelli, B.K., Lloyd, S.M., Kalladka, D., Moreton, F.C., Siddiqui, A., Ford, I., Muir, K.W.: Alteplase versus tenecteplase for thrombolysis after ischaemic stroke (ATTEST): a phase 2, randomised, open-label, blinded endpoint study. Lancet Neurol. **14**(4), 368–376 (2015)
3. MacDougall, N.J., McVerry, F., Huang, X., Welch, A., Fulton, R., Muir, K.W.: Post-stroke hyperglycaemia is associated with adverse evolution of acute ischaemic injury. In: Cerebrovascular Diseases, vol. 37, p. 267, Karger Allschwilerstrasse, Basel (2014)
4. Wardlaw, J.M., Muir, K.W., Macleod, M.J., Weir, C., McVerry, F., Carpenter, T., Shuler, K., Thomas, R., Acheampong, P., Dani, K., Murray, A.: Clinical relevance and practical implications of trials of perfusion and angiographic imaging in patients with acute ischaemic stroke: a multicentre cohort imaging study. J. Neurol. Neurosurg. Psychiatry **84**(9), 1001–1007 (2013)
5. Dabbah, M.A., et al.: Detection and location of 127 anatomical landmarks in diverse ct datasets. In: SPIE Medical Imaging, p. 903415. International Society for Optics and Photonics (2014)
6. Lisowska, A., Bereridge, E., Muir, K., Poole, I.: Thrombus detection in CT brain scans using a convolutional neural network. In: Proceedings of the 10th International Joint Conference on Biomedical Engineering Systems and Technologies (BIOSTEC 2017), Bioimaging, vol. 2, pp. 24–33. Scitepress (2017)
7. Lisowska, A., O'Neil, A., Dilys, V., Daykin, M., Beveridge, E., Muir, K., Mclaughlin, S., Poole, I.: Context-aware convolutional neural networks for stroke sign detection in non-contrast CT scans. In: Valdés Hernández, M., González-Castro, V. (eds.) MIUA 2017. CCIS, vol. 723, pp. 494–505. Springer, Cham (2017). https://doi.org/10.1007/978-3-319-60964-5_43
8. Wolterink, J.M., Leiner, T., Viergever, M.A., Išgum, I.: Automatic coronary calcium scoring in cardiac CT angiography using convolutional neural networks. In: Navab, N., Hornegger, J., Wells, W.M., Frangi, A.F. (eds.) MICCAI 2015. LNCS, vol. 9349, pp. 589–596. Springer, Cham (2015). https://doi.org/10.1007/978-3-319-24553-9_72
9. Chollet, F.: Keras (2015). https://github.com/fchollet/keras
10. Theano Development Team: Theano: a Python framework for fast computation of mathematical expressions. arXiv e-prints abs/1605.02688, May 2016
11. Kingma, D., Ba, J.: Adam: a method for stochastic optimization. arXiv preprint arXiv:1412.6980 (2014)

12. Lin, T.Y., Goyal, P., Girshick, R., He, K., Dollár, P.: Focal loss for dense object detection. arXiv preprint arXiv:1708.02002 (2017)
13. Mair, G., Boyd, E.V., Chappell, F.M., von Kummer, R., Lindley, R.I., Sandercock, P., Wardlaw, J.M.: Sensitivity and specificity of the hyperdense artery sign for arterial obstruction in acute ischemic stroke. Stroke **46**(1), 102–107 (2015)
14. Campbell, B.C., Donnan, G.A., Mitchell, P.J., Davis, S.M.: Endovascular thrombectomy for stroke: current best practice and future goals. Stroke Vascu. Neurol. **1**(1), 16–22 (2016)

Tracking Anterior Mitral Leaflet in Echocardiographic Videos Using Morphological Operators and Active Contours

Malik Saad Sultan[1](✉), Nelson Martins[1,2], Eva Costa[2], Diana Veiga[2], Manuel João Ferreira[2,3], Sandra Mattos[4], and Miguel Tavares Coimbra[1]

[1] Instituto de Telecomunicações,
Faculdade de Ciências da Universidade do Porto, Porto, Portugal
{msultan,mcoimbra}@dcc.fc.up.pt
[2] Neadvance - Machine Vision, S.A., Braga, Portugal
{nmartins,ecosta,dveiga,mferreira}@neadvance.com
[3] Centro Algoritmi, University of Minho, Guimarães, Portugal
[4] Círculo do Coração de Pernambuco, Recife, PE, Brazil
ssmattos@cardiol.br

Abstract. Rheumatic heart disease is the result of damage to the heart valves, more often the mitral valve. The heart valves leaflets get inflamed, scarred and stretched which interrupts the normal blood flow, resulting into serious health condition. Measuring and quantifying clinically relevant features, like thickness, mobility and shape can help to analyze the functionality of the valve, identify early cases of disease and reduce the disease burden. To obtain these features, the first step is to automatically delineate the relevant structures, such as the anterior mitral valve leaflet, throughout the echocardiographic video. In this work, we proposed a near real time method to track the anterior mitral leaflet in ultrasound videos using the parasternal long axis view. The method is semi-automatic, requiring a manual delineation of the anterior mitral leaflet in the first frame of the video. The method uses mathematical morphological techniques to obtain the rough boundaries of the leaflet and are further refined by the localized active contour framework. The mobility of the leaflet was also obtained, providing us the base to analyze the functionality of the valve (opening and closing). The algorithm was tested on 67 videos with 6432 frames. It outperformed with respect to the time consumption (0.4 s/frame), with the extended modified Hausdorff distance error of 3.7 pixels and the improved tracking performance (less failure).

Keywords: Ultrasound images · Medical image processing
Active contours · Segmentation and tracking · Mitral valve

N. Peixoto et al. (Eds.): BIOSTEC 2017, CCIS 881, pp. 146–162, 2018.
https://doi.org/10.1007/978-3-319-94806-5_9

1   Introduction

1.1   Motivation

Mitral valve diseases are widespread and are commonly affected by Rheumatic Heart Disease (RHD) [1]. RHD is an autoimmune disease that usually begins in childhood. It starts as a strep throat infection that is caused by the streptococci. If the strep throat infection is untreated, it results into rheumatic fever. The repeated episodes of rheumatic fever slowly damages the heart valves.

Following one of the most relevant published studies [2,3], about 15.6 million people are affected globally from RHD, and require medical follow-up, being responsible for 233,000 deaths per year. Heart valve diseases create a massive economic burden on health authorities. The average surgery cost to treat mitral regurgitation was 24.871 ± 13.940 dollars per patient in Europe [4–6]. The heart valve treatments and operations are not only expensive, but also a highly risky cardiac process [7].

The literature suggests the cost effective solution of using penicillin in the early stage [8]. It reduces the probability of recurrence of the rheumatic fever, resulting less risk of damage to the heart valves. Therefore, earlier detection is considered vital to control disease progression and to estimate disease burden in low-resource regions of the world [1].

RHD thickened the Anterior Mitral Leaflet (AML) that directly affects the shape and mobility of the leaflet, resulting into pathologies like stenosis and regurgitation. Quantifying the degree of change in morphological features helps to identify early cases and to control disease progression.

The key benefits of using the Echocardiography modality are its non-ionizing, non-invasive property and is able to analyze fast moving structures like AML in real time. It is a low cost modality and is available as a portable device that makes it the most appropriate choice to use it in low resource areas [9].

The Parasternal Long Axis view provides the most suitable window to measure and quantify the clinically relevant parameters of the mitral valve such as, thickness, mobility and valvular anatomy (Fig. 1) [10]. To achieve this the first step is to segment and track the structures throughout the cardiac cycle. Manual segmentation is undesirable, given its impracticality, subjectivity and expert knowledge required. Automatic and semi-automatics methods to identify and track mitral valve structures can improve the diagnostic process, providing quick and objective measurements of clinically relevant parameters, even without any expert cardiology knowledge.

1.2   State of the Art

Active contour models were used to delineate the objects with deformable shapes and were extensively used by the research community for segmentation and tracking of the structures in medical images. The reason to adopt this kind of approach is their robustness against image noise and shape fragmentation, ability to track non-rigid motion and its capability to incorporate geometric

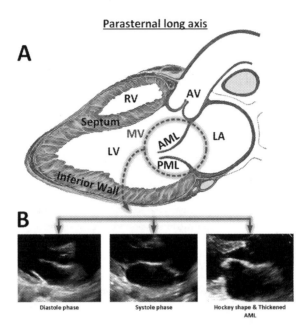

Fig. 1. Parasternal long axis view, (adapted from [24]) (A): showing Mitral valve (MV), Anterior Mitral Leaflet (AML), Posterior Mitral Leaflet (PML) and other structures. (B): Shows the MV in Diastole/Systole phase, the thickened and hockey shape leaflet.

constraints, such as the expected shape [11]. Optical flow was integrated in the active contour framework to segment and track the AML in echocardiography [12]. The limitations of the proposed method are, incapability to track large frame to frame displacement of AML, require manual initialization in the first frame and was computationally expensive to process a single cardiac cycle (20 m). In another work, transformation fitting was used to obtain initial boundaries that are further refined by the two connected active contours [13]. The proposed method requires initialization, parameter adjustment, failed in high displacement ($\geq$10 pixels) and is computationally expensive with 1.8 s/frame for the ten iterations. A fully automatic and unsupervised method was based on outlier detection in a low rank matrix to track the region of the AML, in both 2D and 3D ultrasound images [14]. Despite the fact that it is fully automatic, it is very sensitive rank and noise. Literature review demands a real time segmentation and tracking algorithm with less user interaction and the ability to efficiently track the mitral valve when faced with a large frame to frame displacements [11–14].

Mathematical morphology is widely used in image processing for analysis of shapes, geometrical and topological structures. They were previously used to segment the left ventricle [15], myocardium, ischemic viable and non-viable in echocardiography [16].

1.3   Objectives and Contributions

The objective of this work is to obtain robust and real-time tracking of the AML in ultrasound videos.

Our key contribution in this work is the novel use of combined morphological operators and active contours to address robust AML tracking in frames with large displacement.

The remainder of the paper is organized as follows. Section 2 provides the methodology adopted in this paper. In Sect. 3 we report the results that demonstrate the accuracy of the proposed algorithm and finally Sect. 4 concludes the paper with a discussion on the problem, our contribution to it and the future work.

2   Methodology

In the first step, echocardiography video is read, followed by contrast stretching to normalize the illumination of the image. In this work, we assumed the perfect segmentation (manual) in the first frame and is provided in priori. In each step, two successive frames are iteratively selected. Since AML is a thin region that shows fast motion, the thin regions of the successive images are extracted followed by the regions with large displacement, using basic mathematical morphological techniques. These regions are subsequently merged with the segmentation result of the preceding frame and filtered, in the candidate region module. Obtained regions are classified by taking into account their shapes and geometrical properties. The obtained boundaries of the AML with morphological operator are not well localized. Therefore localized active contour model is used to refine the obtained boundaries. After having the segmentation results, we proceed to the post processing step of AML analysis. A summary of the proposed processing pipeline is depicted in Fig. 2, and each step will now be discussed in detail.

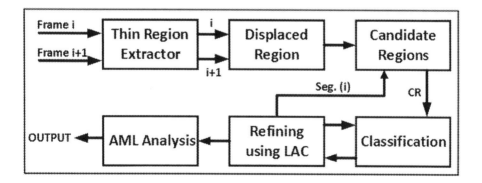

Fig. 2. AML tracking pipeline (adapted from [24]).

2.1   Thin Region Extractor

In this stage, two consecutive frames were extracted iteratively until the whole cardiac cycle was covered. The basic mathematical morphological operations were used that requires, the input image and the structuring element of suitable size and shape. These morphological operations can be used for both binary and grayscale images. For the resolution of the videos used in this papers experiments the maximum recorded thickness of the AML was 24 pixels. Following this, we used the grayscale images with the disk shape structuring element of width 24 pixels, to extract the potential regions.

Finally, The thin AML region (Fig. 3C) is extracted by taking the difference between the grayscale input image (Fig. 3A) and the grayscale opened image (Fig. 3B) with the flat disk shape structuring element of 24 pixel diameter.

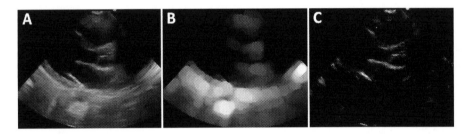

Fig. 3. (A) Grayscale image (B) Morphological opening (C) Top-hat transform (adapted from [24]).

2.2   Displaced Region

Based on the analysis of the AML in the PLAX view, the thin AML region shows a very large displacement in successive frames, compare to other regions in an image. Other regions such as, septum, inferior wall (Fig. 1) do not show significant displacement in successive frames and thus the regions are overlapped. This prior information is meaningful to overcome the problem of tracking in frames with large AML displacement.

The focus of this module is to extract region that showed large displacement from frame $t-1$ to frame t. That can simply be achieved by taking the difference of successive frames followed by selecting only the positive intensity values (Fig. 4). Hard threshold is then applied to get the binary image.

$$Disp^t_{gray} = [I_t(x,y) - I_{t-1}(x,y)] \quad Disp^t_{gray} < 0 \tag{1}$$

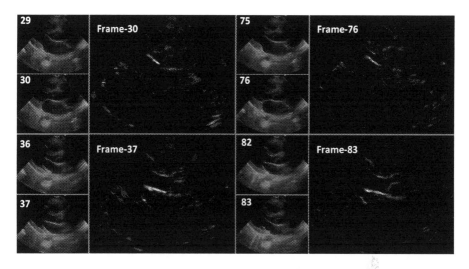

Fig. 4. Regions with high displacement at four different times (frames)   (adapted from [24]).

2.3 Candidate Image

The segmented region obtained at the time $t-1$ is filtered to remove the regions which belong to the blood pool (black region) in frame at time t. The filtered region is then summed up with the results of the displaced region module. Small discontinuities (with a distance of 2 pixels or less) were merged by a morphological closing using a disk shape structuring element with a radius of 2. The obtained results are shown in Fig. 5.

2.4 Region Classification

The regions extracted from the last module are classified as the AML or the outliers, based on the morphological features such as area, centroid, minor axis length, major axis length. These features provides the structural and locality information to assign the probability of being the AML or outlier.

These basic morphological features do not typically change significantly in successive frames. In ideal conditions, these features should be constant throughout the cardiac cycle. The features obtained from the manual segmentation in the first frame is used as a reference for the upcoming frame. After processing each frame, the reference features are automatically updated with the average, by using the feedback channel (Fig. 6).

An error matrix is designed that compute the relative error compare to the segmentation in previous frames. The error matrix consist of four vectors, area error: computes the change in area, centroid error: computes the change in location, major/minor axis length error: computes the change in length and width. Next, the region with the minimum overall error is classified as the AML and other as outliers.

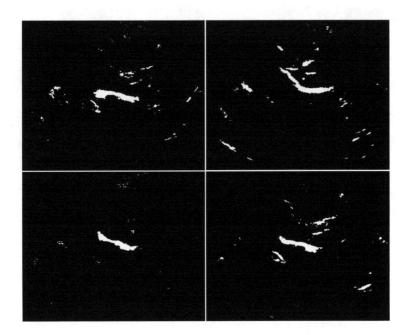

Fig. 5. Candidate image for final AML classification (adapted from [24]).

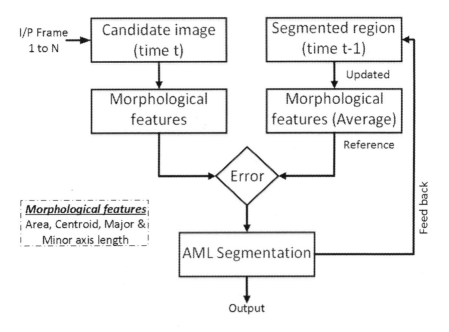

Fig. 6. Classification scheme (adapted from [24]).

2.5   Refining Using Active Contours

The active contour framework has been widely used for the purpose of image segmentation and tracking [17]. The contour deforms under the internal and external energy to segment the desired object. The active contours can be broadly divided as, the edge based and the region based [18,19].

The edge based active contours [18] uses the image gradient (edges) to attract the contour towards the desired boundary. Active contour framework requires the placement of contour close to the object and is sensitive to the image noise. However, it work reasonably well in images with heterogeneous regions.

The region based active contours [19] uses the global intensity statistics of the regions to evolve the contour, until find the optimum choice. They are not sensitive to initial placement of the contour and is insensitive to noise.

Automatic Initialization. The boundaries of the AML obtained by the mathematical morphological techniques are used to initialize the active contour framework. Initial boundaries are close to the real boundaries, but are not well localized. Therefore, analyzing local regions can provide robust and well defined boundaries, with a few iterations.

Localized Active Contours. Ultrasound images are very noisy and frequently contain heterogeneous regions, and as such neither edge based contours, nor region based contours are a suitable choice. In this situation, we need a model that take the benefits from both edge and region based active contours. A localized region-based active contour (LAC) framework [20] were proposed to address this problem. This hybrid region-based curve evolution is robust to noise and doesn't rely on the global configuration of the image.

The rough boundaries of the AML obtained from the morphological operators were used to initialize the LAC framework, to refine the leaflet boundaries. The algorithm is based on the analysis of the local circular regions with five pixels radius, at each point on the curve. At each point the algorithm locally identifies the background and foreground optimally by their mean intensities. The formulation of the local energy function along the curve is defined as:

$$
\frac{\partial \phi}{\partial t}(x) = \delta\phi(x) \int_{\Omega_y} B(x,y)\, \delta\phi(y) \cdot ((I(y) - u_x)^2 \\
- (I(y) - v_x)^2) dy + \lambda \delta\phi(x) div\left[\frac{\nabla\phi(x)}{|\nabla\phi(x)|}\right]
\tag{2}
$$

Here, δ is the Dirac function, $B(x,y)$ represents a region that locally defines the interior and the exterior of the region at point x and the radius of the local region is specified by the user. The uniform modelling energy is used as an internal energy [19]. The localized version of the internal energy is defined as the local interior regions and exterior regions at each point on the curve. (v_x, ν_x) are the localized version of means at each point x. The second term is the normalization term that keeps the curve smoother. It penalizes the arc length based on the weights λ tuned by the user.

2.6 AML Analysis

Skeletonization. Prior to perform the analysis, the shape of the AML is simplified by using skeletonization. The morphological thinning is used to get a line of one pixel width, while preserving the topological characteristics of the AML. Skeletonization works in the same way as morphological operators, convolving the structuring element (template) on the binary image. The Mark-and-Delete based templates were found very reliable and effective for thinning algorithms and thus used in this work [21]. Ultrasound images are usually affected by the speckle noise resulting into irregular boundaries, producing superfluous minor branches of the skeleton. These branches are filtered out to extract the fundamental part of the skeleton. This can be done by computing the Euclidian distance between the branch and the end points. All those branches whose length are less than the defined threshold (6 pixels) are discarded.

Motion Patterns. The focus of this module is to compute the motion pattern of the AML and analyze to extract the meaningful information. The mean motion of the X and Y coordinates of the skeleton was computed. The motion of the AML in X-axis was small and doesn't provide any meaningful information. However, the motion of the AML in Y-axis has shown large motion with a unique pattern. The mean of the y-coordinates of the AML skeleton for each frame is plotted against time, showing the motion pattern of the AML (Fig. 7). The cardiac cycle is divided into systole and diastole phase based on the maximum and minimum of the peaks of the obtained motion pattern. The classification helps to label the AML as open or close and will be useful for the analysis such as, computing the thickness when the valve is open. Further work can help to classify frames in early filling and late filling phase (Fig. 7). The late filing will be useful to extract frames in which the AML is perpendicular to the ultrasound beam. This is the best position to measure the thickness of the AML tip, which provides a strong clue regarding the presence or not of diseases.

Shape. The hockey stick like appearance of the AML in PLAX view is an indicator of stenosis. A condition in which the heart valve leaflets get restricted (narrowed, blocked) resulting into interruption in the normal blood flow. In order to identify this condition, we proposed the measurement of the local curvature on the skeleton of the AML. A template based method is used to measure the local bending of the AML [22]. We tested two template based methods, the trigonometrical and crossover point method (Fig. 8).

   The trigonometrical approach relates the crossover angle with the curvature (Eq. 3). The crossover angle is the angle between the crossover point, where the curve intersect the disk mask and the X-axis of the disk. This approach is sensitive to noise to estimate the precise angle of the crossover points.

$$K_{tr} = \frac{2sin\theta_c}{1 - sin^2\theta_c} \tag{3}$$

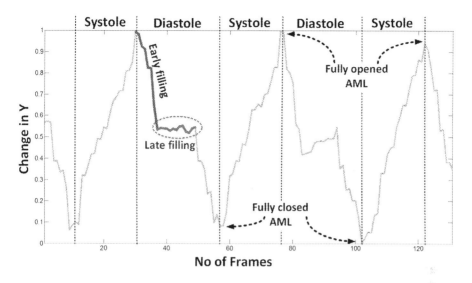

Fig. 7. Motion patterns generated by AML (adapted from [24]).

The crossover point approach approximate the curvature by computing the area between curve and the disk, and is related to the crossover angle (θ_c) [22]. The squared area covered by the curve and disk are inversely proportional to the curvature (Eq. 4).

$$K_{cp} = \frac{1}{A^2} \tag{4}$$

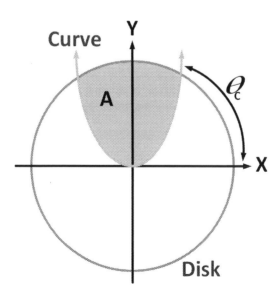

Fig. 8. Curvature approximation using area and crossover angle θ_c.

The obtained area is large for the small curvature. Thus the reciprocal of squared area is close to zero that increase the confidence by avoiding infinity and the reliability of the approach.

The experiments has shown that the area based method is less sensitive to speckle noise and provide smoother results, and thus used for this analysis. For each frame, we measured the local curvature at each point on the AML skeleton, followed by computing the overall mean to obtain the global curvature. In stenosis, the leaflet is restricted and can be identified by the curvature (shape) change.

We observed that the motion pattern of the AML and the pattern of the global curvature change are correlated. When the valve opens the curvature of the AML tends to decrease showing the straightness of the leaflet and when the valve opens the curvature start increasing, suggesting the bending of the leaflet. This motion shape relation might help in future by providing a clue to identify pathological condition.

For a better visual representation of the motion and curvature pattern, we first smoothed the curved and then normalize to restrict it in the range (0–1) (Fig. 9).

3   Results

3.1   Materials

An initiative from the Real Hospital Português, in Recife, Brazil lead to the screening of 1203 childrens and pregnant women, looking for cardiac pathologies. All patients were tested regarding the presence of streptococcal infection and short mitral valve videos were recorded. The data were collected using different ultrasound devices (M-Turbo, Edge II model by SonoSite, Vivid my model

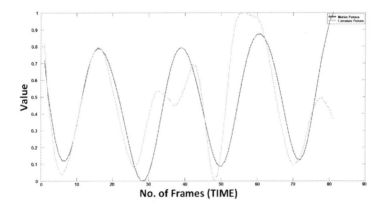

Fig. 9. Motion and curvature pattern of AML, red: motion pattern, green: curvature pattern. (Color figure online)

by GE healthcare and $CX50$ model by Philips), with a wide range of transducers, frequency and scanning depths. Sixty seven of these exams was manually annotated by the doctors using Osirix software and were used to test the novel method proposed in this work. These sixty seven videos include a total of 6432 frames with a dimensions of 422×636 pixels. The proposed method has been implemented using $MATLAB$ R2016b.

3.2 Extended Modified Hausdorff Distance (E-MHD)

The Modified Hausdorff Distance [23] was proposed to obtain a distance measure to match two objects. In this work, we extended this approach by categorizing the segmented region as false positive, false negative and true positive. We assumed that the nearest point between Automatic Segmentation (AS) and Ground Truth (GT) with Euclidean distance smaller than 2 pixels are true positives. The part of the AS that is falsely segmented as AML were considered false positives and the parts of the GT that were missed by the automatic segmentation were considered as false negatives, always using 2 pixels distance as reference T (Fig. 10).

$$
\begin{aligned}
d_{AS \rightarrow GT} &= min\left\{AS, SEG\right\} \ FP = d > T \ TP = d < T \\
d_{GT \rightarrow AS} &= min\left\{AS, SEG\right\} \ FN = d > T \ TP = d < T \\
D_{MHD} &= max\left[avg\left(d_{AS \rightarrow GT}\right), avg\left(d_{GT \rightarrow AS}\right)\right]
\end{aligned}
\tag{5}
$$

3.3 Segmentation and Tracking

In this section, we analyze and compare the tracking ability of the proposed algorithm on 67 cases in 2D ultrasound videos, obtained from the PLAX view. To validate the algorithm, we compared the results of the proposed algorithm with the doctors annotation. Results were also compared with the reference state of the art algorithm [25]. The reference algorithm used the modified internal energy

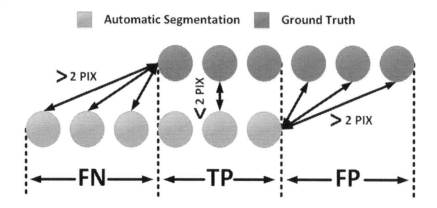

Fig. 10. Region classification (adapted from [24]). (Color figure online)

(open-ended contour) and external energy (added Harris cornerness measure), to track the AML in ultrasound. We used the E-MHD error to compute the relative Euclidean distance between AS and GT.

In this work, we assumed perfect segmentation (manual annotation) in the very first frame of the video, followed by defining the region of interest. It helps to removes the irrelevant structures from the right and left of the AML.

3.4 Quantification

The performance metric used are: the E-MHD error, the number of failures and the processing time. The morphological operators are relatively fast to obtain the boundaries of the AML, spending on average 0.4 s/frame, however the reference algorithm consumes 1.2sec/frame. To refine the obtained boundaries, we used the LAC that consumes about 0.7 s/frame. The boxplot is used for the statistical analysis of the mean E-MHD and the number of failure in each video. The E-MHD error was computed for each frame of the video and the mean E-MHD error was saved in a vector for visual inspection.

The boxplot of E-MHD error (Fig. 11) shows that the median E-MHD error of our method is smaller than the reference algorithm, 3.7 and pixels 5.2 respectively. The most frequent error for our method lies between 3.14 to 4.6 pixels. However, the reference algorithm covers the comparatively large range from 4.6 to 6.6 pixels. The overall range of our method is also improved, from 2.12 to 5.54, whereas the reference covers the higher values from 3.32 to 8.06 pixels. In the Fig. 10, the red dots shows the outliers.

Proposed method has shown an improvement in tracking, with a median number of failure in each video of 2 (Fig. 12). The reference method failed twice as much than proposed method (median of 4). The most frequent range of failure

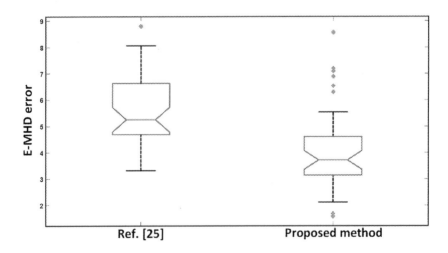

Fig. 11. Extended modified Hausdorff distance error, 67 cases.

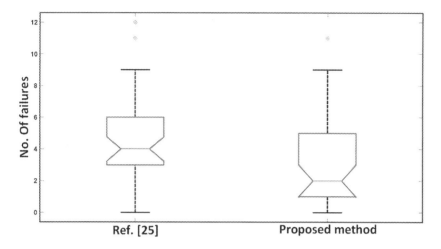

Fig. 12. Number of failure in each video, 67 cases.

in proposed method is between 1 to 5 failures. On the other side, the reference method shows lies between 3 to 6 failures.

Proposed algorithm has performed reasonably well, with respect to time consumption, E-MHD and the number of failures. The limitation of the work are the incapability of the algorithm to avoid segmenting the neighbor regions. The algorithm is robust to segment the whole leaflet with a sensitivity of 85% and a recall of 72%.

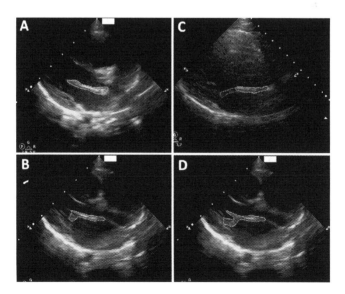

Fig. 13. Segmentation results, red: doctors's annotation, green: proposed method. (Color figure online)

The segmentation results were plotted for better problem understanding. The Fig. 13A, B shows the reasonable results with fully segmented AML and with the small region falsely segmented as the AML. However, in Fig. 13C we have the discrete regions in an image and thus missed by the proposed algorithm and is one of the reason, why the proposed method fails. In Fig. 13D, the proposed method has segmented not only the AML, but also segmented the chordae tendineae and the posterior aorta. These missing and over-segmented regions are the responsible of having large E-MHD, with low sensitivity and recall.

4   Discussion and Future Work

In this work, a new tracking approach is proposed that uses morphological operators to predict the location and boundaries of the AML. To obtain more precise boundaries, the localized active contour framework is adopted. The algorithm is found robust to track in the difficult situations when the valve opens with the mean AML displacement of about 35 pixels. In such situation, the active contours often fails to segment the boundaries (edges) that are far from the contour. The proposed algorithm outperform the reference algorithm with respect to time, however it is still slow to get the real time performance of the algorithm.

The main limitation of the algorithm is its incapability to avoid segmenting the neighbor regions (chordae tendineae, cardiac walls, septum etc.). It happens because the intensity and texture of the neighbor regions are similar. The chordae tendineae and the posterior aorta are directly connected with the AML, containing the same features. So we dont have any reliable feature that identify starting and ending of the leaflet. In this work, we define the region of interest that minimize this problem, however we need an automatic system that robustly define the region of interest and impose the shape constraints in the active contour frame work to further improve the segmentation performance.

Another limitation of the proposed algorithm is its incapability to recover from the failure. This is the situation that occur frequently due to low quality of the image and due to the missing structures in several frame of the ultrasound video.

In future, we will focus to overcome the limitations such as, the time consumption, reduce failure, minimize segmenting irrelevant regions, and finally to estimate and quantify morphological features to identify pathological cases.

Acknowledgements. This article is a result of the project NORTE-01-0247-FEDER-003507-RHDecho, co-funded by Norte Portugal Regional Operational Programme (NORTE 2020), under the PORTUGAL 2020 Partnership Agreement, through the European Regional Development Fund (ERDF). This work also had the collaboration of the Fundação para a Ciência a e Tecnologia (FCT) grant no: PD/BD/105761/2014 and has contributions from the project NanoSTIMA, NORTE-01-0145-FEDER-000016, supported by Norte Portugal Regional Operational Programme (NORTE 2020), through Portugal 2020 and the European Regional Development Fund (ERDF).

References

1. Bisno, A., Butchart, E.G., Ganguly, N.K., Ghebrehiwet, T., et al.: WHO Expert Consultation on Rheumatic Fever and Rheumatic Heart Disease, Geneva (2004)
2. WHO: World Heart Federation, World Stroke Organization. Global atlas on cardiovascular disease prevention and control (2011). ISBN 9789241564373
3. WHF (2012). http://www.world-heart-federation.org/fileadmin/user_upload/docu ments/Fact_sheets/2012/RHD.pdf
4. Trochu, J.N., Tourneau, T.L., Obadia, J.F., Caranhac, G., Beresniak, A.: Economic burden of functional and organic mitral valve regurgitation. Arch. Cardiovasc. Dis. **108**, 88–96 (2015)
5. Ribeiro, G.S., Tartof, S.Y., Oliveira, D.W.S., Guedes, A.C.S., Reis, M.G., Riley, L.W., Ko, A.I.: Surgery for valvular heart disease: a population-based study in a Brazilian urban center. PLoS One **7**(5), e37855 (2012)
6. The economic cost of cardiovascular disease from 2014–2020 in six European economies. Centre for Economics and Business Research, London (2014)
7. Mirabel, M., Iung, B., Baron, G., Messika-Zeitoun, D., Dtaint, D., Vanoverschelde, J.-L., Butchart, E.G., Ravaud, P., Vahanian, A.: What are the characteristics of patients with severe, symptomatic, mitral regurgitation who are denied surgery? Eur. Heart J. **28**, 1358–1365 (2007)
8. Colquhoun, S.M., Carapetis, J.R., Kado, J.H., Steer, A.C.: Rheumatic heart disease and its control in the Pacific. Expert Rev. Cardiovasc. Ther. **7**(12), 1517–1524 (2009)
9. Remnyi, B., Wilson, N., Steer, A., Ferreira, B., Kado, J., Kumar, K., Lawrenson, J., Maguire, G., Marijon, E., et al.: World Heart Federation criteria for echocardiographic diagnosis of rheumatic heart diseasean evidence-based guideline. Nat. Rev. Cardiol. **9**(5), 297–309 (2012)
10. Omran, A.S., Arifi, A.A., Mohamed, A.A.: Echocardiography of the mitral valve. J. Saudi Heart Assoc. **22**, 165–170 (2010)
11. Sheng, C.: Segmentation in echocardiographic sequences using shape-based snake model. Comput. Inf. **27**, 423–435 (2008)
12. Mikic, I., Krucinski, S., Thomas, J.D.: Segmentation and tracking in echocardiographic sequences: active contours guided by optical flow estimates. IEEE Trans. Med. Imaging **17**(2), 274–284 (1998)
13. Martin, S., Daanen, V., Chavanon, O., Troccaz, J.: Fast segmentation of the mitral valve leaflet in echocardiography. In: Beichel, R.R., Sonka, M. (eds.) CVAMIA 2006. LNCS, vol. 4241, pp. 225–235. Springer, Heidelberg (2006). https://doi.org/ 10.1007/11889762_20
14. Zhou, X., Yang, C., Yu, W.: Automatic mitral leaflet tracking in echocardiography by outlier detection in the low-rank representation. In: IEEE Conference on Computer Vision and Pattern Recognition, pp. 972–979. IEEE Computer Society, Washington, DC (2012)
15. Yun-gang, L., Jacky, K.K., Shi, L., Guan, Y., Linong, L., Qin, J., PhengAnn, H., Winnie, C.C., Defeng, W.: Myocardial iron loading assessment by automatic left ventricle segmentation with morphological operations and geodesic active contour on T2* images, Scientific reports (2015)
16. Lascu, M., Lascu, D.: A new morphological image segmentation with application in 3D echographic images. WSEAS Trans. Electron. **5**(3), 72–82 (2008)
17. Noble, J.A., Boukerroui, D.: Ultrasound image segmentation: a survey. IEEE Trans. Med. Imaging **25**(8), 987–1010 (2006)

18. Kass, M., Witkin, A., Terzopoulouse, D.: Snakes : active contour model. Int. J. Comput. Vis. **1**(4), 321–331 (1988)
19. Chan, T., Vese, L.: An active contour model without edges. In: Nielsen, M., Johansen, P., Olsen, O.F., Weickert, J. (eds.) Scale-Space 1999. LNCS, vol. 1682, pp. 141–151. Springer, Heidelberg (1999). https://doi.org/10.1007/3-540-48236-9_13
20. Lankton, S., Tannenbaum, A.: Localizing region-based active contours. IEEE Trans. Image Process. **17**(11), 2029–2039 (2008)
21. Zhang, T.Y., Suen, C.Y.: A fast parallel algorithm for thinning digital patterns. Commun. ACM **27**(3), 236–239 (1984)
22. Masoud, A.S., Pourreza, H.R.: A novel curvature-based algorithm for automatic grading of retinal blood vessel tortuosity. IEEE J-BHI **20**(2), 586–595 (2016)
23. Dubuisson, M.-P., Jain, A.K.: A Modified hausdorff distance for object matching. In: Proceedings of International Conference on Pattern Recognition, Jerusalem, Israel, pp. 566–568 (1994)
24. Sultan, M.S., Martins, N., Costa, E., Veiga, D., Ferreira, M., Mattos, S., Coimbra, M.: Real-time anterior mitral leaflet tracking using morphological operators and active contours. In: Proceedings of International Joint Conference on Biomedical Engineering Systems and Technologies, Porto, Portugal (2017)
25. Sultan, M.S., Martins, N., Veiga, D., Ferreira, M.J., Coimbra, M.T.: Tracking of the anterior mitral leaflet in echocardiographic sequences using active contours. In: EMBC, pp. 1074–1077 (2016)

Convolutional Neural Network Based Segmentation of Demyelinating Plaques in MRI

Bartłomiej Stasiak[1], Paweł Tarasiuk[1], Izabela Michalska[2],
Arkadiusz Tomczyk[1(✉)], and Piotr S. Szczepaniak[1]

[1] Institute of Information Technology, Lodz University of Technology,
Wolczanska 215, 90-924 Lodz, Poland
{bartlomiej.stasiak,pawel.tarasiuk,arkadiusz.tomczyk,
piotr.szczepaniak}@p.lodz.pl
[2] Department of Radiology, Barlicki University Hospital,
Kopcinskiego 22, 91-153 Lodz, Poland
izabela.anna.michalska@gmail.com

Abstract. In this paper a new architecture of convolutional neural networks is proposed. It is a fully-convolutional architecture which allows to keep the size of the processed image constant. This, in consequence, allows to apply it for image segmentation tasks where for a given image a mask representing sought regions should be produced. An additional advantage of this architecture is its ability to learn from smaller images which reduces the amount of data that must be propagated through the network. The trained network can be still applied to images of any size. The proposed method was used for automatic localization of demyelinating plaques in head MRI sequences. This work was possible, which should be emphasized, only thanks to the manually outlined plaques provided by radiologist. To present characteristic of the considered approach three architectures and three result evaluation methods were discussed and compared.

Keywords: Multiple sclerosis · Segmentation · Machine learning
Convolutional neural networks

1 Introduction

In recent years, thanks to the technological progress (computations with GPU) and growing access to large amount of labeled data, convolutional neural networks (CNN) achieved outstanding success in automatic analysis of the images containing scenes from the surrounding world. However, in the case of specialized, e.g. medical, images the advance is not that evident. The main reason is the lack of sufficiently large annotated training sets. Gathering of such data is hard because the group of domain experts able to annotate images is relatively small and the amount of data that must be analyzed may be bigger than it is

© Springer International Publishing AG, part of Springer Nature 2018
N. Peixoto et al. (Eds.): BIOSTEC 2017, CCIS 881, pp. 163–188, 2018.
https://doi.org/10.1007/978-3-319-94806-5_10

in the case of traditional images (e.g. 3D sequences). It is even harder in case of image segmentation task where every structure needs to be described with details which makes this process extremely time-consuming [1,2]. That is why it must be emphasized that research presented in this paper was only possible thanks to the hard work of radiologist who precisely outlined the regions of interest, demyelinating plaques, on every slice of head MRI sequence.

A typical application of CNNs is the whole image content classification task. In the case of image segmentation two basic approaches can be found in the literature. First one is a modified sliding window technique where CNN is used as a part of the classifier. In this case, however, the label is not assigned to the whole image but to the selected regions of that image (in particular to the regions representing neighbourhood of a given pixel). Consequently also to train such a classifier smaller image fragments, cut from the images manually annotated by an expert, are taken. Such a method was used, for example, in segmentation of anatomical regions in MRI images [3]. The second approach is so-called fully convolutional approach [4]. Here, the whole image constitutes the network input and as an output the mask, of the same size as an input image, describing object localization is expected. To gain such a result some modification must be made in CNN structure. Typical architecture contains convolutional and pooling layers which reduce the size of the intermediate results. That is why some new, upscaling (deconvolutional) layers need to be added to restore the original image size. And although this approach requires CNN modifications its advantage is fact that it can be trained using whole input images and expected masks without the need of cutting them into smaller fragments. This kind of approach was successfully used in e.g. analysis of transmitted light microscopy images [5] and MRI prostate examinations [6]. The latter approach is particularly interesting since it considers 3D convolution and the 3D MRI sequence is processed by CNN as a whole.

The solution proposed in this work to some extent possesses features of both above approaches. On the one hand, it tries to train CNN to act as a non-linear filter capable of indicating areas of interest. Consequently the output is the image of the same size as the input. In this case, however, no upscaling (deconvolutional) layers are required. On the other hand, it allows to train such a network using smaller image fragments without the necessity of processing as large amount of data as needed for the training based on the whole images.

The paper is organized as follows: the second section describes the considered dataset and medical background justifying the importance of demyelinating plaques localization, in the third section the proposed method is discussed and in the fourth and the fifth section the obtained results and their analysis are presented. Finally, the last section contains a short summary of the conducted research.

2   Medical Background

Multiple sclerosis (MS) is a common, chronic disease involving the central nervous system and leading progressively to different degrees of neurological disability. In multiple sclerosis cells of the human immune system attack myelin sheaths of the nerve fibres which represent white matter in the brain and spinal cord. The consequence of the myelin damage is inflammation in the affected areas and then creating scar tissue. This process is known as demyelination and the afflicted areas within the nerves' sheaths are called demyelinating plaques. To diagnose MS the combination of clinical symptoms, typical history, cerebrospinal fluid examination and magnetic resonance imaging (MRI) of the central nervous system is required. MRI plays an important role in diagnosing MS as it enables not only to confirm the diagnosis and defining its pattern but also to assess the progress of the disease and the response to treatment. It is essential to know which areas of the brain are affected because the process of demyelination as well as some other lesions in the white matter could also be present in different neurological disorders. White matter lesions in MS occur in some characteristic locations. Thus most of the lesions appear typically in juxtacortical regions (that is close to the brain cortex), periventricularly (that is around the ventricles and these lesions tend to lay perpendicularly to the long axis of the lateral ventricles), in corpus callosum, cerebellum (within hemispheres and cerebellar peduncles) and peripherally in brainstem (that is in cerebral peduncles, pons and medulla oblongata).

T2-weighted images (T2WI) are MR scans which are the most sensitive in showing the white matter lesions that are presented as areas of a high signal (that means they are hyperintense and appear white on the images) in regard to normal white matter. More sensitive than conventional T2WI in detecting juxtacortical and periventricular lesions are FLAIR (fluid-attenuated inversion recovery) sequences because they suppress the signal of fluid, including cerebrospinal fluid which fills the ventricles and subarachnoidal space. As a result the cerebrospinal fluid has a low signal and appears black on the scans obtained in FLAIR technique, as compared to the white matter abnormalities which remain hyperintense. On conventional T2WI cerebrospinal fluid presents high signal like demyelinating lesions in the white matter thus it may be difficult to recognize plaques localized in the vicinity of the ventricles and juxtacortical areas. On the FLAIR images the contrast between cerebrospinal fluid and the white matter lesions disposed in its proximity is more clearer and makes the plaques can be better detected.

The present study is based on indicating demyelinating lesions in the white matter on head MR images. All MR scans chosen to the study were performed in FLAIR sequences, in axial plane, with 3 to 5 mm slices using 1,5 Tesla scanner. The study comprised a hundred patients with confirmed diagnosis of MS, including fifty men and fifty women in the age range between 19 and 66 years old and in various stages of the disease. All noticeable changes of the signal intensity within the white matter were considered as demyelinating lesions.

3   Method

Convolutional neural networks are biologically inspired [7] machine learning techniques, where the input has a form of a finite-dimensional linear space range.

They can be treated as a modification of multi-layer perceptron (MLP) with weights sharing and reduced connections between layers. As opposed to MLP, where the permutation of inputs does not influence the training process, in CNN the structure of input data is important and remains unaffected while processing. This and proper weights sharing cause that processing in CNN is translation invariant. Typically in CNN as an input images are given after optional initial preprocessing (scaling, normalization, etc.) [8]. The outputs of the hidden layes are called *feature maps* [9,10] since they the describe actual localization of some image features.

An usual application area of CNN is image classification. A typical approach assumes that CNN performs some reduction of input image size which gives image representation that is later processed by some general-purpose classifier - MLP is preferred here since the whole CNN+MLP architecture can be trained at the same time using gradient based optimization methods [10]. Many of the winning solutions in ImageNet Large Scale Visual Recognition Challenge [11] are based on such architectures [8,12,13]. Some of those solutions were later successfully applied for other image recognition tasks [14]. And although classification is a typical application, there are also research works where CNN acts as a feature extractor [15] or is used directly for object localization [16,17].

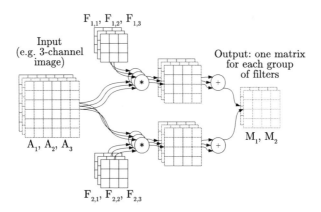

Fig. 1. Structure of the convolutional layer. Sample input matrices A_1, A_2, A_3 are processed with 2 groups of $F_{i,j}$ filters (3 filters in each group). The results produced by each filter group are summed up constituting separate output matrices: M_1, M_2. Image originally published in [18].

Taking into account structure of feature maps, it is possible to define object localization as a task of generating a specific feature map. It requires, however, pure convolutional architecture without a classifier, since it destroys information about spatial structure. Moreover, to obtain such a feature map, which can be easily interpreted as an object localization mask, it must be ensured that input and output dimensions are the same. That is why the approach proposed in this work, instead of reducing the size of feature maps, keeps their dimensions constant. The details and consequences of that approach are described in Sect. 3.2. Thanks to the normalization of the CNN output (e.g. using unipolar sigmoid function), a fuzzy mask is created where the value assigned to each point can be interpreted as a probability of its belonging to the object. Further processing (noise removal, thresholding) leads to a binary mask which is useful in some applications. Our approach to thresholding is described in Sect. 3.3.

3.1   Formal Description

To describe a *convolutional layer*, the basic unit of CNN, let us denote the input data as a tuple of matrices $A_1 \ldots A_p$ of a fixed $n_a \times m_a$ size (for the first layer it could be for example a multi-channel digital image). The key element of the layer are q *filter groups* where each group is a tuple of p matrices of $n_f \times m_f$ size ($F_{i,j}$ for $i = 1 \ldots p$, $j = 1 \ldots q$). The output is a tuple of *feature maps* $M_1 \ldots M_q$ where for each $i = 1 \ldots q$

$$M_i = Z_i + \left(\sum_{j=1}^{p} \right) A_j * F_{i,j}.$$

The Z_i used in the formula above is a bias matrix of the same size as M_i. Matrix convolution $A_j * F_{i,j}$ is a matrix of elements $(A_j * F_{i,j})_{r,c}$ for $r = 1 \ldots (n_a) - (n_f) + 1$, $c = 1 \ldots (m_a) - (m_f) + 1$ such that

$$(A_j * F_{i,j})_{r,c} = \left(\sum_{d_n=0}^{n_f-1} \right) \left(\sum_{d_m=0}^{m_f-1} \right) (F_{i,j})_{(n_f-d_n),(m_f-d_m)} \cdot (A_j)_{(r+d_n),(c+d_m)}.$$

The resulting M_i matrices size is $n_a - n_f + 1 \times m_a - m_f + 1$ (Fig. 1).

Since the output is a tuple of matrices it can be processed by the next convolutional layer. However, since the matric convolution with a fixed $F_{i,j}$ is a linear transformation, it is recommended to apply some non-linear activation function between those layers for every element of the output matrices. Although the sigmoid-like functions are known to work here, it is recommended to use ReLU (rectified linear unit) [8] or PReLU (parametrized extension of ReLU) [19] functions. Additionally, in typical applications, the maximum- or average-pooling layers are used between the convolutional layers. This reduces the matrix dimensions by a certain factor [9]. In our task this would be counterproductive, and that is why such pooling layers are not used.

If the size of filters is other than 1×1, A_j matrices have different size than M_i. To overcome that problem we add zero-padding to the A_j to increase the input size to $(n_a + n_f - 1) \times (m_a + m_f - 1)$. This, of course, does not lead to any information loss since using padding of the proposed size makes it possible to construct the identity operator ($F_{i,j}$ of odd dimensions with 1 in a central element and 0 everywhere else). Moreover, the padding size (adding $(n_f - 1)$

rows and $(m_f - 1)$ columns) is independent from the input size – it is related only to the filter size.

Each element of convolutional layer output is a result of processing some $n_f \times m_f$ rectangle taken from each A_j. For the first feature map, $n_f \times m_f$ is a size of *visual field* [7]. For further layers, the size of visual fields can be easily calculated by tracking down the range of CNN input pixels affecting each output element. Should the network consist of convolutional layers and element-wise operations only, the visual field size would be $n_z \times m_z$ where $n_z = (n_{f_1} + \ldots + n_{f_t}) - t + 1$ and $m_z = (m_{f_1} + \ldots + m_{f_t}) - t + 1$. In these formulas t denotes a number of convolutional layers and $n_{f_w} \times m_{f_w}$ is w-th layer filter size for $w = 1 \ldots t$.

3.2   Detector Training and Usage

The proposed CNN architecture is a superposition of: zero-padding (of a size which will keep the feature map size constant) [20], convolutional layers and element-wise activation functions. Such a network can be trained to associate inputs $A_1 \ldots A_p$ with the resulting maps representing object localization binary masks. Naturally, to obtain satisfactory training results, the neighboring pixels that represent the context of the analysed regions must be also taken into account.

Thanks to the translation invariance of CNN, if the object location on the image changes and context remains sufficient, the proposed solution guarantees that output will be translated as well. It makes application of CNN easier, than it would be for a naive solution which would require techniques such as sliding window.

The advantage of the described approach goes even further than that. Consider image $B_1 \ldots B_p$, similar to $A_1 \ldots A_p$ but of different size. For example $B_1 \ldots B_p$ could be a bigger image including some objects to be detected. If it is used as an input of it can be remarked that still:

– padding and convolution layer keep the image size unchanged, since no parameters depend on input size;
– convolution is possible to calculate as long as feature maps are larger than filters (which is automatically satisfied if B_j are larger than A_j);
– element-wise functions are independent of the map sizes.

Consequently, the output map would still show the proper mask of a detected object [17]. In other words, without any additional utilities – after training on the small samples (which is remarkably faster than processing a big image with a small object) we get an object detector with support of any greater input size, as it is shown in Fig. 2. Detecting multiple objects works out of the box as well. If there is some space between the objects to detect, so the visual fields do not intersect, the process becomes equivalent to the detection of a single object.

Using some context around the object in the training images already prevents CNN from picking any points of the included background, but it leaves the network unprepared for any phenomena that occur only in greater distance

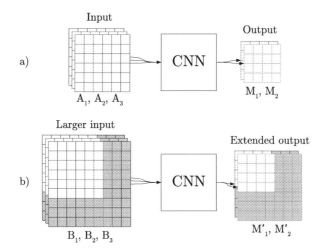

Fig. 2. For each additional row/column of input matrices, you get one more row/column of the output: (a) - the original configuration, (b) - the extended input. In (b) for a rectangle of the same size as A_j matrices results are similar to (a) configuration (it would work in this way for the white pixels of B_j and M'_i). Image originally published in [18].

from the detected objects. In order to avoid such problems with input regions appearing in the bigger image but not present in smaller training samples, the training set should include negative samples as it is described in Sect. 4.1.

3.3   Evaluation

As mentioned above, the size of the feature maps is kept constant from layer to layer in the proposed neural network. We also do not use MLP layers at the output and the goal of the training is regression instead of, as it would be typical for CNNs, image classification. The raw MR scans are put on the CNN input, and we expect the output to take a form of the same-sized image, clearly marking the MS lesions as white regions, surrounded by black, neutral background. In practice, however, the output image will not be truly black-and-white, and the intensity of a given output pixel may be interpreted in terms of the probability that it is a part of a lesion. Therefore, we have to apply thresholding in order to make the final decision and to obtain a black-and-white result that may be directly compared to the expert-generated ground-truth mask.

The value of the threshold $T \in [0,1]$, used for this purpose, determines the standard evaluation measures of a binary classifier: *precision* and *recall*. Low threshold means that many brighter regions of the output image will be interpreted as sufficiently bright to represent demyelinating lesions, thus increasing the recall. For the lowest possible threshold value, $T = 0$, the *whole* image will be regarded as a brain tissue lesion, and hence every actual ground-truth lesion will be marked as properly detected (100% recall). The precision of this detection, however, will be very low. On the other hand, using high value of T will result in the opposite: only the most outstanding regions will be detected as lesions, yielding high precision, but many actual lesions will not have sufficient intensity and they will remain undetected, yielding low recall. Therefore, the frequently applied "balanced" measure of classification efficacy is to compute the harmonic mean of precision and recall, known as the *F-measure*.

In our approach the F-measure is used to find the optimal value of the threshold T. After the training is finished, we threshold the output images (obtained for the input images from the training set) with several values of T, recording the resulting F-measure values. The value of T maximizing the F-measure then becomes the final threshold, which we subsequently use to compute the classification results on a separate set of images (the testing set).

However, it should be noted that the exact method of computation of precision and recall may be defined in various ways. Below we will present 3 approaches that were used in the present study to obtain different evaluations of the classification results.

Per-Pixel Evaluation (PPE). In the first evaluation method we measure the coincidence between the regions detected by the network and the ground-truth annotations by means of simple raw pixel count. For this purpose, we define three sets of pixels – the *true positive* pixels (TP), the *false positive* pixels (FP) and the *false negative* pixels (FN). The pixel at coordinates (x, y) belongs to one of these sets under one of the following conditions:

$$\text{TP} : (I_{thres}(x, y) = 1) \wedge (I_{targ}(x, y) = 1),$$
$$\text{FP} : (I_{thres}(x, y) = 1) \wedge (I_{targ}(x, y) = 0),$$
$$\text{FN} : (I_{thres}(x, y) = 0) \wedge (I_{targ}(x, y) = 1),$$

where I_{thres} and I_{targ} denote the image obtained at the network output (subjected to thresholding) and the target ground-truth image provided by the human expert, respectively. Having computed the number of pixels in each set, the precision and the recall are defined as:

$$\text{precision} = \frac{|\text{TP}|}{|\text{TP}| + |\text{FP}|} = \frac{|\text{TP}|}{|\text{P}|},$$
$$\text{recall} = \frac{|\text{TP}|}{|\text{TP}| + |\text{FN}|} = \frac{|\text{TP}|}{|\text{T}|},$$

where $|\text{X}|$ denotes the cardinality of the set X. The precision is hence defined as the proportion of the number of TP pixels (correctly reported within the lesion areas) to all of the *actually detected* pixels (*positive* pixels, P). Similarly, the recall is the proportion of TP to all the pixels that *should be reported* (*true* pixels, T) [18].

Connected Component Evaluation (CCE). The pixel-based approach described above is straightforward and unambiguous. However, it tends to underestimate the results, even when all the lesions have been properly found, in the case of significant mismatch of their shape or size. Counting pixels seems a bit simplistic here. It is also counterintuitive – we typically want to give more priority to finding the lesions than to marking their exact shape, especially when we consider the limited precision of the manually generated annotations. The conducted experiments revealed that the lesions marked in the output images were often much smaller than expected, due to relatively high values of the threshold T. Naturally, lowering the threshold would make them bigger – and closer in size to the corresponding annotations – but on the cost of generating many false-positive lesions, which would eventually decrease the precision significantly.

Therefore, in order to concentrate more on the number of detected lesions, instead of on the number of pixels, we decided to construct a different evaluation measure on the basis of the connected components (CC) representing regions identified in the thresholded output image and in the target image. Similarly to the pixel-based approach, we define several sets (of connected components in this case) and we compute the proportions of their respective sizes. Four sets are necessary here: the set of all *true* CCs in the ground-truth image (T), the set of all *positive* CCs in the thresholded output image (P), the set of all "matched" true CCs (MT) and the set of all "matched" positive CCs (MP), where the latter two are defined as:

$$MT = \{cc_0 \in T : \exists(cc_1 \in P)\ cc_0 \cap cc_1 \neq \emptyset\},$$
$$MP = \{cc_0 \in P : \exists(cc_1 \in T)\ cc_0 \cap cc_1 \neq \emptyset\}.$$

In other words, the output region is matched if it contains at least one pixel coincident to a lesion region in the ground truth image and similarly for the matched regions in the target image. It should be noted that we need the distinction between MP and MT, because several different CCs in the target image may be matched by a single connected component in the thresholded output image and vice versa. The precision and recall are then defined as:

$$precision = \frac{|MP|}{|P|},$$
$$recall = \frac{|MT|}{|T|}.$$

Region-of-Interest Evaluation (RIE). The CCE approach, as defined above, operates on a higher level of image representation (connected components instead of the pixels). Matching the lesions irrespective of their size and shape seems appealing, but it also has some drawbacks, unfortunately. The problem is that even the smallest regions, including single isolated pixels appearing in the thresholded output image are now considered separate CCs, having equal importance to bigger "visually relevant" regions. This often leads to a significant, yet quite "artificial" increase of the number of the positive regions (P) followed by the drop of the precision value.

In order to overcome this and to make our evaluation more intuitive, we decided to introduce the third evaluation, based on post-processing of the thresholded output images. We aim at defining regions of interest (ROI) within them, so that a single ROI may cover several nearby connected components. This is done in several steps. First, we draw a bounding rectangle around every connected component found in the thresholded output image. Every bounding box is then padded (enlarged) by 10 pixels from all the four sides and this enlarged rectangle is filled with foreground (white) pixels. After that, it is possible, that individual nearby CCs got merged, so we repeat the search of connected components obtaining the final set of detected regions. On this "second-level" representation we compute the standard evaluation measures (precision, recall and F-measure) in the same way as in the CCE approach.

Additionally – for visualization purposes – we draw the bounding rectangle around every of those enlarged and merged "second-level" regions. In this way we obtain a very practical and useful outcome, that may be directly used by a specialist to immediately spot the regions of interest, potentially containing the demyelinating lesions in the MRI scan (Fig. 3).

4   Experiments

4.1   Dataset Preparation

The initial data set consisted of 100 scans from different patients. In order to guarantee the consistent image format, with fixed image resolutions and number of scan levels for each patient, data from 4 scans was discarded. The processed data was split into the set used for training and validation purposes (77 patients) and the test set (19 patients). This means that the evaluation on the test set

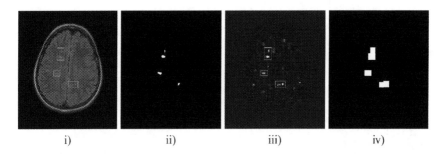

i)   ii)   iii)   iv)

Fig. 3. Illustration of Region-of-Interest Evaluation. From left to right: an input image with the detected regions marked by the bounding rectangles (i), the target ground-truth image (ii), the raw output of the network (before thresholding) with the detected regions marked by the bounding rectangles (iii) and the filled rectangles of the individual connected components (iv).

is based only on the patients that were not known during the stages of weights adaptation and model selection. MR scans taken from the patients were converted to sets digital images, 448×512 pixels each. The scans that contained demyelinating plaques were used in the further processing. This yielded 982 training-and-validation images and 242 test images.

The 982 images selected for training and validation purposes were further processed in order to provide the training set where a significant part of surface consists of the plaques of demyelination. Instead of the whole images, selected 50×50 pixel tiles were used. The objective of this step was to reduce the computational complexity of training when compared to the full-resolution images, since the tile surface is 90 times smaller that the surface of the whole image. What is more, selecting tiles where the demyelinating plaques were overrepresented was intended to prevent the stochastic gradient-based training from reaching the local minima of parameters that yielded "all-zero" results, erroneously indicating that every analyzed scan is completely free of MS symptoms. The initial approach was to use only tiles with centered occurrences of demyelinating plaques. The initial attempts to create the working solution revealed that this method of building the training set does not cover all the phenomena visible in the MRI scans. In the result, bright objects that were underrepresented in the training set, such as skull bones, adipose body of the orbit and paranasal sinuses resulted in falsely-positive labeling of the MS lesions. In order to provide the model that recognizes such cases, additional tiles from the other regions of the scans were included in the training set as well (Figs. 4 and 5).

The selected data sets can be summarized in the following way:

– **Training set** – 7856 tiles of 50×50 size picked from the 982 training-and-validation images. Tiles were selected in a pseudo-random way, but areas with high average brightness or contrast were preferred. Approximately one tile out of three contained only healthy tissues, without demyelinating plaques. In case of MS lesions that were positioned close to the image boundaries, the image was extended appropriately. This data set is used for the weights adaptation in the presented neural networks.
– **"Quasi-validation set"** – 982 full-sized (448×512) images. This set serves similar purpose to the typical validation set, but due to limited amount of labeled data, it is not separate from the training set. It must be emphasized, however, that this set contains remarkably more data than the training set. The quasi-validation set is used for monitoring the learning progress and selection of additional parameters of the final solution, such as threshold level.
– **Test set** – 242 full-sized (448×512) images, separate from all the other data sets not only in terms of images extracted from MRI scans, but in terms of the set of patients that were examined. This set is used only for the final benchmarks of the selected models.

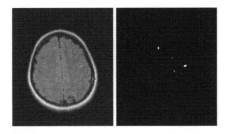

Fig. 4. Example of the MRI scan used in the test set (left) and the corresponding reference demyelinating plaques mask (right).

4.2   CNN Architecture

The structure of the network, i.e. the number of layers, the number of neurons, the size of the receptive fields and the non-linearity types as well as different training procedures were the subject of intensive experiments in the presented study. Three selected solutions are described below.

All the experiments were done with Caffe deep learning framework on a cluster node with Tesla K80M GPU accelerator. The training set of 7856 50×50 tiles was fed to the network in mini-batches of 199 tiles each. The proposed solution is a CNN composed of convolutional layers only (no MLP layers), which makes it behave like an image *filter*, which accepts input images of any size, without any changes to the architecture or the weights. This mechanism was explained in detail in Sect. 3.2. This property makes it possible to calculate mean square error (Euclidean loss) between the network outputs and the ground-truth masks achieved for the full-sized scans ("quasi-validation set"). This error value was used as the indicator of the training progress. The "quasi-validation set" set contained 982 images of 448×512 size from which training tiles were cut.

Basic Architecture. In order to provide a full description of the neural network architecture and the training process, a vast number of parameters needs to be decided manually. The series of trial-and-error attempts lead us to some general remarks about the optimal values of certain parameters. Six convolutional layers make the neural network deep enough to recognize complex objects and allow the back-propagation training to adapt all the weights in the network. Greater amount of consequent layers would make it difficult to train the filters of the initial layers (closer to the data input) because of the vanishing gradient. Standard momentum rate od 0.9 and the learning rate of 0.00001 seem to provide stable and effective training for the selected architecture. Images were processed by the neural network in batches, each containing 199 images to be processed simultaneously.

The specific architecture of the "basic" experiment is illustrated in the diagram 6. The standard approach involved using PReLU (parametric rectified linear units) activation functions between the layers and the unipolar sigmoid

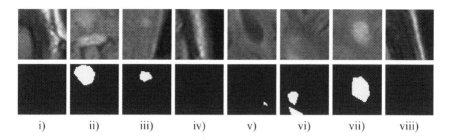

i)   ii)   iii)   iv)   v)   vi)   vii)   viii)

Fig. 5. Example of tiles cut from the training-and validation set (top) with the corresponding lesion masks (bottom). Both tiles and the masks were cut from the full-resolution images of the same format as it was illustrated in Fig. 4. Note, that tiles (i), (iv), (viii) do not contain the lesions. Tiles (i) and (iv), however, present some of the great number of possible big, bright structures that are likely to cause false positives when detecting the lesions.

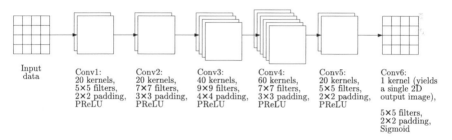

Input data

Conv1:
20 kernels,
5×5 filters,
2×2 padding,
PReLU

Conv2:
20 kernels,
7×7 filters,
3×3 padding,
PReLU

Conv3:
40 kernels,
9×9 filters,
4×4 padding,
PReLU

Conv4:
60 kernels,
7×7 filters,
3×3 padding,
PReLU

Conv5:
20 kernels,
5×5 filters,
2×2 padding,
PReLU

Conv6:
1 kernel (yields
a single 2D
output image),

5×5 filters,
2×2 padding,
Sigmoid

Fig. 6. The sequence of layers used in the convolutional neural network used in the basic architecture.

activation function on the output of the final convolutional layer. The final layer yields a single matrix, which can be later compared to the expected mask with marked demyelinating plaques.

The slow, but stable convergence in terms of mean squared error on quasi-validation set is presented in the top plot of Fig. 7. For as long as 24 millions of image propagations in the training process, the error on the quasi-validation set clearly decreases. The network learns to detect lesions on the training tiles, and the result is general enough to apply to the full-sized images. The minimum of mean squared error is **199.0**.

In order to provide a practical verification of the network effectiveness, the network output was thresholded to obtain the binary image, which can be compared directly to the target mask. The value of the threshold selected in order to maximize the F-measure, as described in Sect. 3.3. It should be noted, however, that the characteristics of the training set, which was composed of small tiles, were so different from the testing set containing the full scans. The appropriate way to select the most useful threshold was to maximize the F-measure on the quasi-validation set.

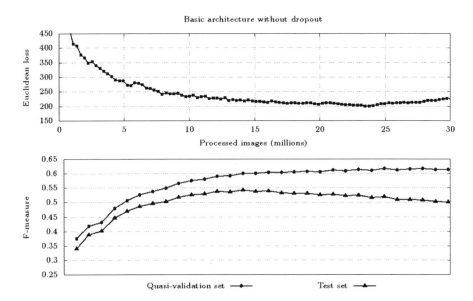

Fig. 7. Training of the basic architecture without dropout. Top: learning curve (Euclidean loss) on quasi-validation set; bottom: F-measure on the quasi-validation set and the testing set. The unit on the horizontal axis corresponds to 10^6 tiles, which were grouped in batches of 199 images.

The maximum F-measure value on the test set is 0.551, but we have no formal way of selecting that exact model. The best F-measure on the quasi-validation set is 0.622, but the corresponding model is visibly overtrained and yields onle 0.496 on the test set. Following the lowest mean squared error would result in selecting a model that yields F-measure values of **0.617** on the quasi-validation set and **0.545** on the test set.

The per-pixel F-measure value observed on the quasi-validation set keeps growing as well, as we can see int he bottom plot of Fig. 7. The second curve presented in that plot, however, describes the dynamics of F-measure on the test set. This result starts decreasing much earlier than the MSE from the top plot – the generalization error becomes visible after processing 14 millions images. The network is apparently getting overtrained, as the result keeps losing its general properties. It must be emphasized, however, that this effect happens only after the whole training set was iterated over for almost 1800 times, which corresponds to ca. 26 h of training.

Basic Architecture with Dropout. The proposed extension to the architecture from the previous section involves a basic application of the dropout mechanism [21]. As it is presented in Fig. 8, the additional layer with $p = 50\%$ dropout probability was added directly before the final convolutional layer. In order to compensate for the reduced amount of data in the training phase

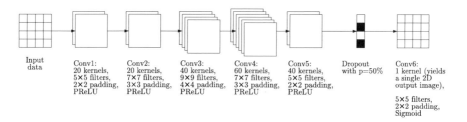

Input
data

Conv1:
20 kernels,
5×5 filters,
2×2 padding,
PReLU

Conv2:
20 kernels,
7×7 filters,
3×3 padding,
PReLU

Conv3:
40 kernels,
9×9 filters,
4×4 padding,
PReLU

Conv4:
60 kernels,
7×7 filters,
3×3 padding,
PReLU

Conv5:
40 kernels,
5×5 filters,
2×2 padding,
PReLU

Dropout
with p=50%

Conv6:
1 kernel (yields
a single 2D
output image),

5×5 filters,
2×2 padding,
Sigmoid

Fig. 8. The sequence of layers used in the convolutional neural network used in the basic architecture with dropout mechanism.

(half of the input values for `Conv6` layer were replaced with zeros), the number of filters in `Conv5` layer was increased twofold. The change involved only one level of the network, so the resulting training speed decrease amounted for only 15% when compared to the basic architecture.

As we can see in the plots from Fig. 9, the effects of network overtraining in the architecture with dropout are remarkably less intense than in the basic architecture. The minimum of minimal square error on the quasi-validation set occurred after ca. 24 millions of image propagations, which is similar to the previous experiment. The rate of error increase in the overtraining stage, however, is much lower than it was without dropout. Similar remark can be observed in the bottom plots of Figs. 7 and 9. The F-measure on the quasi-validation has similar dynamics in both cases. The F-measure on the test set, however, reaches the minimum notably later in case of the model with dropout (after 20 million images instead od 15 million), and does not start to drop as rapidly as it did in the previous experiment. The minimum of mean squared error is **195.7**, which is slightly lower than it was without dropout.

In order to compare the F-measure values to the previous model, we use the model that minimizes the mean square error again. This model, when used with the optimal threshold, generates F-measure values of **0.620** on the quasi-validation set and **0.539** on the test set, which is comparable to the previous experiment.

Improved Architecture. After the series of experiments on Tesla K80M GPU accelerator, the CNN architecture presented in Fig. 10 was proposed. The specific design of this architecture is supposed to take advantage from the fact that larger filters are easier to adapt when they are closer to the network output, because of the vanishing gradient making it difficult to adapt the convolutional layers close th the network input. Similar remark was a reason for increasing the number of filters in the first convolutional layer – since the filters are small and difficult to adapt, using the increased number of randomly-initialized filters is intuitively desirable. What is more, the dropout mechanism was used even more extensively than in the "basic architecture with dropout" – there were two levels of layers where some of the data (30% and 50%, respectively) was dropped out. The architecture with multiple dropouts means increased amount of necessary time

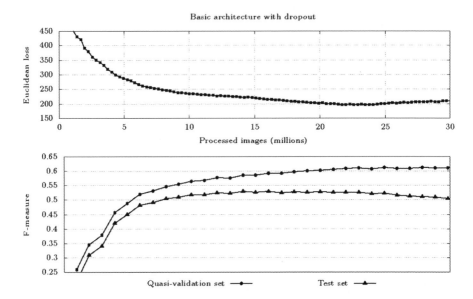

Fig. 9. Training of the basic architecture with dropout. Top: learning curve (Euclidean loss) on quasi-validation set; bottom: F-measure on the quasi-validation set and the testing set. The unit on the horizontal axis corresponds to 10^6 tiles, which were grouped in batches of 199 images.

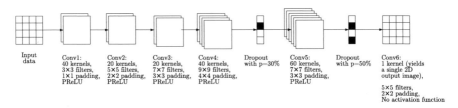

Fig. 10. The sequence of layers used in the convolutional neural network used in the new, improved architecture.

per processed image, which makes the training of this model almost 35% slower than the basic architecture.

The plots presented in Fig. 11, indicate that the general properties are similar to the basic architecture with dropout – the overtraining effects are not nearly as intense as in the basic architecture without dropout, but occur nonetheless. The number of processed images related to the mean square loss and F-measure optima is similar to the basic architecture with dropout as well. The achieved minimum of the mean squared error function, however, is the best amongst the three models, assuming value of **189.5**.

In order to compare the F-measure values to the previous model, we use the model that minimizes the mean square error again. This model, when used with the optimal threshold, generates F-measure values of **0.620** on the

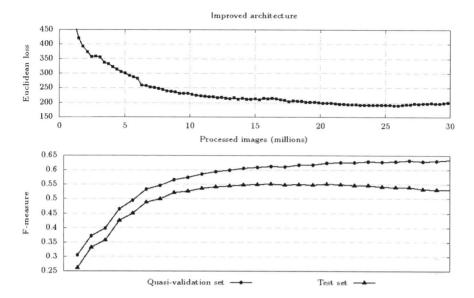

Fig. 11. Training of the improved architecture. Top: learning curve (Euclidean loss) on quasi-validation set; bottom: F-measure on the quasi-validation set and the testing set. The unit on the horizontal axis corresponds to 10^6 tiles, which were grouped in batches of 199 images.

quasi-validation set and **0.542** on the test set. This is apparently slightly better than the basic architecture with dropout, but not necessarily than the basic architecture. The three proposed solutions, despite of the differences, yielded vastly similar F-measure values.

4.3   Threshold Selection

Obtaining the final classification results required thresholding of the raw network output images, as described in Sect. 3.3. The threshold selection was based on the results obtained on the quasi-validation set, which in turn depended both on the network model (basic, basic with dropout, improved) and on the evaluation measure (PPE, CCE, RIE). This generated 9 possible experiment settings, and the threshold was computed for each of them individually. The obtained thresholds were quite similar, although some differences were evident between the pixel-based evaluation scheme and CC-based evaluation scheme (including also RIE). The representative plots are presented in Figs. 12 and 13.

As may be observed, the obtained threshold was higher for the measure based on the connected-components. This may easily be explained, if we consider that in the case of the CCE even a single pixel is enough to have the corresponding ground-truth lesion "matched". We may therefore increase the threshold, removing more pixels (which in the case of the PPE approach would be punished), reducing also the number of false positive regions and boosting the precision in this way.

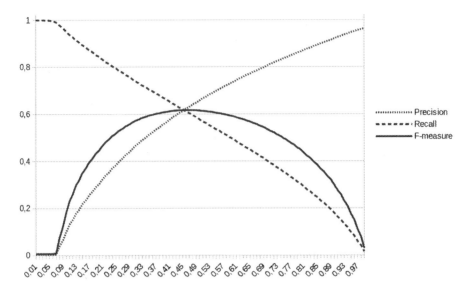

Fig. 12. Threshold selection for the PPE measure.

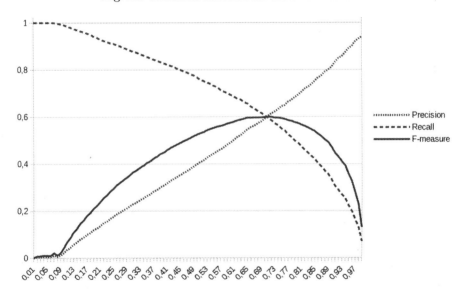

Fig. 13. Threshold selection for the CCE measure.

4.4   Sample Results

The results reported hereby have been obtained on the test set, with the three presented network models (basic, basic with dropout, improved), and the three evaluation methods (PPE, CCE and RIE). The threshold value was computed individually for each of the nine experiment settings on the quasi-validation set, as described above. Table 1 presents the precision, recall and F-measure values for all the three network architectures and the PPE evaluation scheme. Similarly, Tables 2 and 3 show the results for the connected-component-based approaches. It should be noted the reported numbers of pixels and regions are counted across the whole test dataset (292 images).

Table 1. Experiment 1 (PPE) – the results.

Model	Threshold	T	P	TP	Precision (TP/P)	Recall (TP/T)	F-measure
Basic	0.46	143207	150444	80045	0.5321	0.5589	0.5452
Basic + Dropout	0.54	143207	148367	78595	0.5297	0.5488	0.5391
Improved	0.51	143207	156686	81362	0.5193	0.5681	0.5426

The results are generally quite similar, in terms of the obtained F-measure values. Interestingly, the evaluation scheme involving the connected components introduces only very small improvement over the pixel-based approach, although it is based on completely different assumptions. Only the region-based method is quite significantly better, exceeding 60%, probably due to the additional enlargement and merging of the connected components.

Table 2. Experiment 2 (CCE) – the results.

Model	Threshold	T	P	MT	MP	Precision (MP/P)	Recall (MT/T)	F-measure
Basic	0.71	1022	1319	605	711	0.5390	0.5920	0.5643
Basic + Dropout	0.77	1022	1341	620	704	0.5250	0.6067	0.5629
Improved	0.74	1022	1416	615	709	0.5008	0.6018	0.5466

Table 3. Experiment 3 (RIE) – the results.

Model	Threshold	T	P	MT	MP	Precision (MP/P)	Recall (MT/T)	F-measure
Basic	0.71	1022	912	675	514	0.5636	0.6605	0.6082
Basic + Dropout	0.78	1022	910	664	501	0.5505	0.6497	0.5960
Improved	0.75	1022	976	666	504	0.5164	0.6517	0.5762

Example images where the quality of lesion detection was remarkably good (Table 5), remarkably poor (Table 7) and acceptably successful (Table 4) were presented in the tables that consist of: the input image, the demyelinating plaques mask (ground-truth annotations), and the results of all the three neural networks presented in this paper. Additionally, the successful image, which can be considered easy in terms of lesion labeling, is used to demonstrate that the presented methods need to be intelligent even in order to solve the simplest tasks. Simple thresholding can be considered as an alternate method of marking "bright, important points" in the image. However, when compared to the neural network, such a simplistic attitude is likely to act remarkably poor, as it is shown in Table 6.

Table 4. Example image: acceptable detection of multiple small demyelination plaques.

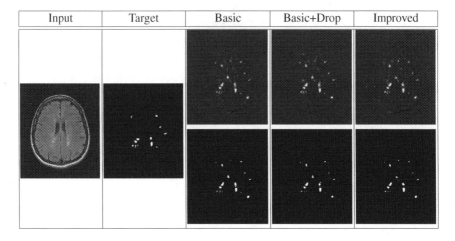

Table 5. Example image: remarkably successful detection in case of all models.

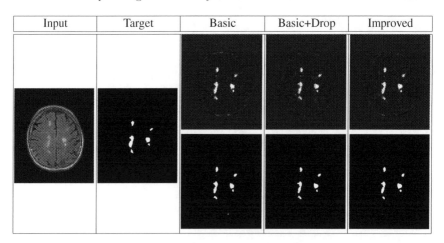

Table 6. Successful detection compared to simple thresholding.

Target	Improved	Threshold 50%	Threshold 55%	Threshold 60%

Table 7. Example image: selected difficult case.

Input	Target	Basic	Basic+Drop	Improved

5   Analysis

The sample results shown in the previous section are intended to demonstrate the general possibilities of CNNs application for the image detection task. The detection of typical demyelinating lesions was successful often enough to consider the achieved results promising. It must be emphasized that the ability to detect the demyelinating plaques is not only based on their intensity, but on their shape and the characteristics of the surrounding tissue as well. This property can be illustrated by the comparison of the results from Tables 5 and 6, where the same sample is processed with the proposed neural network and with a simple threshold operator.

It can be observed that the threshold of 50% is too low to detect only the lesions, as it marks some other points between the cerebral hemispheres as well. Higher threshold values, however, result in heavily reducing (55%) or totally omitting (60%) one of the lesions. At the same time, even the threshold level of 60% is not sufficient to ignore the skull. Convolutional neural networks, however, have no problem with labeling all of the demyelinating lesions contained in this sample and with ignoring the skull. This specific sample is, apparently, easy enough to process by all the proposed models.

The general result of F-measure remaining around the range of 55%–60% even in the most optimal of the presented solutions is sufficient to be considered useful, yet far from the perfect outcome. The reasons for this can be investigated in more detail in order to formulate possible ways to improve this result.

One of the problems is related to the structures such as bones and meninges being the sources of false positives. As it was described in Sect. 4.1, the problem can be partially addressed by extending the training set with additional samples where no demyelinating plaques are present, and the average brightness and contrast are relatively high. As it was shown in Tables 5 and 4, omitting the skull is a simple problem. Structures such as eyes, which are present only in some of the scans, are more likely to cause problems. Scans close to the top of the skull are difficult to process as well, as the bones of the calvaria are not perpendicular to the projection plane. This special case makes the bones appear too thick to be properly recognized as unrelated to the lesions – example of this phenomenon is visible in Fig. 5.

One of the possible solutions is to increase the number of training samples containing such structures, in order to make the network train directly to solve the task of recognizing them. Another remedy worth considering would be to increase the size of tiles. The 50×50 images that are included in the training set are insufficient to contain some of the brain tissues with enough context to train the CNN to ignore the bright regions of great surface, such as eyes. Both suggested solutions lead to increase of the overall area of training data unrelated to the lesions. This property is, however, undesirable – it makes the network more likely to learn to generate plain black output images. The "all-zero" outputs are usually related to the local minimum of the cost function used in the learning process. The greater the percentage of black points in the reference output is, the more difficult it is to force the network to do anything else. More promising direction is therefore to use some external tools to remove the irrelevant parts of the input MR scans. Some automatic or semi-automatic solution can be applied prior to the training and testing with CNN-based solutions. Such an approach would make the whole solution less universal, but it would let the CNN concentrate on the cerebral tissue only – and that is where we are expected to find MS lesions.

Another problem that has proven to have negative influence on the obtained results is the quality and quantity of the collected scans. The training set is small, and in order to use as much data as possible, the quasi-validation set was not separate from the training set. Greater number of patients in the database would be likely to improve not only the result, but the overall possibility to use the most proper experimental methods as well. The remark on quality of the data set is related to the visibility of some of the lesions. While the most of the demyelinating plaques are clearly visible in the scans, there are many small or very faint lesions present in the scans as well. Lesions like that are likely to pose problems in the task of unequivocal identification as MS plaques. The problems with overtraining and generalization, indicated in Figs. 7, 8, 9, 10 and 11 suggests that it would be advantageous to use a significantly bigger set of the training images. More consistent standards of image annotation, perhaps involving several independent specialists, would undoubtedly improve the quality of the data set as well.

Yet another issue worth mentioning is related to the precision of defining the actual shape of the lesions by human annotators. It must be emphasized, that in terms of per-pixel F-measure, even if all the lesions were properly detected in the output image, the size and shape provided by the neural network is likely to differ from the ground-truth mask. This issue was partially solved by the connected component-based approach presented in this paper. The suggested approach to splitting/joining of adjacent lesions is still dependent on the size of the plaques suggested by the human annotator, but it is a notable step towards the more credible quality measure of the suggested solutions.

6   Conclusions and Future Work

Diagnosis of the MS requires careful and time-consuming analysis of the brain MRI scans. The final interpretation and decision about the treatment always belongs to the human expert with appropriate medical knowledge. This process, however, can be assisted with an automatic tool which is prepared with the techniques of machine learning. The phenomenon of "demyelinating plaques" that are visible in the MRI scans is precisely defined and well known to the radiology specialists, but it is difficult to imagine any explicit, concise mathematical formula that describes a plaque. The presented work is intended to provide the best possible suggestions that can be obtained with the convolutional neural networks.

The data set used in this paper consisted of MRI scans of 100 patients. The groups was intended to be representative, so it included patients from different age groups. Multiple slices from each MRI scans were stored in digital images of relatively high resolution, which is 448×512 pixels. Images of that size were cut into 50×50 for the purpose of CNN training. Multiple neural network models proposed in this paper were trained from scratch, starting with randomly initialized filter contents. Due to the specific architecture which was based solely on convolutional layers, the solution was able to process images of different sizes, as it was described in Sect. 3.2. This means that the network trained with 50×50 tiles could be used for full-resolution 448×512 images without any changes to the architecture or the weights that were achieved through the network training.

One of the goals of this paper was to analyse alternative methods of evaluation of the classification results. In addition to the approach used in previous works [18], based on counting individual pixels, two additional methods have been tested in the present study. Analysis of the connected components brought about a very moderate increase of the reported results, while defining the regions of interest from the enlarged and merged connected components enabled to present the detected areas of demyelination in a potentially useful and visually appealing way.

The best results in terms of per-pixel F-measure were close to the 55% on the test set. While this result is not perfect, it can be considered as sufficient to get the general location of the most of the plaques, which is already useful when the task of diagnosis assistance is considered. The expected masks used in both training and evaluation of the neural networks consisted of polygons, which were marked approximately by the medical specialists. Repeating the same polygon shapes is virtually impossible – either for the neural network or for another expert. Some of the significant sources of errors were related to the large bright areas resulting in the false positives. This includes temporal bones and optic nerves. Another common source of errors was related to the small regions of noise that were erroneously detected as demyelinating plaques. Additional consideration was devoted to the points that were detected in a general area of the MS lesions – the proposed modifications to the measure of the object detection quality provides us with some deeper insight into the results analysis.

The obtained result is promising, but the further room for improvement remains apparent. The crucial room for improvement is related to the data set size – greater number of training samples, covering better variety of cases, would be likely to improve the result. The selected size of the training samples, which is 50×50, is another parameter that might require further discussion. Larger tile size would make it easier to include the whole temporal bones and optic nerves in the training samples. Greater tile size, however, makes the training additionally difficult, because generating plain black outputs becomes a remarkable local minimum of the neural network cost function. This problem can be addressed either by cost function modification or manual region growing on the expected outputs that would increase the number of white points. Alternatively, the irrelevant parts of the input images – namely, everything but the cerebral tissue – can be removed manually by the separate tool.

The general field of the CNNs application for the medical image processing is usually affected by the difficulty with collecting the sufficient data sets. Unsurprisingly, this problem is visibly present in our work as well. Our analysis, however, can be considered as an initial step towards even more efficient solutions. Object localization based solely on convolutional layers, dynamic threshold selection, and detailed description of the results involving F-measure and connected components are some ideas, that – when used together – form an elegant solution that can be applied to the great diversity of object localization problems.

Another way to improve the proposed method is to involve some well-known pretrained CNN models instead of starting from the random weights. Neural networks such as AlexNet [8] or VGG [22] consist of carefully trained weights that are known to be useful in detection and classification of multiple normal, real life objects. The mentioned networks are usually used as classifiers, but application to the scale-preserving object localization solution is possible as well. Using parts of the network with maximum-pooling layers is not necessarily impossible in this task – the problem of restoring original resolution can be addressed with techniques such as deconvolutional neural networks [12].

Acknowledgements. This project has been partly funded with support from National Science Centre, Republic of Poland, decision number DEC-2012/05/D/ST6/03091.

Authors would like to express their gratitude to the Department of Radiology of Barlicki University Hospital in Lodz for making head MRI sequences available.

References

1. Tomczyk, A., Spurek, P., Podgórski, M., Misztal, K., Tabor, J.: Detection of elongated structures with hierarchical active partitions and CEC-based image representation. In: Burduk, R., Jackowski, K., Kurzyński, M., Woźniak, M., Żołnierek, A. (eds.) Proceedings of the 9th International Conference on Computer Recognition Systems CORES 2015. AISC, vol. 403, pp. 159–168. Springer, Cham (2016). https://doi.org/10.1007/978-3-319-26227-7_15

2. Tomczyk, A., Szczepaniak, P.S.: Adaptive potential active contours. Pattern Anal. Appl. **14**, 425–440 (2011)

3. de Brebisson, A., Montana, G.: Deep Neural Networks for Anatomical Brain Segmentation. ArXiv e-prints arXiv:1502.02445 (2015)

4. Shelhamer, E., Long, J., Darrell, T.: Fully Convolutional Networks for Semantic Segmentation. ArXiv e-prints arXiv:1605.06211 (2016)

5. Milletari, F., Navab, N., Ahmadi, S.A.: V-Net: Fully Convolutional Neural Networks for Volumetric Medical Image Segmentation. ArXiv e-prints arXiv:1606.04797 (2016)

6. Ronneberger, O., Fischer, P., Brox, T.: U-Net: Convolutional Networks for Biomedical Image Segmentation. ArXiv e-prints arXiv:1505.04597 (2015)

7. Hubel, D.H., Wiesel, T.N.: Receptive fields and functional architecture in two nonstriate visual areas (18 and 19) of the cat. J. Neurophysiol. **28**, 229–289 (1965)

8. Krizhevsky, A., Sutskever, I., Hinton, G.E.: ImageNet classification with deep convolutional neural networks. In: Pereira, F., Burges, C.J.C., Bottou, L., Weinberger, K.Q. (eds.) Advances in Neural Information Processing Systems 25, pp. 1097–1105. Curran Associates, Inc. (2012)

9. LeCun, Y., Bengio, Y.: Convolutional networks for images, speech, and time-series. In: Arbib, M.A. (ed.) The Handbook of Brain Theory and Neural Networks. MIT Press, Cambridge (1995)

10. Cireşan, D.C., Meier, U., Masci, J., Gambardella, L.M., Schmidhuber, J.: Flexible, high performance convolutional neural networks for image classification. In: Proceedings of the Twenty-Second International Joint Conference on Artificial Intelligence, IJCAI 2011, vol. 2, pp. 1237–1242. AAAI Press (2011)

11. Deng, J., Dong, W., Socher, R., Li, L.J., Li, K., Fei-Fei, L.: ImageNet: a large-scale hierarchical image database. In: CVPR 2009 (2009)

12. Zeiler, M.D., Fergus, R.: Visualizing and understanding convolutional networks. CoRR abs/1311.2901 (2013)

13. Nguyen, T.V., Lu, C., Sepulveda, J., Yan, S.: Adaptive nonparametric image parsing. CoRR abs/1505.01560 (2015)

14. Cheng, G., Zhou, P., Han, J.: Learning rotation-invariant convolutional neural networks for object detection in VHR optical remote sensing images. IEEE Trans. Geosci. Remote Sens. **54**, 7405–7415 (2016)

15. Mopuri, K.R., Babu, R.V.: Object level deep feature pooling for compact image representation. CoRR abs/1504.06591 (2015)

16. Matsugu, M., Mori, K., Mitari, Y., Kaneda, Y.: Subject independent facial expression recognition with robust face detection using a convolutional neural network. Neural Netw. **16**, 555–559 (2003)

17. Dai, J., He, K., Sun, J.: Convolutional feature masking for joint object and stuff segmentation. CoRR abs/1412.1283 (2014)

18. Stasiak, B., Tarasiuk, P., Michalska, I., Tomczyk, A., Szczepaniak, P.: Localization of demyelinating plaques in MRI using convolutional neural networks. In: Proceedings of the 10th International Joint Conference on Biomedical Engineering Systems and Technologies (BIOSTEC 2017), BIOIMAGING, vol. 2, pp. 55–64. SCITEPRESS (2017)
19. He, K., Zhang, X., Ren, S., Sun, J.: Delving deep into rectifiers: surpassing human-level performance on ImageNet classification. CoRR abs/1502.01852 (2015)
20. LeCun, Y., Bottou, L., Bengio, Y., Haffner, P.: Gradient-based learning applied to document recognition. In: Proceedings of the IEEE, pp. 2278–2324 (1998)
21. Srivastava, N., Hinton, G., Krizhevsky, A., Sutskever, I., Salakhutdinov, R.: Dropout: a simple way to prevent neural networks from overfitting. J. Mach. Learn. Res. **15**, 1929–1958 (2014)
22. Simonyan, K., Zisserman, A.: Very deep convolutional networks for large-scale image recognition. CoRR abs/1409.1556 (2014)

Bioinformatics Models, Methods and Algorithms

Compositional Analysis of Homeostasis of Gene Networks by Clustering Algorithms

Sohei Ito[1(✉)], Kenji Osari[2], Shigeki Hagihara[3], and Naoki Yonezaki[4]

[1] National Fisheries University, Shimonoseki, Japan
ito@fish-u.ac.jp
[2] Yahoo Japan Corporation, Tokyo, Japan
[3] Tohoku University of Community Service and Science, Sakata, Japan
[4] Tokyo Denki University, Inzai, Japan

Abstract. In this work we present a compositional approach to qualitatively analyse homeostasis of gene networks. The problem of analysing homeostasis of gene networks is 2EXPTIME-complete in the sizes of the network specifications. Due to this high complexity of the problem, only small networks consisting of a few genes were successfully analysed. Since the analysis of homeostasis of gene networks is based on the technique of *realisability* checking of Linear Temporal Logic formulae, we can apply a compositional algorithm devised to mitigate the computational difficulty in realisability problems. For this, we develop a clustering algorithm to divide network specifications in suitable sizes to utilise the compositional algorithm. We report the experimental results of analyses of homeostasis of several gene networks with our proposed method. Our experiments show a fair improvement especially in the analyses of larger networks.

Keywords: Gene regulatory network · Systems biology
Homeostasis · Temporal logic · Realisability · Formal method

1 Introduction

Homeostasis of biological systems is an important property of life. This property emerges from the elaborate interaction among several components in cells. To understand the mechanisms of homeostasis, therefore, we should investigate not only individual components but also how they work in collaboration with other components. The latter research discipline is called *systems biology*.

There are two paradigms in systems biology - qualitative and quantitative - to model target biological systems. Quantitative approaches enable us analysing real-valued properties such as response times or predicting a time-series of concentration values of a certain molecular species. However, the quantitative parameters to construct such precise model are not commonly available. In qualitative approaches, we cannot analyse such real-valued properties. Instead, it can be applied to biological systems with incomplete information under parameter uncertainty, which are common in most of organisms.

© Springer International Publishing AG, part of Springer Nature 2018
N. Peixoto et al. (Eds.): BIOSTEC 2017, CCIS 881, pp. 191–211, 2018.
https://doi.org/10.1007/978-3-319-94806-5_11

The authors have developed qualitative framework to model and analyse gene networks [15,16]. In our framework, gene networks are represented as logical specifications that constrain their possible behaviours. Since behaviours of gene networks are formally modelled as infinite sequences of sets of propositions, the logical constraints are given in Linear Temporal Logic (LTL) [8]. This framework is closely connected to the paradigm of verification of *reactive system* specifications. Thanks to this close connection, we formulated homeostasis of gene networks as the *realisability* in reactive system specifications and analysed homeostasis of some gene networks using realisability checkers [11,13].

The computational complexity of realisability problem for LTL is known to be quite expensive: 2EXPTIME-complete in the size of a formula [1,21]. In our framework, the size of specification of a gene network is proportional to the size of a network. This indicates that only modest size of gene networks can be successfully analysed of their homeostasis. To tackle this issue, there are two possibilities - one is to approximately analyse the homeostasis, which was reported in our previous work [12]. The other is to utilise compositional approach in which a logical specification is divided into several sub-specifications and are analysed individually. The final outcome is obtained by merging the results of each sub-specification. One of promising compositional method for realisability problem is developed by Filiot et al. [10].

The non-trivial problem in compositional analysis is how to divide a formula, which is critical to the performance of analysis. Therefore, in this paper, we present a method for dividing the logical specifications of gene networks so that the compositional method will be effective. Our approach is to develop a new clustering algorithm which divides clauses (a piece of formula) into clusters based on a 'score' which evaluates how good the clustering is. We demonstrate our approach by analysing homeostasis of several gene networks varying in size.

The rest of the paper is organised as follows. Section 2 introduces LTL and reviews how we model gene networks in LTL. Section 3 introduces how we formulate the notion of homeostasis using *realisability* of reactive system specifications. Section 4 introduces the compositional analysis of realisability. We show how we divide a network specifications to compositionally analyse homeostasis. Section 5 shows and discusses the experimental results of compositional analysis. In Sect. 6, we discuss related work. Section 7 offers conclusion and discusses some future directions.

This work is the extended version of the authors' previous work [17] in the sense that the paper structure is reorganised, the algorithm is modified and the analysis of experimental results are augmented and the new experimental data are presented.

2 Qualitative Framework for Modelling and Analysing Gene Networks Using Linear Temporal Logic

A gene network is represented as a directed graph whose nodes and edges (labelled by $+/-$) represent genes and regulation relations (activation/inhibition) among them, respectively. In Fig. 1 we show an example of a

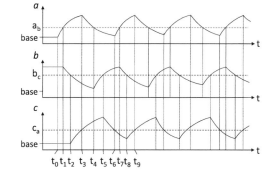

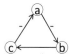

Fig. 1. Simple circadian clock. The transcription product of gene a inhibits gene b, gene b similarly inhibits gene c and finally gene c inhibits gene a. This network produces periodic expression pattern of each gene.

Fig. 2. Time series of expression levels of gene a, b and c in the network Fig. 1.

gene regulatory network which is known as a circadian clock [7]. A behaviour of a gene network is represented as a time series of expression profiling of the genes in the network. Figure 2 shows an example time series of the network Fig. 1. In this behaviour the value a_b is the threshold level of gene a to inhibit gene b, b_c the threshold level of gene b to inhibit gene c and c_a the threshold level of gene c to inhibit gene a. At the beginning, only gene b is expressed. At time t_0, gene a begins to be expressed and its expression level begins to grow. At time t_1 gene a crosses the threshold a_b, thus gene b becomes OFF due to the negative effect from gene a. At time t_2 the expression level of gene b falls below b_c, thus gene c begins to be expressed since the negative effect from gene b is stopped. Then gene c is expressed beyond the level c_a at time t_3, and gene a becomes OFF and finally falls below a_b at time t_4. Thus gene b begins to be expressed and crosses the level b_c at time t_5, then gene c becomes OFF. At time t_6 gene c falls below c_a, and gene a begins to be expressed. In this way, each gene is periodically expressed.

Our start point is to symbolically represent a time series of a behaviour of a gene network. In the above verbal expression of the behaviour, there are a few facts which we used to describe the behaviour – whether each gene is expressed or not (ON or OFF) and whether the expression level of each gene is beyond the threshold. To represent such atomic facts, we introduce the following propositions.

- on_a, on_b, on_c: whether genes a, b and c are ON or OFF respectively.
- a_b, b_c, c_a: whether the expression level of gene a, b and c are beyond the threshold a_b, b_c and c_a respectively[1].

---

[1] Threshold values are written in roman while propositions are written in italics.

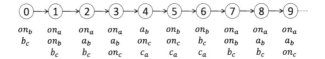

Fig. 3. Symbolic representation of the time series of Fig. 2.

We can use these propositions to capture a state of the gene network, e.g. between time t_1 and t_2 the propositions $\{on_a, a_b, b_c\}$ are true, which means that gene a is ON, gene a is expressed beyond a_b and gene b is expressed beyond b_c (but gene b is OFF). Using these propositions, we now have the symbolic representation of the behaviour as depicted in Fig. 3 which consists of states (represented as circle) and transitions (represented as arrows). The propositions listed below the states represent the facts that are true in the states. We call this symbolic representation of a behaviour as *linear time structure*. We easily see that state 0 represents the state of the network at the beginning, state 1 represents the state between t_0 and t_1, state 2 between t_1 and t_2, and so on.

In general, there are many behaviours which can be produced by a single network. Our purpose is to analyse a biological property for a given gene network, e.g. whether the network can produce the behaviour in which gene a, b and c oscillate. To solve this problem, we must characterise the set of possible behaviours and check that a certain behaviour (e.g. genes oscillate) is contained in the possible behaviours. To characterise (or model) the behaviours of a network, we need some mathematical representation. In quantitative approach, ordinary differential equations (ODEs) are widely used. In the current setting, we do not handle a numerical time series but a symbolic time series of a behaviour (a linear time structure). To characterise and reason about such structures, linear temporal logic (LTL) is the suitable mathematical language. LTL can be seen as propositional logic equipped with temporal operators such as G (Globally), F (Future) and U (Until). $G\phi$ means ϕ is always true, $F\phi$ means ϕ is eventually true, and $\phi U \psi$ means ϕ is true until ψ is true. The formal syntax and semantics are shown in Appendix A.

We are to characterise the set of possible behaviours (linear time structures) for a given network. This can be done by specifying an LTL formula ϕ_G for a given network G such that the set of possible behaviours of a network is characterised as $\{\sigma \mid \sigma \models \phi_G\}$, i.e. all linear structures which satisfy the behaviour specification ϕ_G. The problem of analysing network behaviours, e.g. checking whether there is a behaviour which satisfies a certain property ψ (also written in LTL), can be solved by finding σ such that $\sigma \models \phi_G \wedge \psi$, i.e. checking *satisfiability* of the formula $\phi_G \wedge \psi$. Thus analysing a gene network is reduced to satisfiability checking of LTL. Once we have a formula $\phi_G \wedge \psi$, the analysis can be automatically done by LTL satisfiability checkers.

Now the question: how do we specify ϕ_G which characterises possible behaviours of a given network G? The key idea is the following qualitative principles of gene network behaviours:

- A gene is ON when its activators are expressed beyond some thresholds.
- A gene is OFF when its inhibitors are expressed beyond some thresholds.
- If a gene is ON, its expression level increases.
- If a gene is OFF, its expression level decreases.

By expressing these principles in LTL, we have a characterisation of possible behaviours of a gene network.

First we determine the set of atomic propositions AP for a given network. As we have seen in the network of Fig. 1, we have the propositions $on_x, on_y, \ldots$ for each gene $x, y, \ldots$ that mean whether genes $x, y, \ldots$ are ON or OFF, respectively. In addition, for each threshold x_i of each gene x, we have the propositions x_i that means whether the expression level of gene x exceeds the threshold x_i.

A timing when a gene becomes ON or OFF depends on its regulator genes. Positive regulators activate its expression and negative regulators inhibit its expression. For example, let us consider that gene x has three regulators – gene u and v as the activators and gene w as the inhibitor. Considering the meaning of activation and inhibition, if gene u and v exceeds the threshold u_x and v_x respectively, and gene w is not expressed over w_x, gene x will be ON. Similarly, if gene w exceeds the threshold w_x, and neither gene u nor gene y is expressed beyond the thresholds, gene x will be OFF. These constraints are described in LTL as:

$$G(u_x \wedge v_x \wedge \neg w_x \rightarrow on_x),$$
$$G(\neg u_x \wedge \neg v_x \wedge w_x \rightarrow \neg on_x).$$

What about the case that both activators and inhibitors are effective? If we know a special bias that the inhibition prevails the activation, that knowledge is easily described as $G(w_x \rightarrow \neg on_x)$, which means that only the fact that w_x is true is sufficient to turn gene x off. For the case that the activation prevails the inhibition, we can handle the case similarly. If we do not assume any bias, we do not need to add any clause, i.e. gene x can be ON or OFF in that case.

If a gene is ON, its expression level increases over time. To express this fact, we use propositions for the expression levels of a gene. Suppose that gene x has three thresholds x_1, x_2 and x_3 in this order. This order relation can be described in LTL as follows:

$$G(x_3 \rightarrow x_2) \wedge G(x_2 \rightarrow x_1).$$

Recall that the proposition x_3 means that gene x is expressed *beyond* the level x_3, and since x_3 is greater than x_2, gene x is expressed beyond x_2, i.e. proposition x_2 is true. Similarly, if gene x exceeds x_2, it also exceeds x_1.

The increase of expression levels when gene x is ON can be described as:

$$G(on_x \rightarrow F(x_1 \vee \neg on_x)), \tag{1}$$
$$G(on_x \wedge x_1 \rightarrow (x_1 W \neg on_x)), \tag{2}$$
$$G(on_x \wedge x_2 \rightarrow (x_2 W \neg on_x)), \tag{3}$$
$$G(on_x \wedge x_3 \rightarrow (x_3 W \neg on_x)). \tag{4}$$

Formula (1) corresponds to the case that the current expression level of gene x is basal. Then, gene x will exceed x_1 in a future, otherwise gene x will become OFF. Formula (2) corresponds to the case that the level is beyond x_1, which means 'if gene x is ON and the current expression level of gene x is above x_1, gene x *at least* keeps its level as long as gene x is ON'. Since this formula only prohibits that the expression level of gene x falls down below x_1 even though gene x is expressed, it is possible for gene x to attain the next level x_2 in some future. Thus, by this formula, we ensure that the level of gene x will increase (or keep its level) when gene x is expressed. Formulas (3) and (4) are similar to Formula (2). Note that, in formula (4), since the maximum level of gene x is x_3, it only says that gene x will keep its level as long as gene x is ON.

If a gene is OFF, its expression level decreases over time. We have the symmetric formulae to the above:

$$G(\neg on_x \rightarrow F(\neg x_3 \vee on_x)),$$
$$G(\neg on_x \wedge \neg x_3 \rightarrow (\neg x_3 W on_x)),$$
$$G(\neg on_x \wedge \neg x_2 \rightarrow (\neg x_2 W on_x)),$$
$$G(\neg on_x \wedge \neg x_1 \rightarrow (\neg x_1 W on_x)).$$

Behaviour specification ϕ_G for a given network G is the conjunction of all the clauses obtained from the above rules for each gene in G.

Example 1. For a network depicted in Fig. 1, we introduce the set of propositions $\{on_a,\ on_b,\ on_c,\ a_b,\ b_c,\ c_a\}$. Using these propositions, we have the following behaviour specification.

$$G(a_b \leftrightarrow \neg on_b) \wedge G(b_c \leftrightarrow \neg on_c) \wedge G(c_a \leftrightarrow \neg on_a)\wedge$$
$$G(on_a \rightarrow F(a_b \vee \neg on_a)) \wedge G(on_a \wedge a_b \rightarrow (a_b W \neg on_a))\wedge$$
$$G(\neg on_a \rightarrow F(\neg a_b \vee on_a)) \wedge G(\neg on_a \wedge \neg a_b \rightarrow (\neg a_b W on_a)) \wedge \ldots.$$

For this network let us check the property 'each gene oscillates', which is written in LTL as:

$$G(F on_a) \wedge G(F \neg on_a) \wedge G(F on_b) \wedge G(F \neg on_b) \wedge G(F on_c) \wedge G(F \neg on_c).$$

We check the satisfiability of the conjunction of the above formulae. We used T^3-builder [2] to check it and had the answer 'Yes'. Thus we formally analysed that the circadian clock of Fig. 1 surely oscillates.

3   Formulating Homeostasis with Realisability

In this section we present[2] how we formulate homeostasis of a gene network by the notion of realisability [20].

---

[2] The definition is based on our previous publication [11].

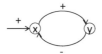

Fig. 4. A gene network consisting of two genes x and y. Gene x receives positive input from environment. (Source: [17]).

First we introduce reactive systems and realisability. A *reactive system* is defined as a triple $\langle X, Y, r \rangle$, where X is a set of events caused by the environment, Y is a set of events caused by the system and $r : (2^X)^+ \rightarrow 2^Y$ is a reaction function. The set $(2^X)^+$ denotes the set of all finite sequences on subsets of X, that is to say, finite sequences on a set of environmental events. Let $AP = X \cup Y$ be a set of atomic propositions. We denote a time structure σ on AP as $\langle x_0, y_0 \rangle \langle x_1, y_1 \rangle \ldots$ where $x_i \subseteq X$, $y_i \subseteq Y$ and $\sigma[i] = x_i \cup y_i$. Let φ be an LTL specification. We say $\langle X, Y, \varphi \rangle$ is *realisable* if there exists a reactive system $RS = \langle X, Y, r \rangle$ such that

$$\forall \tilde{x}. behave_{RS}(\tilde{x}) \models \varphi,$$

where $\tilde{x} \in (2^X)^\omega$ and $behave_{RS}(\tilde{x})$ is the infinite behaviour determined by RS, that is,

$$behave_{RS}(\tilde{x}) = \langle x_0, y_0 \rangle \langle x_1, y_1 \rangle \ldots,$$

where $\tilde{x} = x_0 x_1 \ldots$ and $y_i = r(x_0 \ldots x_i)$.

Intuitively, a specification φ is realisable if for any sequence of external events there exists a system which controls its internal events such that its behaviour satisfies the specification φ.

Now we consider the homeostasis of gene networks. Homeostasis is informally stated as the tendency of a system to maintain its internal condition desirable against any situation or stimulus. In other words, the problem of analysing homeostasis of a gene network is to check whether a network satisfies a given property against *any external input sequence*. The purpose of this section is to present a formal definition for this problem.

A gene network can be regarded as reactive systems, since it reacts to external inputs (e.g. from environment or other cells) and determines its internal states.

In Sect. 2, we show how we specify possible behaviours of a given network in LTL. Then we can regard behaviour specification of a network (say φ) as a reactive system specification. Thus a gene network behaves according to the specification φ in reaction to external inputs. To consider a gene network as a reactive system, we also need to divide the propositions occurring in φ into internal propositions (i.e. output propositions) and external propositions (i.e. input propositions). For example, let us consider the example network depicted in Fig. 4.

In this network, gene x accepts positive inputs from environment. To capture this, we introduce two propositions in_x and e_x. The proposition in_x represents whether the input is coming to gene x. The proposition e_x represents whether the level of the input is beyond the threshold e_x above which gene x is activated. As a result, we have the following propositions: $\{in_x, on_x, on_y, e_x, x_y, y_x\}$. The division of external propositions E and internal propositions I is as follows: $E = \{in_x\}$, $I = \{on_x, on_y, e_x, x_y, y_x\}$. Note that the environment only controls in_x, which means that the environment is only able to determine whether it inputs to gene x or not. Whether the level of the input exceeds the level e_x is determined by the behaviour specification. Thus e_x is internal propositions. Note, however, that through the behaviour description, environment can indirectly control the truth of e_x. The specification for change of levels of inputs is the same as that of genes:

$$G(in_x \rightarrow F(e_x \vee \neg in_x))$$
$$G(in_x \wedge e_x \rightarrow (e_x W \neg in_x))$$
$$G(\neg in_x \rightarrow F(\neg e_x \vee in_x))$$
$$G(\neg in_x \wedge \neg e_x \rightarrow (\neg e_x W in_x))$$

Here we introduce a network property ψ (specified in LTL) of a given network that we are to check. Example network properties are: 'certain gene is always ON', 'when a gene is ON, it will later be OFF' and so on. These properties are easily specified by LTL.

The problem of checking whether a network whose behaviours are specified by φ satisfies ψ for any input sequence is formally stated as follows.

Definition 1. *Let E be the set of external propositions, I be the set of internal propositions and E and I are disjoint. Let $AP = E \cup I$ be the set of atomic propositions. A property ψ is* homeostatic *with respect to a behaviour specification of a network $\langle E, I, \varphi \rangle$ if $\langle E, I, \varphi \wedge \psi \rangle$ is realisable. Here φ and ψ are written in LTL with AP.*

In some situation it is reasonable to consider a homeostasis of a network against not all input sequences but *some* input sequences. Here we introduce a *generalised homeostasis* of gene networks:

Definition 2. *Let E be the set of external propositions, I be the set of internal propositions and E and I are disjoint. Let $AP = E \cup I$ be the set of atomic propositions. A property ψ is* homeostatic *with respect to a behaviour specification of a network $\langle E, I, \varphi \rangle$ under the environmental assumption ξ if $\langle E, I, \xi \rightarrow \varphi \wedge \psi \rangle$ is realisable. Here φ and ψ are written in LTL with AP, and ξ is written in LTL with E.*

Definition 1 is a special case of Definition 2 in which $\xi = \top$.

Example 2. Let φ be a network specification of the network depicted in Fig. 4, where the switching condition on gene x is described as

$$G(e_x \wedge \neg y_x \rightarrow on_x),$$

which says that if the input level is beyond the threshold e_x and gene y is not expressed beyond the threshold y_x (i.e. proposition y_x is false; $\neg y_x$ is true), then gene x is ON, and the switching condition on gene x is described as

$$G(x_y \leftrightarrow on_y).$$

Then, this network is homeostatic with respect to a property 'whenever gene x becomes ON, the expression of gene x will be suppressed afterwards'. This property is described in LTL as follows:

$$G(on_x \to F(\neg on_x \wedge \neg x_y)).$$

Let φ be a behavioural specification of the network (partly shown in the previous section). This is verified by checking realisability of the specification

$$\langle \{in_x\}, \{on_x, on_y, x_y, y_x, e_x\}, \varphi \wedge G(on_x \to F(\neg on_x \wedge \neg x_y)) \rangle.$$

This property is also homeostatic if we put an environmental assumption 'the input to x is always ON' which is described as:

$$Gin_x.$$

That is to say, the specification $\langle \{in_x\}, \{on_x, on_y, x_y, y_x, e_x\}, Gin_x \to \varphi \wedge \psi \rangle$ is realisable (where ψ represents the above property).

This definition reduces the problem of checking homeostasis to the problem of checking realisability of reactive system specifications. Therefore we can use realisability checkers [4, 9, 18, 19] to solve the homeostasis problems.

The complexity of realisability checking of LTL is 2EXPTIME-complete in the size of formulae [21]. In our framework, the size of a formula obtained from a gene network is proportional to the size of the network. Due to the high-complexity of realisability checking, direct analyses of large networks are generally intractable. In the next section we introduce a compositional method to ease the analysis of large networks.

4   Compositional Analysis of Homeostasis

First we briefly describe the underlying realisability checking algorithm that is later leveraged in the compositional algorithm [10]. Let φ be a given LTL formula whose realisability we are to check. Then the algorithm (called *monolithic* algorithm) proceeds as follows:

1. Translate φ to a universal co-Büchi automaton A_φ.
2. Translate A_φ to a safety game $G(A_\varphi)$.
3. Compute the winning strategy of the game $G(A_\varphi)$.

Among these steps, the first step is known to be the bottleneck, since known algorithms to translate LTL formulae into equivalent automata run in exponential time with respect to the sizes of formulae. For large LTL formulae, the algorithm often fails in the first step.

The compositional algorithm is devised to overcome the difficulty in the first step. Without loss of generality, reactive system specifications are written as $\varphi = \varphi_1 \wedge \varphi_2 \wedge \cdots \wedge \varphi_n$ [3]. In compositional approach, each sub-formula φ_i is translated into automaton A_{φ_i} and thus translated into a local game $G(A_{\varphi_i})$, then the winning strategy is computed for each $G(A_{\varphi_i})$. Thanks to the nice property of safety games, the winning strategy for $G(A_{\varphi})$ – the strategy for the original game – can be computed from the winning strategies for each local game $G(A_{\varphi_i})$. Since each φ_i is much smaller than the original φ, the automata construction for each φ_i is much less demanding. Note that, however, we have to pay extra cost to merge the winning strategies for local games, which we do not in the monolithic (i.e. non-compositional) algorithm. If we manage to divide φ into a suitable set of sub-formulae, we will gain much benefit from the compositional algorithm.

This compositional algorithm is implemented in the tool Acacia+ [5]. According to the experiments reported, the compositional algorithm outperforms the monolithic algorithm. However, the formulae are divided heuristically by hand. There is no guideline how to obtain a good division.

To facilitate applying compositional algorithm, we invent a new clustering algorithm that suitably divide LTL specifications. Here the clauses are to be distributed into several clusters $c_1, c_2, \ldots, c_k$, i.e. $\varphi = (\bigwedge c_1) \wedge (\bigwedge c_2) \wedge \cdots \wedge (\bigwedge c_k)$ where $\bigwedge c_i = \bigwedge_{\phi \in c_i} \phi$.

The basic idea how to divide LTL specification is based on the following observation. Let us assume that we have 20 clauses and are distributing them into 2 clusters. Consider two clusterings: (1) to put 1 clause into one cluster and 19 clauses into the other, (2) to put 10 clauses into each cluster. Intuitively, the second clustering seems better, since in such uneven clustering as the first one, the 19 clauses cluster will be a bottleneck and the efficiency may not improve as a whole. Thus a good clustering distributes clauses into clusters as equally as possible. However, the number of clauses may not be a good criterion, since the sizes of formulae are not the same; in an extreme situation, the size of a certain formula might be equal to the size of the rest. Thus we distribute clauses into clusters whose sizes are as equal as possible.

To facilitate the winning strategy computation of each local game, it is desirable to obtain small automata. The size of automata A_{φ} is determined by the number of sub-formulae in φ. To compute the number of sub-formulae for each clause is not realistic because it is exponential to the size of the formula. For example, for a formula $(a \wedge \neg b) \rightarrow Fb$, we have the following variations of sub-formulae: $a, b, \neg b, Fb, a \wedge \neg b$ and $(a \wedge \neg b) \rightarrow Fb$. The plausible criterion is the number of variations of propositions – the more variations of propositions we have, the more will be the number of sub-formulae. For example, $(a \rightarrow b) \wedge (a \rightarrow c)$ has

---

[3] Our network specifications actually conform to this form.

the following sub-formulae: $a, b, c, a \rightarrow b, a \rightarrow c, (a \rightarrow b) \wedge (a \rightarrow c)$. Meanwhile, $(a \rightarrow b) \wedge (c \rightarrow d)$ has $a, b, c, d, a \rightarrow b, c \rightarrow d, (a \rightarrow b) \wedge (c \rightarrow d)$. Thus we also take the variation of propositions in a cluster into consideration, in addition to the size of a cluster.

Before formalising the above idea, we clarify the case where an LTL specification is of the form $\xi \rightarrow \varphi$ where ξ is an environmental assumption. In this case, we only consider how to divide φ into clusters $c_1, \ldots, c_k$. However, when we translate each sub-formula into the corresponding automaton, it should be translated from the formula $\xi \rightarrow \bigwedge c_\ell$.

Now we formalise our idea. Let $C = \{c_1, \ldots, c_k\}$ be an arbitrary clustering of a specification $\langle E, I, \xi \rightarrow \bigwedge_{1 \leq i \leq n} \varphi_i \rangle$, that is, each cluster c_ℓ consists of some φ_is. Let $N(\chi)$ and $V(\chi)$ respectively denote the number of propositions and the variations of propositions in a formula χ. We introduce the evaluation function $\mathcal{F}$ of clustering C as follows:

$$\mathcal{F}(C) = \sum_{1 \leq i \leq k} \mathcal{E}(\xi \rightarrow \bigwedge_{\varphi \in c_i} \varphi), \qquad \text{(Source: [17])}$$

where $\mathcal{E}(\chi) = N(\chi)^2 + V(\chi)^2$

The function $\mathcal{E}$ represents the evaluation of a single formula χ based on the size of χ and the variation of propositions in χ. Due to the squared terms in the function $\mathcal{E}$, we can easily see that a clustering consists of two clusters of the sizes 5 and 5 is better than that of 9 and 1. A good clustering is the one which minimises the value of this function.

The number of possible clustering of n clauses into k clusters is $S(n, k)$, i.e. the Stirling number of the second kind that is a huge number. Thus the naïve algorithm to find the optimal cluster is not realistic in general. Thus we introduce a suboptimal algorithm whose complexity is $O(kn)$ which we show in Algorithm 1.

This algorithm starts with the initial clustering where c_1 contains all clauses $\varphi_1, \ldots, \varphi_n$ and the others with empty clusters. Beginning from the first clause in c_1, we move it to the cluster that gives the best evaluation of the clustering. Outermost loop is executed n times and for each iteration of the outermost loop, the inner loop is executed k times. Therefore, this algorithm runs in time $O(kn)$. We implemented the algorithm in OCaml and confirmed that this suboptimal algorithm computes a clustering whose evaluation well approximates the optimal clustering.

5   Experimental Results and Discussion

In this section, we present experimental results of homeostasis analysis performed on several networks varying in size. All network specifications are realisable because compositional analysis is available for only realisable specifications.

As we noted in the previous section, we aim to reduce the cost of translating LTL formulae into automata (and then safety games) by means of the compositional algorithm,. Instead, we need an extra computational cost to merge

---

Algorithm 1. Suboptimal clustering algorithm. (Modified from [17]).

Input: $\{\varphi_1,\ldots,\varphi_n\}$ (specification), k (the number of the clusters)
Output: $C = \{c_1,\ldots,c_k\}$
  $c_1 \leftarrow \{\varphi_1,\ldots,\varphi_n\}$
  for $i = 2$ to k **do**
    $c_i \leftarrow \emptyset$
  end for
  $C \leftarrow \{c_1,\ldots,c_k\}$
  $min \leftarrow \mathcal{F}(C)$
  for $i = 1$ to n **do**
    for $j = 2$ to k **do**
      $C' \leftarrow \{c_1\backslash\{\varphi_i\},\ldots,c_j\cup\{\varphi\},\ldots,c_k\}$
      $f \leftarrow \mathcal{F}(C')$
      if $f < min$ **then**
        $C \leftarrow C'$
        $min \leftarrow f$
      end if
    end for
  end for

---

the winning strategies for each local game. This cost will grow as the number of clusters increases. Although the number of clusters may affect the overall performance, we have no idea how to estimate the best number of clusters in advance. Hence, we demonstrate our clustering method with several number of clusters so that we can see the impact of the number of clusters.

The networks that we used in this experiment are depicted in Figs. 5, 6, 7, 8, 9, 10 and 11. The network 'bistable switch' is the network that consists of two genes x and y where x activates y, y activates x and x receives negative input from environment (Fig. 5). The network 'bistable switch2' is the same as 'bistable switch' except both gene x and y receive negative inputs from environment (Fig. 6). The networks 'anti-stress response (a)(b)(c)' are the stress response networks studied in [23] (Fig. 7). The networks '3 genes' to '6 genes' are depicted in Figs. 8, 9, 10 and 11. They are artificially synthesised for the experiment. The homeostatic properties we analysed are tendency to ease stress (described as $G(stress \rightarrow F\neg stress)$) for anti-stress response networks and stability of a certain gene expression (described as Gon) for the others. We impose as environmental assumptions the following formulae that says every input is oscillating: $G((input \rightarrow F\neg input) \wedge (\neg input \rightarrow F input))$.

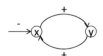

Fig. 5. A bistable switch. (Source: [17]).

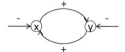

Fig. 6. A bistable switch with additional inputs. (Source: [17]).

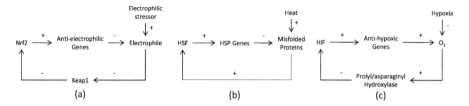

(a)   (b)   (c)

Fig. 7. Anti-stress networks. (Source: [17]).

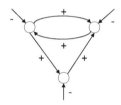

Fig. 8. A network consisting of 3 genes. (Source: [17]).

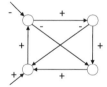

Fig. 9. A network consisting of 4 genes. (Source: [17]).

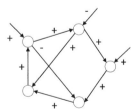

Fig. 10. A network consisting of 5 genes. (Source: [17]).

We show the results of experiments in Table 1. These experiments are carried out on a computer with Intel Core i7-3820 3.60 GHz CPU and 32 GB memory. The realisability checker used is Acacia+ [5].

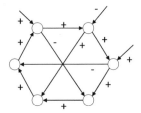

Fig. 11. A network consisting of 6 genes. (Source: [17]).

Table 1. Experimental results. Columns 'E' and 'I' respectively show the numbers of external propositions and internal propositions. Column 'S' shows the size of formula. (i.e. number of connectives and propositions). The columns 'Time(s)' show the total time of the verification for various number of clusters (k). '$k = 1$' means non-compositional analysis. For '$k \geq 1$' the times include computation of clustering. (Source: [17]).

Network	E	I	S	Time(s)					
				$k = 1$	$k = 2$	$k = 3$	$k = 4$	$k = 5$	$k = 6$
Bistable switch	1	6	232	0.40	0.07	0.08	0.10	0.10	0.07
Bistable switch2	2	8	353	206.81	0.81	0.41	0.42	0.51	0.53
Anti-stress response (a)	1	9	289	0.48	0.31	0.35	0.41	0.47	0.51
Anti-stress response (b)	1	7	237	0.22	0.12	0.13	0.15	0.16	0.18
Anti-stress response (c)	1	9	288	0.39	0.31	0.38	0.41	0.47	0.51
3 genes	3	10	418	1617.87	5.03	5.43	6.08	5.82	6.30
4 genes	2	12	444	>3600	4.07	4.48	5.16	5.69	6.21
5 genes	3	15	547	>3600	173.31	123.80	192.17	135.77	194.75
6 genes	3	18	646	>3600	2676.37	2792.61	2877.03	2942.62	3087.91

The figures shown in the table for $k \geq 2$ include the computational times of clustering. They are less than 0.01 regardless of the number of clusters for any network except for '6genes' at $k = 6$ (0.011 s). We can see that the compositional algorithm ($k \geq 2$) outperforms the monolithic algorithm ($k = 1$). The improvement by the compositional algorithm increases as the size of the network grows.

Next, we compare our method to random clustering. For each network specification, we generate 50 random clusterings. The way to generate random clusterings is that we first randomly choose the size of each cluster, in other words, we first determine how many clauses each cluster should include. Then, we randomly distribute the clauses of the original formula to each cluster according to the determined size.

We show the results of random clustering in Table 2. The figures shown in the table are the average of the verification times for 50 random clusterings. During the experiment on random clusterings, the realisability checking for some clusterings did not finish within 1 h. Such clusterings are considered to be verified in 3600 s for the sake of convenience. We marked the figures with stars on such figures in the table. Thus the real averages must be greater than them.

Table 2. Results of random clustering. It shows average verification times of 50 randomly clustered specs. The figures show the time (in seconds) to check homeostasis. The stars on the figures show that some trials failed due to time out of 1 h. Such clusterings are treated as finished in 3600 s for the sake of expedience. (Source: [17]).

Network	$k = 2$	$k = 3$	$k = 4$	$k = 5$	$k = 6$
Bistable switch	0.11	0.11	0.11	0.11	0.12
Bistable switch2	12.20	4.39	2.24	1.62	1.23
Anti-stress response (a)	0.36	0.38	0.43	0.44	0.47
Anti-stress response (b)	0.13	0.14	0.15	0.16	0.17
Anti-stress response (c)	0.35	0.37	0.40	0.43	0.46
3 genes	81.80	29.44	50.88	10.44	10.94
4 genes	687.47*	441.53*	166.43*	45.99	130.66
5 genes	1746.24*	845.6*	772.39*	841.6*	842.74*
6 genes	3220.6*	2953.01*	2767.81*	2830.68*	2641.21*

Table 3. Standard deviation of the results of random clustering. (Source: [17]).

Network	$k = 2$	$k = 3$	$k = 4$	$k = 5$	$k = 6$
Bistable switch	0.05	0.03	0.02	0.01	0.01
Bistable switch2	23.00	12.1	4.51	3.74	2.30
Anti-stress response (a)	0.09	0.08	0.13	0.04	0.04
Anti-stress response (b)	0.02	0.02	0.01	0.01	0.01
Anti-stress response (c)	0.06	0.09	0.03	0.04	0.05
3 genes	183.01	138.24	273.49	13.04	22.63
4 genes	1239.13*	1021.42*	618.16*	218.94	377.97
5 genes	1593.59*	1318.82*	1183.29*	1295.33*	1270.92*
6 genes	700.55*	763.89*	835.77*	819.86*	989.15*

For larger specifications such as 'bistable switch2', '3genes', '4genes' and '5genes', we can clearly see that our method outperforms random clustering. However, the random clustering seems to be as good as or even outperform our clustering algorithm for '6genes'. As we remarked above, however, the figures are not real ones. we treated timed-out samples as 3600 s when averaging the results. If we set time out more than 1 h, the figures will be worse.

For smaller specifications such as 'bistable switch' and 'anti-stress response' networks, the difference between random clustering and our clustering algorithm cannot be seen clearly. However, as we show later, considering the standard deviations and the relative standings, our clustering algorithm works well especially for smaller k.

Table 4. Relative standing of the verification time with our method within the run-times of random clusterings. The value 'best' means that our method was the best. (Source: [17].)

Network	$k = 2$	$k = 3$	$k = 4$	$k = 5$	$k = 6$
Bistable switch	10%	14%	39%	43%	best
Bistable switch2	38%	13%	15%	41%	41%
Anti-stress response (a)	27%	17%	64%	88%	88%
Anti-stress response (b)	31%	45%	70%	70%	92%
Anti-stress response (c)	23%	86%	68%	92%	92%
3 genes	14%	26%	47%	27%	27%
4 genes	17%	8%	34%	38%	43%
5 genes	19%	12%	43%	15%	35%
6 genes	14%	26%	41%	44%	50%

Table 5. The automaton construction times for our clustering method.

Network	Time(s)				
	$k = 2$	$k = 3$	$k = 4$	$k = 5$	$k = 6$
Bistable switch	0.05	0.05	0.06	0.05	0.02
Bistable switch2	0.56	0.12	0.12	0.13	0.12
Anti-stress response (a)	0.08	0.07	0.06	0.06	0.07
Anti-stress response (b)	0.06	0.06	0.07	0.06	0.07
Anti-stress response (c)	0.08	0.07	0.07	0.06	0.08
3 genes	1.14	0.67	0.59	0.54	0.57
4 genes	0.27	0.17	0.17	0.16	0.17
5 genes	4.92	1.75	1.26	1.09	1.05
6 genes	13.49	3.49	2.18	1.85	1.75

Readers might wonder why '4genes' for $k = 5$ is considerably smaller than others in random clustering. Plausible explanation is that the random sampling happened to give biased clusterings. However, even so our method is much better.

Now we show the standard deviations of the random clustering in Table 3. As we can see from the table, the standard deviations are high for larger specifications. This means that our evaluation function is actually a statistically meaningful criterion, because random clustering ranges from better to worse. Our clustering algorithm tactfully chooses better ones.

We also show the relative standings of our results (the values shown in Table 1) within the run-times of random clusterings. In other words, the percentile ranks of our results in the random clusterings in Table 4. As we can see, for $k = 2$ or 3 our algorithm gives good scores. For $k \geq 4$, however, this table shows that our clustering algorithm is not so effective compared to $k \leq 3$. This

Table 6. The averages of automaton construction times for 50 random clusterings. The stars on the figures show that some trials failed due to time out of 1 h.

Network	Time(s)				
	$k = 2$	$k = 3$	$k = 4$	$k = 5$	$k = 6$
Bistable switch	0.09	0.07	0.08	0.07	0.07
Bistable switch2	11.95	4.13	1.95	1.3	0.88
Anti-stress response (a)	0.13	0.11	0.12	0.09	0.10
Anti-stress response (b)	0.08	0.07	0.07	0.07	0.07
Anti-stress response (c)	0.12	0.10	0.09	0.09	0.09
3 genes	78.18	25.36	46.75	6.23	6.48
4 genes	684.28*	437.44*	162.09*	40.93	125.57
5 genes	1666.97*	731.27*	643.03*	713.69*	716.28*
6 genes	2478.64*	1515.71*	1205.51*	1400.31*	894.75*

Table 7. The winning strategy computation times for our clustering method.

Network	Time(s)				
	$k = 2$	$k = 3$	$k = 4$	$k = 5$	$k = 6$ -
Bistable switch	0.02	0.03	0.04	0.05	0.05
Bistable switch2	0.25	0.29	0.3	0.38	0.41
Anti-stress response (a)	0.23	0.28	0.35	0.41	0.44
Anti-stress response (b)	0.06	0.07	0.08	0.10	0.11
Anti-stress response (c)	0.23	0.31	0.34	0.41	0.43
3 genes	3.89	4.76	5.49	5.28	5.72
4 genes	3.80	4.31	4.99	5.52	5.68
5 genes	168.39	122.04	190.90	134.67	193.69
6 genes	2662.88	2789.11	2874.84	2940.76	3086.15

is because if we increase the number of clusters, the size of formulae in each cluster tends to be small, so that the automata construction time decreases and becomes less important in the verification process. Thus the larger k tends to relatively impair the impact of the difference of clustering algorithm.

To look into this matter further, we prepare the tables for automaton construction times and the winning strategy computation times separately for our clustering algorithm and the random clustering. They are shown in Tables 5, 6, 7 and 8.

From Tables 5 and 6, we can see that by increasing the number of clusters k, the automaton construction times are decreasing in both algorithms. Meanwhile, the winning strategy computation time does not change so much when we increase k, which can be seen from Tables 7 and 8. Thus increase of k makes

Table 8. The averages of the winning strategy computation times for 50 random clusterings. The stars on the figures show that some trials failed in automaton construction due to time out of 1 h. The averages for such clusters are calculated by ignoring them from the samples.

Network	Time(s)				
	$k = 2$	$k = 3$	$k = 4$	$k = 5$	$k = 6$
Bistable switch	0.03	0.03	0.04	0.04	0.05
Bistable switch2	0.24	0.27	0.29	0.32	0.34
Anti-stress response (a)	0.23	0.28	0.31	0.35	0.38
Anti-stress response (b)	0.06	0.07	0.08	0.09	0.09
Anti-stress response (c)	0.23	0.27	0.31	0.34	0.37
3 genes	3.72	4.09	4.12	4.21	4.46
4 genes	3.55*	4.17*	4.42*	5.06	5.09
5 genes	132.12*	136.11*	150.42*	152.28*	150.55*
6 genes	2181.37*	2343.29*	2297.50*	2236.08*	2226.78*

the effect of clustering less impactful. Furthermore by comparing Tables 7 and 8, the random clustering outperforms our clustering algorithm in the computation of winning strategies in most cases, especially for larger networks. This tendency becomes clear when the number of k increases. This indicates that our clustering algorithm actually improve the automaton construction but does not the winning strategy computation.

We summarise this section. In comparison to monolithic approach, the compositional method with our clustering algorithm improves the efficiency of verification, especially for larger networks. In comparison to random clustering, our approach is generally more efficient, but the difference decreases as we increase the number of clusters. The best performance can be achieved around $k = 2$ or 3 in our method. However, if we increase the number of clusters, the bottleneck seems to shift from automata construction to winning strategy computation. To investigate a method to reduce the time for the winning strategy computation is an interesting future work.

6   Related Work

As for the compositional approach to realisability problems, the tool Unbeast [6] is proposed other than Acacia+ [10]. Unbeast divides a given LTL specification into the part which satisfies *safety* and the other which does not. The advantage of this approach is that the safety part can be easily translated into an automaton. Intuitively, safety means that a system never falls into some undesirable state, and often appears in LTL specifications as $G\neg error$. Since our logical specification mainly consists of non-safety clauses, Unbeast may not be suitable.

As for clustering algorithms, k-means++ [3] and hierarchical clustering with Ward method [22] are well-known and widely used in various domains. To utilise these algorithms in our setting, we somehow need to encode our problem into some vector space. This is an interesting future research direction.

As for compositional analysis of gene networks, we proposed to divide a network into several sub-networks and verify them individually [14,15]. This means we manually divide an LTL formula into several sub-formulae, considering the network structure. We have not discussed any algorithm to divide a network and the corresponding formula. In this paper, our method is based on a syntactic structure of a formula, not on a network structure. Thus it is easy to cluster a formula algorithmically.

7   Conclusion

In this paper we proposed compositional analysis of homeostasis of gene networks, which is formulated in terms of realisability of reactive system specifications. Our approach is to utilise the compositional algorithm for realisability checking where we view an LTL specification as a set of clauses. We introduced a new clustering algorithm which distribute the clauses into several clusters. Our clustering algorithm outputs a clustering in which each cluster is as equally complex as possible with respect to the size of formulae and the variation of propositions. The intention of this clustering criterion is to reduce the cost of the automaton construction in the realisability checking algorithm. The experimental results show that our method drastically improves the performance in analysing larger network specifications. However, the experiment also shows that the increase of the number of clusters does not necessarily mean the improve of performance, since the bottleneck of the realisability checking algorithm shifts from the automaton construction to the winning strategy computation, which is the latter half of the realisability checking algorithm. This experimental results motivate us to investigate another compositional approach which can decrease the cost of winning strategy computation.

A   Linear Temporal Logic

Let A be a finite set. We write A^ω for the set of all infinite sequences on A. We write $\sigma[i]$ for the i-th element of $\sigma \in A^\omega$. Let AP be a set of atomic propositions. A *linear time structure* is a sequence $\sigma \in (2^{AP})^\omega$ where 2^{AP} is the powerset of AP.

The formulae in LTL are defined inductively as follows: (i) $p \in AP$ is a formula, (ii) if ϕ is a formula, $\neg\phi$ is a formula, (iii) if ϕ and ψ are formulae, $\phi \wedge \psi$, $\phi \vee \psi$ and $\phi U \psi$ are also formulae. Now we define the semantics of LTL. Let σ be a linear time structure and ϕ be a formula. We write $\sigma \models \phi$ for ϕ is true in σ and we say σ *satisfies* ϕ. The satisfaction relation $\models$ is defined as follows.

$$\sigma \models p \quad \text{iff } p \in \sigma[0] \text{ for } p \in AP$$
$$\sigma \models \neg\phi \quad \text{iff } \sigma \not\models \phi$$
$$\sigma \models \phi \wedge \psi \text{ iff } \sigma \models \phi \text{ and } \sigma \models \psi$$
$$\sigma \models \phi \vee \psi \text{ iff } \sigma \models \phi \text{ or } \sigma \models \psi$$
$$\sigma \models \phi U \psi \text{ iff } (\exists i \geq 0)(\sigma^i \models \psi \text{ and } \forall j (0 \leq j < i) \sigma^j \models \phi)$$

where $\sigma^i = \sigma[i]\sigma[i+1]\dots$, i.e. the i-th suffix of σ. An LTL formula ϕ is *satisfiable* if there exists a time structure σ such that $\sigma \models \phi$.

We introduce the following abbreviations: $\bot \equiv p \wedge \neg p$ for some $p \in AP$, $\top \equiv \neg\bot$, $\phi \rightarrow \psi \equiv \neg\phi \vee \psi$, $\phi \leftrightarrow \psi \equiv (\phi \rightarrow \psi) \wedge (\psi \rightarrow \phi)$, $F\phi \equiv \top U\phi$, $G\phi \equiv \neg F\neg\phi$, and $\phi W\psi \equiv (\phi U\psi) \vee G\phi$. We assume that $\wedge, \vee$ and U bind more strongly than $\rightarrow$ and unary connectives bind more strongly than binary ones.

Intuitively, $\neg\phi$ means 'ϕ is not true', $\phi \wedge \psi$ means 'both ϕ and ψ are true', $\phi \vee \psi$ means 'ϕ or ψ is true', and $\phi U\psi$ means 'ϕ continues to hold until ψ holds'. $\bot$ is a false proposition and $\top$ is a true proposition. $\phi \rightarrow \psi$ means 'if ϕ is true then ψ is true' and $\phi \leftrightarrow \psi$ means 'ϕ is true if and only if ψ is true'. $F\phi$ means 'ϕ holds at some future time', $G\phi$ means 'ϕ holds globally', $\phi W\psi$ is the 'weak until' operator in that ψ is not obliged to hold, in that case ϕ must always hold.

References

1. Abadi, M., Lamport, L., Wolper, P.: Realizable and unrealizable specifications of reactive systems. In: Ausiello, G., Dezani-Ciancaglini, M., Della Rocca, S.R. (eds.) ICALP 1989. LNCS, vol. 372, pp. 1–17. Springer, Heidelberg (1989). https://doi.org/10.1007/BFb0035748

2. Aoshima, T.: On a verification system for reactive system specifications. Ph.D. thesis, Tokyo Institute of Technology (2003)

3. Arthur, D., Vassilvitskii, S.: K-means++: the advantages of careful seeding. In: Proceedings of the Eighteenth Annual ACM-SIAM Symposium on Discrete Algorithms, SODA 2007, pp. 1027–1035. Society for Industrial and Applied Mathematics, Philadelphia (2007)

4. Bloem, R., Cimatti, A., Greimel, K., Hofferek, G., Könighofer, R., Roveri, M., Schuppan, V., Seeber, R.: RATSY – a new requirements analysis tool with synthesis. In: Touili, T., Cook, B., Jackson, P. (eds.) CAV 2010. LNCS, vol. 6174, pp. 425–429. Springer, Heidelberg (2010). https://doi.org/10.1007/978-3-642-14295-6_37

5. Bohy, A., Bruyère, V., Filiot, E., Jin, N., Raskin, J.-F.: Acacia+, a tool for LTL synthesis. In: Madhusudan, P., Seshia, S.A. (eds.) CAV 2012. LNCS, vol. 7358, pp. 652–657. Springer, Heidelberg (2012). https://doi.org/10.1007/978-3-642-31424-7_45

6. Ehlers, R.: Symbolic bounded synthesis. Formal Methods Syst. Des. **40**(2), 232–262 (2012). https://doi.org/10.1007/s10703-011-0137-x

7. Elowitz, M.B., Leibler, S.: A synthetic oscillatory network of transcriptional regulators. Nature **403**, 335–338 (2000)

8. Emerson, E.A.: Temporal and modal logic. In: van Leeuwen, J. (ed.) Handbook of Theoretical Computer Science, Volume B: Formal Models and Semantics (B), pp. 995–1072. MIT Press, Cambridge (1990)

9. Filiot, E., Jin, N., Raskin, J.-F.: An antichain algorithm for LTL realizability. In: Bouajjani, A., Maler, O. (eds.) CAV 2009. LNCS, vol. 5643, pp. 263–277. Springer, Heidelberg (2009). https://doi.org/10.1007/978-3-642-02658-4_22

10. Filiot, E., Jin, N., Raskin, J.F.: Antichains and compositional algorithms for LTL synthesis. Formal Methods Syst. Des. **39**(3), 261–296 (2011)

11. Ito, S., Hagihara, S., Yonezaki, N.: A qualitative framework for analysing homeostasis in gene networks. In: Proceedings of BIOINFORMATICS 2014, pp. 5–16 (2014)

12. Ito, S., Hagihara, S., Yonezaki, N.: Approximate analysis of homeostasis of gene networks by linear temporal logic using network motifs. In: BIOINFORMATICS 2015 - Proceedings of the International Conference on Bioinformatics Models, Methods and Algorithms, Lisbon, Portugal, 12–15 January 2015, pp. 93–101 (2015)

13. Ito, S., Hagihara, S., Yonezaki, N.: Formulation of homeostasis by realisability on linear temporal logic. In: Plantier, G., Schultz, T., Fred, A., Gamboa, H. (eds.) BIOSTEC 2014. CCIS, vol. 511, pp. 149–164. Springer, Cham (2015). https://doi.org/10.1007/978-3-319-26129-4_10

14. Ito, S., Ichinose, T., Shimakawa, M., Izumi, N., Hagihara, S., Yonezaki, N.: Modular analysis of gene networks by linear temporal logic. J. Integr. Bioinf. **10**(2), 12–23 (2013). https://doi.org/10.2390/biecoll-jib-2013-216

15. Ito, S., Ichinose, T., Shimakawa, M., Izumi, N., Hagihara, S., Yonezaki, N.: Qualitative analysis of gene regulatory networks by temporal logic. Theor. Comput. Sci. **594**(23), 151–179 (2015). https://doi.org/10.1016/j.tcs.2015.06.017. http://www.sciencedirect.com/science/article/pii/S0304397515005277

16. Ito, S., Izumi, N., Hagihara, S., Yonezaki, N.: Qualitative analysis of gene regulatory networks by satisfiability checking of linear temporal logic. In: Proceedings of BIBE 2010, pp. 232–237 (2010). https://doi.org/10.1109/BIBE.2010.45

17. Ito, S., Osari, K., Hagihara, S., Yonezaki, N.: Efficient analysis of homeostasis of gene networks with compositional approach. In: Proceedings of the 10th International Joint Conference on Biomedical Engineering Systems and Technologies (BIOSTEC 2017) - Volume 3: BIOINFORMATICS, Porto, Portugal, 21–23 February 2017, pp. 17–28 (2017). https://doi.org/10.5220/0006093600170028

18. Jobstmann, B., Bloem, R.: Optimizations for LTL synthesis. In: Proceedings of the Formal Methods in Computer Aided Design, FMCAD 2006, pp. 117–124. IEEE Computer Society, Washington (2006)

19. Jobstmann, B., Galler, S., Weiglhofer, M., Bloem, R.: Anzu: a tool for property synthesis. In: Damm, W., Hermanns, H. (eds.) CAV 2007. LNCS, vol. 4590, pp. 258–262. Springer, Heidelberg (2007). https://doi.org/10.1007/978-3-540-73368-3_29

20. Mori, R., Yonezaki, N.: Several realizability concepts in reactive objects. In: Information Modeling and Knowledge Bases IV, pp. 407–424 (1993)

21. Pnueli, A., Rosner, R.: On the synthesis of a reactive module. In: POPL 1989: Proceedings of the 16th ACM SIGPLAN-SIGACT Symposium on Principles of Programming Languages, pp. 179–190. ACM, New York (1989)

22. Ward, J.H.: Hierarchical grouping to optimize an objective function. J. Am. Stat. Assoc. **58**(301), 236–244 (1963)

23. Zhang, Q., Andersen, M.E.: Dose response relationship in anti-stress gene regulatory networks. PLoS Comput. Biol. **3**(3), e24 (2007)

Fast and Sensitive Classification of Short Metagenomic Reads with SKraken

Jia Qian, Davide Marchiori, and Matteo Comin[(✉)]

Department of Information Engineering, University of Padova, Padua, Italy
comin@dei.unipd.it

Abstract. The major problem when analyzing a metagenomic sample is to taxonomically annotate its reads in order to identify the species and their relative abundances. Many tools have been developed recently, however they are not always adequate for the increasing database volume. In this paper we propose an efficient method, called SKraken, that combines taxonomic tree and k-mers frequency counting. SKraken extracts the most representative k-mers for each species and filter out less representative ones. SKraken is inspired by Kraken, which is one of the state-of-art methods. We compare the performance of SKraken with Kraken on both real and synthetic datasets, and it exhibits a higher classification precision and a faster processing speed. **Availability:** https://bitbucket. org/marchiori_dev/skraken.

1 Introduction

Metagenomics is a study of the heterogeneous microbes samples (e.g. soil, water, human microbiome) directly extract from the natural environment with the primary goal of determining the taxonomical identity of the microorganisms residing in the samples. It is an evolutionary revise, shifting focuses from the individual microbe study to a complex microbial community. As already mentioned in [1,2], the classical genomic-based approaches require the prior clone and culturing for the further investigation. However, not all bacteria can be cultured. The advent of metagenomics succeeded to bypass this difficulty.

The study of metagenomics is far more than just about labeling the species of the microbes. The analysis can reveal the presence of unexpected bacteria and viruses in a microbial sample, also allows the identification and characterization of bacterial and viral genomes at a level of detail not previously possible. For example, in the case of the human body, imbalances in the microbiome are related with many diseases, e.g. inflammatory bowel disease (IBD) [3] and colorectal cancer [4]. Furthermore it may aid the researchers to systematically understand and characterize the microbial communities: how genes influence each others activities in serving collective functions; grasp the collections of communities that composites the biosphere where the humans be a part, etc. It has already been applied in many areas like ecology, medicine, microbiology and some others mentioned in [3–6].

N. Peixoto et al. (Eds.): BIOSTEC 2017, CCIS 881, pp. 212–226, 2018.
https://doi.org/10.1007/978-3-319-94806-5_12

In this paper, we focus on the taxonomic classification, one branch of the metagenomics investigation, with a referenced database. Generally speaking, two techniques could be in consideration for the sake of classification task: (1) sequencing phylogenetic marker genes, e.g., 16S rRNA; (2) next generation sequencing (NGS) of all the genomic material in the sample. The use of marker genes requires amplification steps that can introduce bias in the taxonomic analysis. Moreover, not all bacteria can be identified by traditional 16S sequencing for its divergent gene sequences [7]. Indeed, We believe that the most effective and unbiased method to study microbial samples is via whole-genome NGS. However, the short length of NGS reads poses a number of challenges to the correctness of taxonomical classification for each read. Several methods and software tools are already available, but with the increasing throughput of modern sequencing technologies, the faster and more accurate algorithms are needed. These methods can be broadly divided into three categories: (1) sequence-similarity-based methods, (2) marker-based methods where certain specific marker sequences are used to identify the species. (3) sequence-composition-based methods, which are based on the nucleotide composition (e.g. k-mers usage).

The sequence-similarity-based methods work as searching reads according to the sequence similarity in the reference database, the popular examples are MegaBlast [8] and Megan [9]. They precisely identify reads from genomes within the reference database, while they are generally very slow, especially compared with composition-based methods. Marker-based methods try to use phylogenetic marker genes as a taxonomic reference [10–12]. For example, MetaPhlAn [12] is based on marker genes that are clade specific.

The fastest and most promising approaches belong to the composition-based one. Its trait can be summarized as follows: the genomes of reference organisms are modeled based on k-mers counts; the reads are searched throughout the reduced-version database. The most representative methods located within this category are Kraken [13], Clark [14] and Lmat [15]. As for the precision of these methods, they are as good as MegaBlast [8] (similarity-based method), nevertheless the processing speed is much faster. Thus, these methods are really capable to keep pace with the increasing throughput of modern sequencing instruments.

Recently the paper [16] has shown that Kraken [13] is one of the most promising tool in terms of classifying correctness and speed. It owes to the construction of the reference database, where each genome is expressed by k-mers (a piece of genome with length k), and the a taxonomic tree. More precisely, Kraken constructs a data structure that is an augmented taxonomic tree in which a list of significant k-mers is associated to each node, leafs and internal nodes. Given a node on this taxonomic tree, its list of k-mers is considered representative for the taxonomic label and will be used for the classification of metagenomic reads.

Inspired by this paradigm, in this paper we propose SKraken[1], a tool for metagenomics reads classification that selects the most representative k-mers for each node in the taxonomic tree, though, filtering out uninformative k-mers. The main properties of SKraken can be profiled as: (i) an efficient detection

---

[1] A preliminary version of this manuscript was published in [17].

of representative k-mers over the taxonomic tree; (ii) SKraken improves the precision over Kraken on both simulated and real metagenomic datasets without compromising the recall; (iii) benefit from the downsized database. As a consequence, SKraken requires less memory RAM and the classification speed increases w.r.t. Kraken. In the next section we will give an overview of Kraken and analyze how to improve the classification. SKraken is presented in Sect. 2.2. Both tools are tested on simulated and real metagenomic datasets in Sect. 3 and the conclusions are drawn in Sect. 4.

2   Method

2.1   An Overview of Kraken

In order to better understand our contribution let's briefly present Kraken in the first place. Instead of utilizing the complete genome as reference, Kraken considers only its k-mers, as well as many other tools [14,15], thus a genome sequence is alternatively represented by a set of k-mers, which plays a role of efficiently indexing a large volume of target-genomes database, e.g., all the genomes in RefSeq. This idea is stemmed from alignment-free methods [18] and some researchers have verified its availability in different applications. For instance, the construction of phylogenetic trees, traditionally is performed based on a multiple-sequence alignment technique, the process is be carried out on the whole genomes [19,20], in practice it's difficult to realize due to the improper length of whole genomes. The alignment-free technique with the usage of k-mers is the solver. Recently some variations of k-mers-based methods have been devised for the detection of enhancers in ChIP-Seq data [21–25] and entropic profiles [26,27]. Recently, the assembly-free comparison of genomes and metagenomes based on NGS reads and k-mers counts has been investigated in [28–31]. For a comprehensive review of alignment-free measures and applications we refer the reader to [18].

Considering the taxonomic tree, taken from the complete NCBI taxonomic information, this data structure is extended by annotating each node with k-mers, including leaves and internal nodes. Every node is associated with a list of k-mers that are critical for the future classification. More precisely, given a dataset of target genomes, the construction of this annotated taxonomic tree is carried out by scanning the k-mers of each genome in the dataset. If the k-mer appears only in a given genome, it is associated only to one leaf node J (representing that genome) and the k-mers list of node J is updated. If the k-mer appears in more than one species, the k-mer is erased from those corresponding nodes and moved to the lowest common ancestor of these nodes, see Fig. 1 for an example. At the end of this step each k-mer belongs to only one node in the taxonomic tree.

Once this database of annotated k-mers has been constructed, Kraken can classify reads in a very efficient manner. Figure 2 reports an overview of the classification process. Later when we launch the classification procedure, with a given read, Kraken firstly decomposes the read into a list of its k-mers. Then each

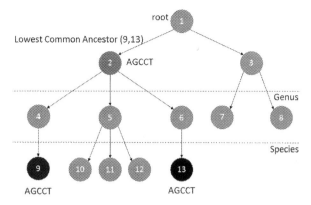

Fig. 1. In this example the k-mer $AGCCT$, that is contained in the species 9 and 13, is moved to the lowest common ancestor, the family node 2 (figure taken from [17]).

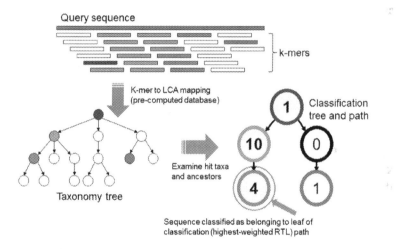

Fig. 2. An overview of the metagenomic reads classification of Kraken (figure taken from [13]).

k-mer is searched in the augmented taxonomic tree, whenever it hits we increase the counter of the corresponding node. After all k-mers have been analyzed, we will classify the read by searching the highest-weight path in the taxonomic tree, from top to button.

2.2 SKraken: Selecting Informative k-mers

The most important step of Kraken is the construction of the augmented taxonomic tree, annotating by a list of k-mers per node in order to implement the classification. In this paper we propose SKraken that has an exclusive procedure, distinguishable from Kraken, we select and filter k-mers instead. Therefore, those uninformative k-mers will be pruned away from the augmented taxonomic tree.

It may occur that one k-mers appears in more than one species, like demonstrated in Fig. 1, sequence "AGCCT" belongs to two species. Kraken adds this k-mers into the ancestor node 2 (representing a taxonomic family) out of node 9 and node 13. Since this k-mers will be used in the classification step, we would like to be informative for the family node 2. However, the majority of species in this family, nodes 10, 11 and 12, do not contain this k-mers.

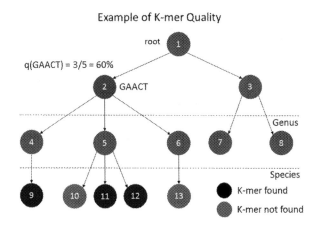

Fig. 3. An example of quality score $q(GAACT)$ (figure taken from [17]).

To address this issue, for each k-mer, we define a scoring function that captures its representativeness within the taxonomic node. We recall that a k-mer is associated with only one node in the tree. Let's define $TaxID(m)$ that indicates the taxonomic node associated with the k-mer m. However, before the upward shift of k-mer, it is possible to occur in more than one species. We define $NumSpecies(m)$ as the number of species that contains m. By construction $TaxID(m)$ is the lowest common ancestor of all these species. Thus the species in which m appears, they are all leaf nodes of the subtree $TaxID(m)$. We define $TotSpecies(n)$ as the total number of species in the subtree routed in the node n. With these values we define $q(m)$ the quality of a k-mer m as (equation from [17]):

$$q(m) = \frac{NumSpecies(m)}{TotSpecies(TaxID(m))}$$

Figure 3 shows an example of the quality $q(GAACT)$. The quality of $GAACT$ can also be interpreted as the percentage of species nodes that contains $GAACT$, i.e. $NumSpecies(GAACT)$, with respect to the family node 2, i.e., $TaxID(GAACT)$, in this case 60%. Similarly, if we consider the example in Fig. 1, the quality of $q(AGCCT) = \frac{NumSpecies(AGCCT)}{TotSpecies(TaxID(AGCCT))} = \frac{2}{5} = 0.4$, that is 40%. We can conclude as, a k-mer has an high quality can be considered representative for a given taxonomic node and the relative sub-tree, thus more likely will be informative for the classification. Based on these observations SKraken tries to screen out the uninformative k-mers by means of their quality value, and prunes the augmented taxonomic tree by removing the k-mers with a quality below a given threshold Q.

In order to compute the quality scores $q(m)$ for all k-mers we have to evaluate $NumSpecies(m)$ and $TotSpecies(n)$ efficiently. Here is our setting: the construction of the augmented taxonomic tree of SKraken is divided into two steps. In the first step, given a set of target genomes, we scan the k-mers of each genome and build the augmented taxonomic tree, similarly to Kraken. Meanwhile, we set a variable to keep tracking $NumSpecies(m)$, as soon as m is found in a new species we increment this variable. However, there can be genomes that are further classified as sub-species of a given species node. In order to compute the correct value of $NumSpecies(m)$, we need to make sure that all genomes of a given species are processed before moving to next species. This can be tackled by scanning the input genomes in a particular order so that all genomes of a species and the sub-species, are processed at once. Another problem is the fact that a k-mer can appear in some sub-species of a given species node. When computing $NumSpecies(m)$ we must ensure not to overcount these occurrences, and thus the corresponding variable is incremented only when m is found for the first time in a given species. All other occurrences of m within the same species will be discarded. At the end of the first step we have computed the augmented taxonomic tree, with all k-mers, and the corresponding values $NumSpecies(m)$.

In the second step SKraken computes the quality values $q(m)$ and filters uninformative k-mers. The number of leaf nodes that are the descendants of n, indicated as $TotSpecies(n)$, can be obtained for all nodes in the tree with a postorder traversal of the taxonomic tree. Consequently all k-mers are processed and the corresponding qualities $q(m)$ are computed. If $q(m)$ is below a given input parameter Q, m is removed from the database.

Note that the size of the taxonomic tree is constant and much smaller with respect to the number of k-mers. The overall process depends only on the total number of k-mers and its size is linear to the input reference genomes. Once the augmented taxonomic tree is build, reads can be classified with the same procedure of Kraken.

3   Results

3.1   Datasets

Before the demonstration of result, we need to build a reference dataset. We conduct the experiments both on real and simulated datasets with different bacterial and archaeal genomes from NCBI RefSeq in order to capture a comprehensive understanding of the performance. The simulated and real datasets are acquired from the original paper of Kraken [13] as well as from other related studies [14,32–34]. The simulated datasets represent five mock communities that are constructed from real sequencing data: MiSeq, HiSeq, Mix1, Mix2, simBA5. MiSeq and HiSeq metagenomes were built using 10 sets of bacterial whole-genome shotgun reads. Mix1 and Mix2 are based on the same species of HiSeq, but with two different abundance profiles.

The MiSeq dataset is particularly difficult to analyze because it contains five genomes from the *Enterobacteriaceae* family (*Citrobacter, Enterobacter, Klebsiella, Proteus and Salmonella*). The high sequence similarity of this family can elevate the difficulty of classification. The metagenome simBA5 was created by simulating reads from the complete set of bacterial and archaeal genomes in Ref-Seq, for a total of 1216 species. It contains reads with sequencing errors caused in the reading process and it was created with the exact purpose of measuring the stability with existing errors in a complex communities.

We also evaluated the performance of SKraken on a real stool metagenomic sample (SRR1804065) from the Human Microbiome Project. Because there is no ground truth for this dataset, we use BLAST with a sequence identity of 95% to find the reads that uniquely mapped to a genome and filter out all other reads. If two paired-end reads do not map to the same genome, we discard them. As a result, the real metagenomic sample contains 775 distinct species and 1053741 reads. A summary of the main characteristics of all simulated and real metagenomics datasets can be found in Table 1.

Table 1. A summary of simulated and real metagenomics datasets (table taken from [17]).

Type	Dataset	Reads	Species	Reads length
Single-end	HiSeq	10000	10	92
Single-end	MiSeq	10000	10	100
Single-end	simBA5	10000	1216	100
Paired-end	Mix1	1000000	10	100
Paired-end	Mix2	1000000	10	100
Paired-end	SRR1804065	1053741	775	100

3.2 Evaluation Metrics

In order to compare the results we used the standard metrics of precision and recall. Given N the number of reads, Y the number of reads classified and X the number of reads correctly classified, we define precision as the fraction of correct assignments over the total number of assignments (X/Y), and recall as the ratio between the number of correct assignments and the number of reads (X/N). Note that our classification task will be unfolded from both genus and species level, where genus level is the parent of species level in the taxonomic tree. If the classification step selected a node at genus level, while we are evaluating the species level, even if the assigned genus-level node is the parent of the correct leaf node, we considered it as mislabeled. On the other hand, when we evaluate the genus-level, if the classification step selected a taxonomic node that is a descendant (leaf node, species level) of the correct (genus-level) node, we consider it to be correct.

When analyzing a metagenomic sample one needs to verify whether the estimated abundance ratios of species is similar to the known profile, here we adopt Pearson correlation that is a technique widely used. If the correlation value is close to 1, which means the estimated abundance ratio perfectly matches the known one. In the next sections, we will test the behavior of SKraken on these three aspects: precision, recall and Pearson correlation.

3.3   Comparison

For a better perception of the performance of Skraken, we comparison it with Kraken, since it is one of the cutting-edge tools as mentioned in [16].

For Kraken we use the default parameter $k = 31$, as suggest by the authors [13], it is the best balance between precision and recall. For SKraken we use the same value $k = 31$ and we test the performance by varying the tuning parameter Q.

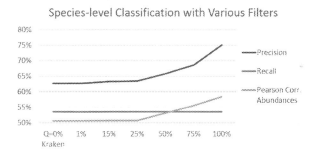

Fig. 4. Results on dataset Mix1 varying the filtering parameter Q, the figure taken from [17].

We devised a series of tests with the variable parameter Q and the taxonomic level at which the classification is evaluated. In the first set we want to test how the filtering parameter Q impact the performance metrics. We run Kraken and SKraken on the dataset Mix1 and evaluate the classification accuracy at the species-level. The results are reported in Fig. 4. If the parameter $Q = 0$ (no filtering) all k-mers are kept as we expected, thus the performance of Kraken and SKraken are identical. As Q grows to 100%, we can see that the precision improves from 63% to 75%, whereas the recall remains constant, which implies the number of mistakenly-classified reads decreases. Another important observation is that the Pearson correlation with the known abundance ratios also increases.

Thus, we use the most stringent filtering ($Q = 100\%$) to classify all dataset at the species-level. Figure 5 shows a summary of precision and recall for all simulated and real metagenomic datasets. This test confirms that SKraken is able to improve the precision on all datasets without compromising the recall. On simulated metagenomes the average precision increases from 73% of Kraken to 81% of SKraken. On the real metagenome, the accuracy of Kraken turns out to be 91%, SKraken achieves 96%.

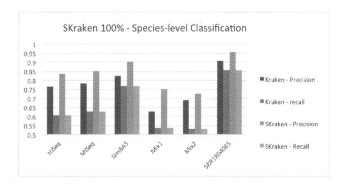

Fig. 5. Precision and recall of species-level classification of Kraken and SKraken ($Q = 100\%$) for all datasets.

In general the study of metagenomic sample requires an analysis based on the component of the genome, and for this reason researchers develop the studies at the lowest taxonomic level, species. However metagenomic reads can be mapped at a higher level, it's also valuable to survey the classification performance at the genus-level. We performed a set of experiments similar to the ones in species-level, considering the genus taxonomic level for classification. At first we set filtering parameter $Q = 100\%$, and the results are shown in Fig. 6. If we observe the performance of Kraken at genus level we can see that are better than those at species level, as expected. Indeed, in the taxonomy tree, when the classification level is more specific (lower), the label assignment is more difficult. Moreover, it is possible that some mislabeled reads exist at species level, while at genus level they are correct due to its loose condition. The average precision of Kraken is 96% at genus-level and 73% at species-level, we may see how great it improves.

When applying $Q = 100\%$, SKraken has a higher precision than Kraken in almost every database, while it's not the case with respect to recall. If we consider a less stringent threshold $Q = 25\%$ (see Fig. 7), we can obtain results that are in line with the previous experiments, with a moderate improvement in the precision and nearly unchanged recall. A possible explanation of the small gain in terms of precision is that the classification at the genus level is relatively easier, and Kraken has already very good performance. Since precision and recall depends on the number of reads classified and on the number of correct assignments, in order to have a complete picture, results are summarized in Table 2.

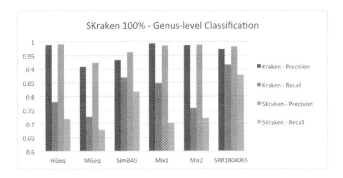

Fig. 6. Precision and recall of genus-level classification of Kraken and SKraken ($Q = 100\%$) for all datasets.

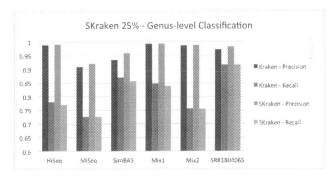

Fig. 7. Precision and recall of genus-level classification of Kraken and SKraken ($Q = 25\%$) for all datasets.

Table 2. Number of reads classified and correct assignments for all datasets and both of the methods.

		Species		Genus	
		Kraken	SKraken	Kraken	SKraken
HiSeq	Correct assignments	6049	6051	7800	7699
	Reads classified	7890	7252	7890	7773
MiSeq	Correct assignments	6260	6256	7258	7254
	Reads classified	7994	7342	7994	7884
SimBA5	Correct assignments	7688	7687	8700	8561
	Reads classified	9327	8513	9327	8929
Mix1	Correct assignments	535809	535798	848221	838720
	Reads classified	854256	713935	854255	844077
Mix2	Correct assignments	529717	529734	756196	754441
	Reads classified	766829	729856	766829	763114
SRR1804065	Correct assignments	902171	902270	966004	965859
	Reads classified	994416	944000	994416	982962

In the last experiment we test the ability to detect the correct abundance ratios in a metagenomic sample, we compared it at both genus level and species level of SKraken and Kraken, as displayed in Fig. 8. Both approaches have an extraordinary result in genus level, in particular, they virtually peaked in dataset HISeq, MIX1, MIX2 and SRR1804065. In dataset simBA5, SKraken increases the score from 0.92 to 0.97, since it is one of the most complex and realistic dataset, with 1216 species. If we compare these Pearson correlations with those of species level classification in general the values decrease confirming that it is more difficult to detect the correct species, rather than the genus. This is the case where the classification accuracy can benefit from a careful selection of discriminative k-mers. In fact in all dataset the correlation of SKraken is better than Kraken. Again, in one of the most difficult metagenome(simBA5) that contains 1216 species, the improvement is substantial from 0.61 of Kraken to 0.77 of SKraken.

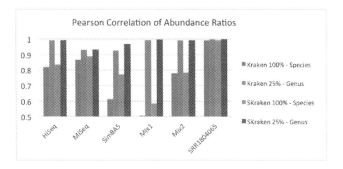

Fig. 8. The Pearson correlation of the estimated abundances with the correct ratios for various level of classification and parameters.

All the results above have shown that SKraken enables to obtain a higher classifying precision without any expense of recall. In other words, more reads are correctly classified, and the estimated abundance ratios have a better match with the known profile. An important property of SKraken is that the impact on these metrics improves as the taxonomic level evaluated in the classification becomes lower and thus more difficult. Moreover, as the number of newly sequenced species grows, the probability that two non-related species share a given k-mer will grow. For this reason we conjecture that SKraken will be able to remove more uninformative k-mers as the number of sequenced genomes increases.

3.4   Memory and Speed

Besides the enhancement of precision, the screening processing has another welcomed "side effect", it reduced the database size since the number of annotated

k-mers decreases. The size of the database produced by Kraken, using all bacterial and archaeal complete genomes in NCBI RefSeq, is about 65 GB and it contains 5.8 billion k-mers. In Fig. 9 we evaluate the percentage of k-mers filtered by SKraken and the impact in memory for different values of threshold Q. As expected, the percentage of k-mers filtered grows with the threshold Q increases and it reaches the maximum of 8.1% with $Q = 100$. By construction, the impact in memory depends linearly on the number of k-mers to be indexed. When $Q = 100$, SKraken requires to index 5.3 billion k-mers in space of 60 GB.

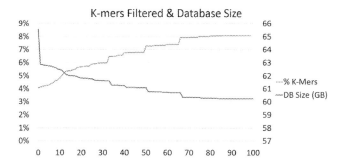

Fig. 9. Percentage of k-mers filtered and database size as a function of the quality threshold Q (taken from [17]).

Table 3. 10^3 reads per minute for various datasets.

	Kraken	SKraken
HiSeq	126	134
MiSeq	210	231
SimBA5	223	241
Mix1	473	498
Mix2	481	522
SRR1804065	694	754

In Table 3 we report the classification speed as reads classified per minute, using these tools on a server equipped by Intel Xeon E5450 (12 MB Cache, 3.00 GHz) and 256 GB RAM, without multithreading. SKraken is tested, as a result being faster than Kraken on all datasets.

4   Conclusion

We have presented SKraken, an efficient and effective method for the genus-level and species-level classifications. It is based from Kraken, with the additional procedure where we detect the representative k-mers and filter the unqualified ones, which produces an improved dictionary. The experimental result has demonstrated that SKraken obtains a higher precision without compromising the recall, moreover it boosts the processing speed. As future direction of investigation it would be interesting to explore alternative way to define the k-mer scores incorporating other topological information of the tree of life.

Acknowledgement. The authors would like to thank the anonymous reviewers for their valuable comments and suggestions. This work was supported by the Italian MIUR project PRIN20122F87B2.

References

1. Felczykowska, A., Bloch, S.K., Nejman-Faleczyk, B., Baraska, S.: Metagenomic approach in the investigation of new bioactive compounds in the marine environment. Acta Biochim. Pol. **59**(4), 501–505 (2012)
2. Mande, S.S., Mohammed, M.H., Ghosh, T.S.: Classification of metagenomic sequences: methods and challenges. Briefings Bioinform. **13**(6), 669–681 (2012)
3. Qin, J., Li, R., Raes, J., et al.: A human gut microbial gene catalogue established by metagenomic sequencing. Nature **464**, 59–65 (2010)
4. Zeller, G., Tap, J., Voigt, A.Y., Sunagawa, S., Kultima, J.R., Costea, P.I., Amiot, A., Böhm, J., Brunetti, F., Habermann, N., Hercog, R., Koch, M., Luciani, A., Mende, D.R., Schneider, M.A., Schrotz-King, P., Tournigand, C., Tran Van Nhieu, J., Yamada, T., Zimmermann, J., Benes, V., Kloor, M., Ulrich, C.M., von Knebel Doeberitz, M., Sobhani, I., Bork, P.: Potential of fecal microbiota for early-stage detection of colorectal cancer. Mol. Syst. Biol. **10**(11), 766 (2014)
5. Human Microbiome Project Consortium: Structure, function and diversity of the healthy human microbiome. Nature **486**(7402), 207–214 (2012)
6. Said, H.S., Suda, W., Nakagome, S., Chinen, H., Oshima, K., Kim, S., Kimura, R., Iraha, A., Ishida, H., Fujita, J., Mano, S., Morita, H., Dohi, T., Oota, H., Hattori, M.: Dysbiosis of salivary microbiota in inflammatory bowel disease and its association with oral immunological biomarkers. DNA Res.: Int. J. Rapid Publ. Rep. Genes Genomes **21**(1), 15–25 (2014)
7. Brown, C., Hug, L., Thomas, B., Sharon, I., Castelle, C., Singh, A., et al.: Unusual biology across a group comprising more than 15% of domain Bacteria. Nature **523**(7559), 208–211 (2015)
8. Zhang, Z., Schwartz, S., Wagner, L., Miller, W.: A greedy algorithm for aligning DNA sequences. J. Comput. Biol. **7**(1–2), 203–214 (2004)
9. Huson, D.H., Auch, A.F., Qi, J., Schuster, S.C.: Megan analysis of metagenomic data. Genome Res. **17**, 377–386 (2007)
10. Caporaso, J.G., Kuczynski, J., Stombaugh, J., Bittinger, K., Bushman, F.D., Costello, E.K., Fierer, N., Pea, A.G., Goodrich, J.K., Gordon, J.I., Huttley, G.A., Kelley, S.T., Knights, D., Koenig, J.E., Ley, R.E., Lozupone, C.A., McDonald, D., Muegge, B.D., Pirrung, M., Reeder, J., Sevinsky, J.R., Turnbaugh, P.J., Walters, W.A., Widmann, J., Yatsunenko, T., Zaneveld, J., Knight, R.: Qiime allows analysis of high-throughput community sequencing data. Nat. Methods **7**(5), 335–336 (2010)

11. Liu, B., Gibbons, T., Ghodsi, M., Treangen, T., Pop, M.: Accurate and fast estimation of taxonomic profiles from metagenomic shotgun sequences. BMC Genomics **12**, P11 (2011)
12. Segata, N., Waldron, L., Ballarini, A., Narasimhan, V., Jousson, O., Huttenhower, C.: Metagenomic microbial community profiling using unique clade-specific marker genes. Nat. Methods **9**, 811 (2012)
13. Wood, D., Salzberg, S.: Kraken: ultrafast metagenomic sequence classification using exact alignments. Genome Biol. **15**, R46 (2014)
14. Ounit, R., Wanamaker, S., Close, T.J., Lonardi, S.: Clark: fast and accurate classification of metagenomic and genomic sequences using discriminative k-mers. BMC Genomics **16**(1), 1–13 (2015)
15. Ames, S.K., Hysom, D.A., Gardner, S.N., Lloyd, G.S., Gokhale, M.B., Allen, J.E.: Scalable metagenomic taxonomy classification using a reference genome database. Bioinformatics **29**, 2253–2260 (2013)
16. Lindgreen, S., Adair, K.L., Gardner, P.: An evaluation of the accuracy and speed of metagenome analysis tools. Sci. Rep. **6**, 19233 (2016)
17. Marchiori, D., Comin, M.: Skraken: fast and sensitive classification of short metagenomic reads based on filtering uninformative k-mers. In: Proceedings of the 10th International Joint Conference on Biomedical Engineering Systems and Technologies (BIOSTEC 2017), pp. 59–67 (2017)
18. Vinga, S., Almeida, J.: Alignment-free sequence comparison-a review. Bioinformatics **19**, 513–523 (2003)
19. Comin, M., Verzotto, D.: Whole-genome phylogeny by virtue of unic subwords. In: 2012 23rd International Workshop on Database and Expert Systems Applications (DEXA), pp. 190–194, September 2012
20. Sims, G.E., Jun, S.R., Wu, G.A., Kim, S.H.: Alignment-free genome comparison with feature frequency profiles (FFP) and optimal resolutions. Proc. Nat. Acad. Sci. **106**, 2677–2682 (2009)
21. Antonello, M., Comin, M.: Fast alignment-free comparison for regulatory sequences using multiple resolution entropic profiles. In: Proceedings of the International Conference on Bioinformatics Models, Methods and Algorithms (BIOSTEC 2015), pp. 171–177 (2015)
22. Comin, M., Antonello, M.: On the comparison of regulatory sequences with multiple resolution entropic profiles. BMC Bioinf. **17**(1), 130 (2016)
23. Comin, M., Verzotto, D.: Beyond fixed-resolution alignment-free measures for mammalian enhancers sequence comparison. IEEE/ACM Trans. Comput. Biol. Bioinf. **11**(4), 628–637 (2014)
24. Goke, J., Schulz, M.H., Lasserre, J., Vingron, M.: Estimation of pairwise sequence similarity of mammalian enhancers with word neighbourhood counts. Bioinformatics **28**(5), 656–663 (2012)
25. Kantorovitz, M.R., Robinson, G.E., Sinha, S.: A statistical method for alignment-free comparison of regulatory sequences. Bioinformatics **23**, i249–i255 (2007)
26. Comin, M., Antonello, M.: Fast computation of entropic profiles for the detection of conservation in genomes. In: Ngom, A., Formenti, E., Hao, J.-K., Zhao, X.-M., van Laarhoven, T. (eds.) PRIB 2013. LNCS, vol. 7986, pp. 277–288. Springer, Heidelberg (2013). https://doi.org/10.1007/978-3-642-39159-0_25
27. Antonello, M., Comin, M.: Fast entropic profiler: an information theoretic approach for the discovery of patterns in genomes. IEEE/ACM Trans. Comput. Biol. Bioinf. **11**(3), 500–509 (2014)

28. Schimd, M., Comin, M.: Fast comparison of genomic and meta-genomic reads with alignment-free measures based on quality values. BMC Med. Genomics **9**(1), 41–50 (2016)
29. Comin, M., Leoni, A., Schimd, M.: Clustering of reads with alignment-free measures and quality values. Algorithms Mol. Biol. **10**(1), 1–10 (2015)
30. Comin, M., Schimd, M.: Assembly-free genome comparison based on next-generation sequencing reads and variable length patterns. BMC Bioinf. **15**(9), 1–10 (2014)
31. Ondov, B.D., Treangen, T.J., Melsted, P., Mallonee, A.B., Bergman, N.H., Koren, S., Phillippy, A.M.: Mash: fast genome and metagenome distance estimation using MinHash. bioRxiv (2016)
32. Girotto, S., Pizzi, C., Comin, M.: Metaprob: accurate metagenomic reads binning based on probabilistic sequence signatures. Bioinformatics **32**(17), i567–i575 (2016)
33. Girotto, S., Comin, M., Pizzi, C.: Metagenomic reads binning with spaced seeds. Theor. Comput. Sci. **698**, 88–99 (2017)
34. Girotto, S., Comin, M., Pizzi, C.: Higher recall in metagenomic sequence classification exploiting overlapping reads. BMC Genomics **18**, 917 (2017)

Computational Identification of Essential Genes in Prokaryotes and Eukaryotes

Dawit Nigatu$^{(\boxtimes)}$ and Werner Henkel

Transmission Systems Group (TrSyS), Jacobs University Bremen,
Bremen, Germany
d.nigatu@jacobs-university.de, werner.henkel@ieee.org

Abstract. Several computational methods were proposed for the identification of essential genes (EGs). The machine learning based methods use features derived from the genetic sequences, gene-expression data, network topology, homology, and domain information. Except for the sequence-based features, the others require additional experimental data which is unavailable for under-studied and newly sequenced organisms. Hence, here, we propose a sequence-based identification of EGs. We performed gene essentiality predictions considering 15 bacteria, 1 archeaon, and 4 eukaryotes. Information-theoretic quantities, such as mutual information, conditional mutual information, entropy, Kullback-Leibler divergence, and Markov models, were used as features. In addition, with the hope of improving the prediction performance, other easily accessible sequence-based features related to stop codon usage, length, and GC content were included. For classification, the Random Forest algorithm was used. The performance of the proposed method is extensively evaluated by employing both intra- and cross-organism predictions. The obtained results were better than most of the previously published EG predictors which rely only on sequence information and comparable to those using additional features derived from network topology, homology, and gene-expression data.

Keywords: Essential genes · Information-theoretic features
Machine learning · Random Forest · Markov model

1 Introduction

If a disruption of a gene is lethal, the gene is defined to be an essential gene (EG) [1,2]. Identification of these genes is not only important for understanding gene function and the relationship between genotype and phenotype, but also has numerous advantages in the fields of synthetic biology and biomedicine. The EGs subset is considered as the minimal requirement to sustain the life of an organism and researchers are re-engineering microorganisms with a minimal genome [3]. EGs of pathogens can also be used as potential drug targets [4,5].

Different knock-out and gene-disruption experimental procedures were used to identify EGs. The methods include single gene knock-out [6,7], transposon

© Springer International Publishing AG, part of Springer Nature 2018
N. Peixoto et al. (Eds.): BIOSTEC 2017, CCIS 881, pp. 227–247, 2018.
https://doi.org/10.1007/978-3-319-94806-5_13

mutagenesis [8], and RNA interference [9]. Recently, the CRISPR (clustered regularly interspaced short palindromic repeats) gene-editing technology has also been used [10–12]. The experimental methods are very accurate. However, they are expensive and time-consuming. Hence, computational methods of EG predictions provide a worthwhile alternative. The earliest computational methods were based on homology mappings [13]. Afterwards, as the EG annotations of many model organisms became available in public databases, machine-learning based methods using features that characterize EGs became popular.

Gene essentiality has been associated with a lot of features. Broadly, the feature types can be classified as features related to sequence composition [14–16], network topology [17–20], subcellular localization [20–22], and gene expression [20,23]. The sequence-based features can be directly obtained from the genetic sequences. These include protein length, GC content, codon bias, amino acid composition, and domain information. In addition, homology information is also based on the genetic sequences. Nevertheless, homology mapping requires a computationally expensive sequence alignment and data base search. Network topology features are obtained from the properties of protein-protein interaction, gene regulatory, or metabolic networks. The most common network based property which is often exploited is degree centrality (EGs are often hubs). Features based on gene-expression data make use of mRNA expression and fluctuation levels.

With the exception of the sequence-based features, computation of the other features rely on the availability of additional experimental data. For the well studied model organisms, gene-expression and interaction networks are available. However, for newly sequenced and understudied species, one needs to perform gene-expression analysis and construct protein/gene networks beforehand. Hence, EG predictions which are based only on sequence information are very important.

Many studies have proposed EG predictors which are sequence-based [14–16,21,22,24–26]. Ning et al. [14] used nucleotide, di-nucleotide, codon, and amino acid frequencies along with codon bias information provided by the analysis software called CodonW (http://codonw.sourceforge.net). The most popular among the CodonW features, which showed a good predictive power and, hence, used by a lot of sequence-based predictors, is Codon Adaptation Index (CAI). CAI measures the relative adaptability of the codon usage in a gene to the codon usage of highly expressed genes [27]. Ning et al. performed cross-validation experiments considering 16 bacteria species. The other very effective EG predictor which uses sequence and sequence-derived properties is Song et al.'s ZUPLS [15]. The features used by ZUPLS are mainly from the so-called Z-curve features and other sequence-based features such as size, CAI, strand, homology, and domain enrichment scores. Cross-organism results were shown using models trained on *E. coli* and *B. subtilis*. Among the sequence-based methods, ZUPLUS seems to be the best method. Palaniappan and Mukherjee [21], in 2011, proposed a machine learning based EG predictor using sequence and pysio-chemical properties, plus cellular localization information. In addition to predictions of EGs between organisms, they showed results at higher taxonomic levels. In 2017, Liu et al. [22], using a feature which measures long-rage correlation (the Hurst exponent) and similar features to [21] made an extensive study on 31 bacteria and presented detailed results. In 2013, a method called Geptop (gene essentiality prediction tool based on orthology and phylogeny) [25] was proposed and due to the high accuracy and the availability of a Web server, it is the most used computational tool. Geptop is based on homology and evolutionary distance features. Using the defined essentiality scores, they performed a threshold-based prediction. Yu et al. [16] and Li et al. [24] used a different set of features based on fractals and inter-nucleotide distance sequences, respectively.

Other machine learning based methods which use sequence information together with network topology and gene expression include the works of Deng et al. [23] and Cheng et al. [20, 28]. Deng et al. [23] followed an integrative approach by combining sequence features with network topology, gene-expression, phylogeny, and domain information. They evaluated the transferability of essentiality annotations among *E. coli, B. subtilis, Acinetobacter baylyi,* and *Pseudomonas aeruginosa,* using a combination of four machine-learning algorithms. Cheng et al. [20] proposed a novel computational method using a combination of network topology, gene expression, and sequence-related features. They performed EG predictions considering 21 species and obtained excellent results.

There were also computational essential gene predictors applied to Eukaryotic species. Chen and Xu [29], in 2005, proposed a protein dispensability prediction based on rates of evolution, protein-protein interaction connectivity, gene-expression, and gene duplication. They used Neural Networks and Support Vector Machines (SVMs) for classifying genes of *Saccharomyces cerevisiae*. Seringhaus et al. [30] investigated the predictability of the EGs of the yeast *S. cerevisiae* using 14 features, which are accessible from the genomic sequence data. They used seven learning algorithms and obtained a positive predictive value (PPV) of 0.69. In addition, EGs of the closely related yeast *S. mikataea* were predicted using a model trained on *S. cerevisiae*. In 2012, Yuan et al. [31] used 491 features derived from the sequence, gene expression, and protein interaction networks and performed lethality phenotype predictions in mice. Their models produced a very good prediction accuracy. Lloyd et al. [32] analyzed relationships between lethality and various gene properties including network connectivity, gene copy number, and gene expression levels in *Arabidopsis thaliana*. Using these features and machine learning models, the EGs of *A. thaliana* were predicted and also cross-organism predictions to transfer essentiality annotations to *Oryza sativa* and *S. cerevisiae* were performed. Recently, Guo et al. [26] showed that using only sequence information, human essential genes can be accurately predicted. They employed an SVM algorithm and used the so-called λ- interval Z-curve features [33], reflecting nucleotide composition and associations.

In a previous study [34], we assessed the predictability of EGs on selected bacterial species using information-theoretic features and the support vector machine (SVM) algorithm. The obtained results were satisfactory and showed that EGs can be identified using only sequence information, without the need of further experimental data. The features we used were common information-theoretic measures such as entropy (Shannon and Gibbs), mutual information (MI), conditional mutual information (CMI), and Markov model based.

Following our study in [35], Shannon and Gibbs entropies were used to characterize the degree of randomness and thermodynamic stability in the gene sequences. MI and CMI has been widely used in the fields of bioinformatics and computational biology for a number of applications, including as a genomic signature [36], metric for phylogeny [37], and for identifying single nucleotide polymorphisms (SNPs) [38]. We used MI and CMI to measure the sequence organizational differences between EGs and NEGs. The Markov features were selected for measuring statistical dependencies in the gene sequences.

In the present work, in addition to the 15 bacterial species, essential gene predictions in Archea and Eukaryotic species were performed. Identification of EGs in four eukaryotes, including humans, and 1 archaeon was performed using a Random Forest classifier. More information-theoretic features, Kullback-Leibler divergence (KLD) between the distribution of k-mers ($k = 1, 2, 3$) in the genes and the background k-mer distributions in the training organism, the total MI, total CMI, and two additional entropy features, were added. Moreover, with the hope of increasing the prediction performance, other non-information-theoretic features, which can be easily obtained from the genetic sequences and known to have a correlation with gene essentiality, were included. The added features are related to optimized stop codon usage, gene length, and GC content. The predictive power of the five feature sets, both individually and collectively, was assessed. In addition to intra-organism predictions where both the training and testing examples are taken from a single species, cross-organismic predictions were also performed based on a pairwise and leave-one-species-out schemes. In the pairwise scheme, models trained on *E. coli* and *B. subtilis* were used to predict the EGs of the other bacteria, while in the leave-one-species-out scheme, EGs of the left out species are predicted using a model trained on the remaining bacteria. The obtained results are with multiple existing and state-of-the-art EG prediction methods.

2   Materials and Methods

2.1   Data Sources

The data for EGs and non essential genes (NEGs) for the 15 bacteria and 1 archaeon were downloaded from the database of essential genes (DEG 13.5). DEG collects a comprehensive list of essential and non-essential genes identified by various researchers through gene knock-out experimental methods [39]. In DEG, although the EGs dataset for eukaryotes are available, the list of NEGs are not included. One way to deal with this is, as done in most of the gene essentiality prediction studies, to regard all other genes as NEGs. Since some studies consider and test a small number of genes (small-scale screenings), taking the untested genes as non-essential could be misleading. Hence, for eukaryotic EG predictions, we used the dataset presented by the database of Online GEne Essentiality (OGEE) [40]. The species used in this study along with the number of EGs and NEGs are listed in Table 1 [34]. The genome sequences were obtained from the NCBI database (ftp://ftp.ncbi.nih.gov/genomes/). We selected the bacterial species studied by Ning et al. [14] to allow easy performance comparisons.

2.2 Information-Theoretic Features

Information-theoretic (IT) quantities enable the measurement and modeling of structural and compositional properties and have been extensively used in computational biology. Here, we used several IT measurements as features for identifying EGs. The IT features are mutual information (MI), conditional mutual information (CMI), entropy (E), Markov (M) model-related, and Kullback-Leibler divergence (KLD). The description of these features was presented in [34]. Here, introduce them again for comprehensiveness. For an additional detailed explanation, we refer the reader to standard information-theory text books [41].

Mutual Information (MI). The mutual information measures the information shared by two random variables. In other words, it is the amount of information one random variable provides about the other. Here, mutual information

Table 1. Names and abbreviations of the species used in this study. The accession numbers along with the number of essential and non-essential genes are listed.

No.	Organism	Abbr.	Accession No.	EGs	NEGs
1	*Acinetobacter baylyi ADP1*	AB	NC_005966	499	2594
2	*Bacillus subtilis 168*	BS	NC_000964	271	3904
3	*Escherichia coli MG1655*	EC	NC_000913	296	4077
4	*Francisella novicida U112*	FN	NC_008601	392	1329
5	*Haemophilus influenzae Rd KW20*	HI	NC_000907	642	512
6	*Helicobacter pylori 26695*	HP	NC_000915	323	1135
7	*Mycobacterium tuberculosis H37Rv*	MT	NC_000962	614	2552
8	*Mycoplasma genitalium G37*	MG	NC_000908	381	94
9	*Mycoplasma pulmonis UAB CTIP*	MP	NC_002771	310	322
10	*Pseudomonas aeruginosa UCBPP-PA14*	PA	NC_008463	335	960
11	*Salmonella enterica serovar Typhi*	SE	NC_004631	353	4005
12	*Salmonella typhimurium LT2*	ST	NC_003197	230	4228
13	*Staphylococcus aureus N315*	SA	NC_002745	302	2281
14	*Staphylococcus aureus NCTC 8325*	SA2	NC_007795	351	2541
15	*Vibrio cholerae N16961*	VC	NC_002505	779	2943
16	*Methanococcus maripaludis S2*	MM	NC_005791	519	1077
17	*Caenorhabditis elegans*	CEL	NC_003280	742	10704
18	*Drosophila melanogaster*	DRO	NT_033779	267	13514
19	*Homo sapiens*	HSA	NC_000015	1632	19897
20	*Mus musculus*	MUS	NC_000081	4289	4592

was used to measure the information between consecutive bases X and Y. It is mathematically defined as

$$I(X,Y) = \sum_{x \in \Omega} \sum_{y \in \Omega} P(x,y) \log_2 \frac{P(x,y)}{P(x)P(y)}, \tag{1}$$

where Ω is the set of nucleotides $\{A, T, C, G\}$, $P(x)$ and $P(y)$ are the marginal probabilities and $P(x,y)$ is the joint probability. In the corresponding gene sequences, the probabilities are estimated from the relative frequencies. In addition to the total mutual information computed according to Eq. (1), for each base pair (x,y), the quantity $P(x,y) \log_2 \frac{P(x,y)}{P(x)P(y)}$ is calculated and used as a feature. Therefore, a total of 17 MI-related features were calculated.

Conditional Mutual Information (CMI). The mutual information between two random variables X and Y conditioned on another random variable Z with a probability mass function (pmf) $P(z)$ is calculated as

$$\begin{aligned} I(X;Y|Z) &= \sum_{z \in \Omega} P(z) \sum_{x \in \Omega} \sum_{y \in \Omega} P(x,y|z) \log_2 \frac{P(x,y|z)}{P(x|z)P(y|z)} \\ &= \sum_{x \in \Omega} \sum_{y \in \Omega} \sum_{z \in \Omega} P(x,y,z) \log_2 \frac{P(z)P(x,y,z)}{P(x,z)P(y,z)} \end{aligned} \tag{2}$$

where $P(x,y,z), P(x,z)$, and $P(y,z)$ are the joint pmfs of the random variables shown in brackets. The three positions in a DNA triplet are regarded as the random variables X, Z, and Y, respectively. In addition to the CMI between X and Y conditioned on Z computed according to Eq. (2), for each possible triplet XZY, the quantity $P(x,y,z) \log_2 \frac{P(z)P(x,y,z)}{P(x,z)P(y,z)}$ was calculated and used as a feature. Hence, in total, 65 CMI-based features were obtained.

Entropy (E). The Shannon entropy [42] quantifies the average information content of the gene sequence from the distribution of symbols. The Shannon entropy is defined as

$$H_N = -\sum_i P_s^{(N)}(i) \log_2 P_s^{(N)}(i), \tag{3}$$

where $P_s^{(N)}(i)$ is the probability of the ith word of block size N. Shannon entropies of the DNA sequences of the genes were determined for block sizes of 2 (base pairs) and 3 (triplets).

Similarly, we used Gibbs' entropy to measure the thermodynamic stability of the genes. Gibbs' entropy is defined as

$$S_G = -k_B \sum_i P_G^N(i) \ln P_G^N(i), \tag{4}$$

where $P_G^N(i)$ is the probability to be in the ith state and k_B is the Boltzmann constant $(1.38 \times 10^{-23} \, \text{J/K})$. Gibbs' entropy is similar to Shannon's entropy except for the Boltzmann constant. Nevertheless, the probability distribution is associated with the thermodynamic stability, which is quantified by the nearest-neighbor free energy parameters. The probability distribution, $P_G(i)$, is modeled by the Boltzmann distribution given by

$$P_G^N(i) = \frac{n_i e^{-\frac{E(i)}{k_B T}}}{\sum_j n_j e^{-\frac{E(j)}{k_B T}}}. \tag{5}$$

T is the temperature in Kelvin and n_i is the frequency of the ith word of block size N. $E(i)$ is the free-energy according to [43]. In [43], the free-energies for base pairs at $37\,^\circ$C are provided. For larger block sizes, the energies can be determined by adding the energies of neighboring di-nucleotides. Shannon and Gibbs entropies for block size of 2 and 3 were calculated.

In addition to Shannon and Gibbs entropies, the relative entropy is computed and used as a feature. The relative entropy, also known as the Kullback-Leibler divergence (KLD) [44] measures the divergence between a probability distribution $P(x)$ and a model distribution $Q(x)$, and it is calculated as

$$KLD = \sum_i P(x) \log_2 \frac{P(x)}{Q(x)}. \tag{6}$$

The frequencies of the nucleotides, di-nucleotides, and tri-nucleotides in a given gene sequence were against the corresponding frequencies in the genome of the organism used for training the model (background distributions). Hence, in total, 7 entropy-related (2 Shannon, 2 Gibbs, 3 KLD) features were generated.

Markov (M). First, assuming that both EGs and NEGs were generated by two separate Markov chains, the correct Markov chain orders, using EGs and NEGs in the training data set, were estimated. Then, two Markov chains ($MC_+(mE)$ and $MC_-(mN)$) of the estimated orders (mE and mN) were constructed. After that, the features are obtained by scoring every gene using the constructed Markov chains.

Numerous Markov chain order estimators have been put forth in the literature. We have assessed the performances of selected estimators [45–49] on DNA sequence data and the estimator proposed by Papapetrou and Kugiumtzis [50] was chosen. The order estimation is based on CMI given in Eq. (2). A Markov chain of order L has the following property.

$$P(x_n | x_{n-1}, \ldots, x_{n-L}, x_{n-L-1}, \ldots) = P(x_n | x_{n-1}, \ldots x_{n-L}). \tag{7}$$

For any $m \le L$, since the nth and $(n-m)^{\text{th}}$ nucleotides are dependent, the CMI between the two conditioned on the $m-1$ bases in the middle will be greater than zero. Conversely, for any $m > L$, two nucleotides are independent and the CMI will be zero. Using this observation, Papapetrou and Kugiumtzis have proposed both parametric and non-parametric significance testing procedures [50,51]. Compared to other approximations, the results of the gamma distribution was better [51]. Hence, we used the gamma distribution based parametric approach for estimating the orders. In a symbol sequence of length N, $\hat{I}(X;Y|Z)$, the estimate of the CMI, is approximated by the gamma distribution as

$$\hat{I}(X;Y|Z) \approx \Gamma(\frac{|Z|}{2}(|X|-1)(|Y|-1), \frac{1}{N\ln 2}). \qquad (8)$$

The gamma distribution is used as the distribution of the null hypothesis, H_0 : $CMI(m) = 0$. Since $CMI \geq 0$ always holds, one-sided parameter testing is performed. Thus, the p-value is computed from the complementary cumulative distribution of the gamma distribution in Eq. 8. H_0 is rejected if the p-value is less than the nominal significance level ($\alpha = 0.05$). Starting from order zero, the null hypothesis is checked and if it is rejected, the next order is checked and the process continues until the null hypothesis is accepted. Using the correct estimated Markov orders, the Markov models are obtained by estimating the transition probabilities from the training sequences.

After the two Markov chains are constructed, the Markov features are computed by scoring the every gene sequences with the two Markov chains. If we represent the sequence as $b_1, b_2, b_3, \ldots, b_L$, the score for an order m is calculated as

$$Score = \sum_{i=1}^{L-m} P(b_i b_{i+1} \ldots b_{i+m}) \log_2(\frac{P(b_{i+m}|b_i b_{i+1} \ldots b_{i+m-1})}{P(b_{i+m})}). \qquad (9)$$

The score measures how likely the sequence is generated by the given mE-th and mN-th order Markov chain. The scores of the gene sequence on the Markov chains $MC_+(mE)$ and $MC_-(mN)$ were used as features. For intra-organism predictions, the Markov orders were estimated from the training sets whereas for cross-organismic gene essentiality predictions, order estimation increased the computational complexity without improving the result. Hence, we decided to use a fixed order Markov chain. After experimenting with orders 1 up to 6, order 1 (i.e., $mE = mN = 1$) was selected.

2.3   Other Simple Sequence-Based Features

To further increase the prediction performances, among the frequently used and easily accessible features, the GC content, length of the protein, and GC3 (GC content in the 3rd position of the codons) were computed. In addition, features related to stop codon usage were included. As in [15,30,31], we calculated the number of "close-to-stop" codons, which are codons a single third-nucleotide substitution away from one of the three stop codons (TAA, TAG, TGA). The five codons differing by a single base to the stop codons are TAC, TAT, TGT, TGC, and TGG. Hence, the total frequency of these codons is used as a feature. The idea is to measure how likely it is for the protein to be terminated when a substitution error occurs. In a similar direction, to include the case where a single insertion or deletion occurs causing a frame-shift, we added a new set of features. We computed the number of stop codons and the position of the first stop codon in the other two reading frames. In total, 8 features are included. For brevity, we call this set of features Stop + Len + GC or non-IT features.

2.4 Classifier Design and Evaluation

We implemented the Random Forest classifier using the data analytics platform Konstanz Information Miner (KNIME 3.3.1) [52] while feature preparation and computations were performed using Python 3.5.2. As a split criteria in the decision trees, information gain was used. Typically, the number of EGs is significantly smaller than that of the EGs. To balance the two classes, various schemes of under- and over-sampling approaches could be taken. Since it was shown in [16] that the choice of a balancing approach does not influence the performance of the classifiers in EG prediction applications, we employed a random undersampling of the majority class.

In cross-organism predictions, classifiers were trained on one (or more) organisms and tested on another, whereas in intra-organism predictions 80% of the data was used for training the models and 20% for testing. The random selections were repeated 100 times, i.e., 100-fold Monte Carlo cross-validation were performed for model establishment.

Typically, the Area Under the Curve (AUC) of the Receiver Operating characteristic Curve (ROC) is used to evaluate a performance of a binary classification. The ROC plots the true positive rate versus false positive rate and shows the trade-off between sensitivity and specificity for all possible thresholds. Other performance evaluation such as F-measure and Accuracy depend on a selected threshold value. Therefore, the AUC score is used for analyzing the performance of the classifier.

3 Results and Discussion

3.1 Prediction of Essential Genes in Bacteria

Intra-organism Predictions. The Bacteria EC, BS, and MP were selected to assess the intra-organism prediction performance in which models are trained and tested on a data obtained from the same species. This setup is typically practical when a portion of the essentiality annotations are performed using an experimental method and machine learning methods are performed to complete the analysis.

EC has 296 EGs and 4077 NEGs. The Random Forest classifier was trained on 80% of the data and the remaining 20% were used to test the model. All five feature groups (MI, CMI, Entropy, Markov, Stop + Len + GC), both individually and collectively, were used and 100 iterations were performed. The average ROC curves are shown in Fig. 1. The combination of all features produced a very good AUC score of 0.86. Equally good results were achieved by using CMI features alone. The results of MI and Markov features were also satisfactory while the entropy and the newly incorporated non-IT features yielded a relatively small prediction accuracy.

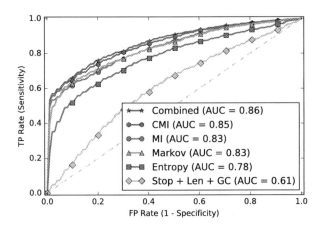

Fig. 1. EG predictions in *E. coli*. The estimated Markov orders were 5 for both EGs and NEGs.

Similarly, the prediction results of our proposed method applied to the bacteria MP are presented in Fig. 2. Using the complete feature set, an AUC score of 0.82 was obtained. Taken separately, all feature groups provided a score greater than 0.72. The result shows that the added non-IT features (Stop + Len + GC) also have the ability to distinguish between essential and non-essential genes with a decent accuracy (0.72). A much higher AUC score of 0.90 was achieved for the bacteria BS (Fig. 3). Both MI and CMI features achieved a score of 0.87, while the entropy and Stop + Len + GC features yielded 0.79 and 0.76, respectively.

Compared to our previous results using the SVM algorithm [34], on average a 4% improvement was obtained, which is due to the additional features. Ning et al. [14] performed a five-fold cross-validation on EC and MP using sequence composition features [14]. Our method improved the results slightly from 0.82 to 0.86 in EC and from 0.74 to 0.82 in MP.

Cross-Organism Predictions. In cross-organism predictions a model trained on the fully annotated genes of a species or set of species is used to predict the EGs of another species. We applied two schemes of cross-organism predictions. The first is a one-vs-one prediction where training and testing was performed between pairs of organisms. Following Song et al.'s [15] approach, models trained on the two well-studied organisms BS (Gram positive) and EC (Gram negative) were used to predict EGs of the other 14 bacteria [15]. The second is a leave-one-out approach in which the classifiers were trained using 14 bacteria and the EGs of the remaining bacteria were predicted.

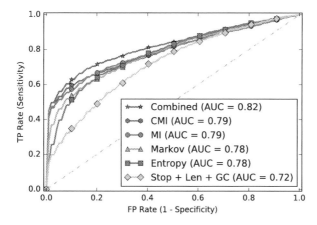

Fig. 2. EG predictions in *M. pulmonis*. The estimated Markov orders were 6 for both EGs and NEGs.

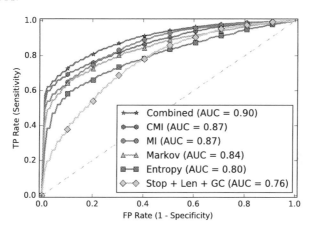

Fig. 3. The average ROC curves of *B. subtilis* EG prediction. The estimated Markov orders were 5 for EGs and 4 for NEGs.

Both models trained on BS and EC resulted in a comparable performance (Fig. 4), averaging to an AUC score of 0.80. The only notable differences were in the prediction of the EGs of MP and PA. A 9% improvement was obtained in predicting MP based on BS rather than EC, whereas the EC model attained a 5% improvement in the prediction of PA. This is due to the phylogenetic relationships, MP is closer to BS and PA is closer to EC. The prediction accuracy of our proposed method is comparable to other published methods, including the ones using network topology and gene-expression features in addition to sequence information. Deng et al. [23] presented a pairwise prediction among AB, BS, and EC using an integrative approach and obtained an average AUC score of 0.83 which is close to our result. The other more successful sequence-based predictor proposed by Song et al. [15] called ZUPLS presented pairwise predictions using models trained with BS and EC. The average AUC score of both models tested on 9 bacteria was 0.86, which is slightly better (4%) compared to our method. However, due to the high computational effort for obtaining the homology- and domain-related features, our method could provide an alternative with a little penalty on the accuracy. We performed an extensive pairwise prediction producing a 15×15 AUC matrix. Similar large-scale pairwise predictions were presented by two research groups, Cheng et al. [28] on 21 species and Liu et al. [22] on 31 species. To compare the performances of the three methods, we plotted the distribution of the pairwise AUC scores of the 15 common species in Fig. 5. Our predictor is significantly better than Liu et al.'s, while Cheng et al.'s predictor is slightly better than ours.

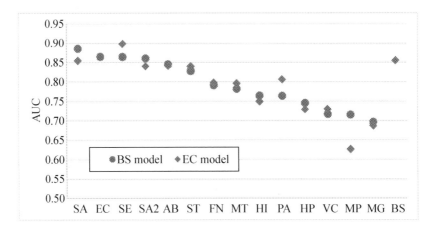

Fig. 4. Pairwise cross-organism predictions results on models trained on EC and BS.

The results of the leave-one-species-out validation are presented in Fig. 6. An average AUC score of 0.81 was obtained. This is similar to the previous results using SVM [34]. The only major improvement is the prediction of MG, where the performance increased from 0.66 to 0.70. Hence, the additional features and the use of a different machine learning algorithm did not affect the result. This shows that the obtained results of the classification are due to the information-theoretic features. A comparison to other EG predictors which presented their results using a leave-one-out approach is shown in Fig. 6. Our method is superior to Liu et al.'s [22] and Palaniappan and Mukherjee's [21]. Geptop [25] is the best and most used among published essential gene prediction tools. Our method yielded a similar performance to Geptop (Fig. 6). However, on the most studied bacteria, such as BS and EC, where the quality of data is much higher, the results of Geptop are outstanding (around a 10% improvement).

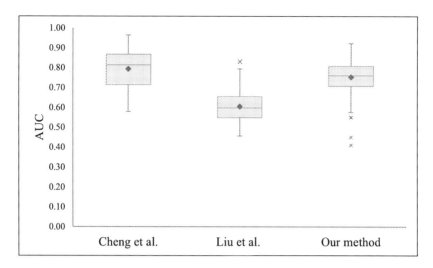

Fig. 5. A comparison between pairwise prediction results of our method and two existing methods, proposed by Cheng et al. [28] and Liu et al. [22]. The diamond markers show the mean values.

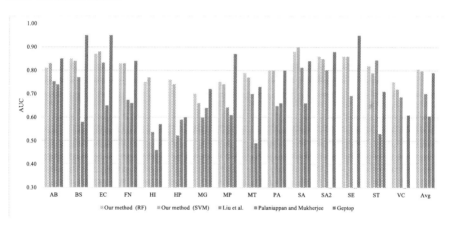

Fig. 6. Leave-one-species-out prediction results using RF and SVM [34]. For comparison, results of three other methods are presented [21,22,25]

3.2   Prediction of EGs in Archaea

Methanococcus maripaludis (MM) is the only archaeon whose EGs and NEGs are available in DEG, generated experimentally by Sarimento et al. [53]. We trained the RF classifier using 80% of the genes, which are randomly selected, and predicted the remaining 20%. The ROC curves of the five feature groups along with their combination are shown in Fig. 7. Using all features, an average AUC score of 0.73 was obtained, which is good but smaller than the values obtained for most of the bacteria. This can be due to the reduced quality of the data. Sarimento et al. could not confidently specify weather 419 genes are essential or non-essential [53]. Hence, most of these genes are regarded as NEGs.

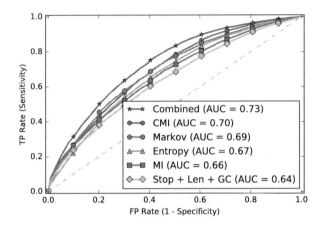

Fig. 7. The average ROC curves of EG prediction in *Methanococcus maripaludis*. The estimated Markov order is 6.

We further predicted the EGs of MM using the known essential and non-essential genes of the bacteria EC and BS. The achieved AUC scores were not satisfactory, 0.59 using EC and 0.64 using BS. The decline in performance is expected because of the inherent differences in the genetic makeup between bacteria and archaea.

3.3   Prediction of EGs in Eukaryots

Genome-scale gene deletion experiments and systematic screens using RNA interference (RNAi) were applied to determine the EGs of relatively simpler eukaryotes, such as yeast and *C. elegans*. However, the RNAi screening technique has not been successful in mammals [54]. Besides, EGs in higher species can only be identified in connection to the indispensability in specific cell types, typically tumor-specific essential genes. The introduction of the CRISPR-Cas9 genome editing method has enabled the identification of human EGs [10–12].

Prediction of EGs in *Homo sapiens*. Experimental studies in human gene essentiality are performed with a purpose of identifying the EGs in different cell lines. Mostly, gene essentiality is determined in relation to the proliferation and viability in various human cancer cell lines, such as ovarian, colon, and chronic myeloid leukemia (CML). Hence, the characterized set of EGs is cell-specific and does not indicate essentiality in all cell types [55]. In the OGEE database, 18 data sets from 7 separate studies are provided. Some of the data sets are small scale and cover only a limited portion of the genes while some of the studies are genome-wide, investigating around 20,000 genes. Since a gene can be designated essential in one data set and non-essential in the other, OGEE adopts a third category named conditionally essential genes (CEG). A specific gene was covered by up to 11 data sets and if all the studies do not agree on the essentiality, it is labeled as CEG.

Out of 21,529 genes, 182 are EGs, 6,985 are CEGs, and 14,362 are NEGs. To categorize the CEGs as essential or non-essential, we adopted a simple majority voting scheme. That is, a CEG is regarded as EG if it is essential in a majority of cell lines. This resulted in 1,632 EGs. We trained RF classifiers for each of the five feature sets and their combinations. The data was split into 80% for training and 20% for testing and 100 trials with different sets were performed. The ROC curves are presented in Fig. 8. Using all the available features, a decent AUC of 0.76 was obtained. Similar to the prokaryotic EG prediction, the mutual information features provided the largest contribution. However, the newly added non-IT features were better than the entropy and Markov features. Guo et al. [26] predicted human EGs utilizing only intrinsic sequence information and obtained an AUC score of 0.89. However, the approach used by Guo et al. is a little bit different. They prepared the positive data set based on a majority decision on essentiality in 11 cell lines. A gene is considered essential if it essential in more than 6 cell lines. Otherwise, the gene is totally discarded rather than taking it as a negative sample. Afterwards, they obtained 1,516 EGs and 10,499 NEGs. Considering that even the CRISPR-based experimental method proposed by Wang et al. [12] yielded a 0.78 AUC score when validated using known EGs of a yeast genome, our results are good.

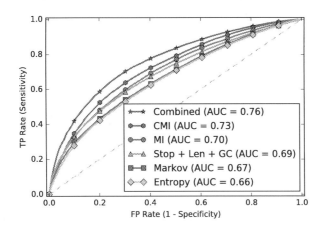

Fig. 8. The average ROC curves of *H. sapiens* EG prediction.

Prediction of EGs in *Drosophila melanogaster*. The other commonly used model organism in developmental biology studies is *Drosophila melanogaster* (DRO). Although there are two data sets providing essentiality annotations for DRO, one of them tested only 437 genes. Hence, we only took the large-scale results obtained using double stranded RNAi on embryonic hemocyte (blood cell) lines. Among the 13781 tested genes, only 267 were found to be EGs. That is the smallest reported percentage of EGs among eukaryotic species. The prediction results are presented in Fig. 9. The combined features yielded a very high AUC score (0.87) and the performances of the individual feature groups are also satisfactory.

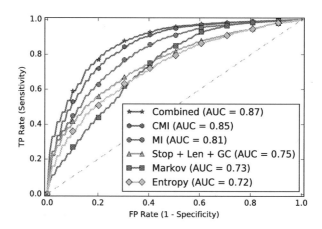

Fig. 9. The average ROC curves of *Drosophila melanogaster* EG prediction.

Prediction of EGs in *Caenorhabditis elegans*. Next, we tested the ability of our method to classify EGs of *Caenorhabditis elegans* (CEL). The CEL dataset in the OGEE database contains 742 EGs and 10704 NEGs. Intra-organism predictions were performed and the ROC curves of 100 iterations are presented in Fig. 10. The prediction scores by all of the feature sets were very high (AUC ≥ 0.74). Taking all the features, an AUC score of 0.85 was obtained.

Prediction of EGs in *Mus musculus*. The *Mus musculus* (MUS) dataset has 4289 EGs and 4592 NEGs. Through a similar validation procedure, we predicted the EGs. The ROC curves are shown in Fig. 11. The combined AUC score was relatively low (0.66). This could be either due to the uncharacteristically almost equal number of EGs and NEGs or the poor predictive power of the used features. We have roughly checked the quality of the annotations by comparing it to another dataset provided by Dickinson et al. [56]. In this dataset, through a developmental gene knock-out study performed on 1751 genes, 410 were found to be lethal genes and 1143 were viable genes. Roughly 124 genes which were regarded as essential in the OGEE dataset are non-essential. This shows that the list of EGs does not reflect the absolute minimal set. Moreover, the mouse genome contains around 23,000 protein-coding genes but only essentiality annotations for 8881 were provided.

Cross-Organism Prediction Between Eukaryotes. To test the transferability of EG annotations among the eukaryotic species, cross-organism predictions

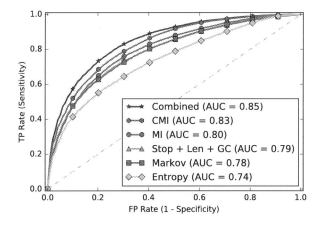

Fig. 10. The average ROC curves of EG predictions in *C. elegans* (worm).

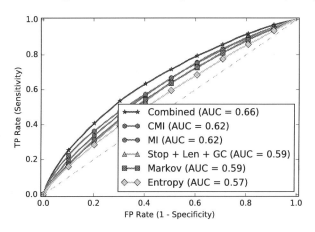

Fig. 11. The average ROC curves of EG prediction in *Mus musculus*.

were performed by training classifiers using DRO, CEL, and HSA data sets. Prediction of CEL using models trained on DRO and HSA yielded an average AUC score of 0.72 and 0.73, respectively. However, our method failed to predict human EGs using both DRO and CEL models. Prediction of DRO EGs using a classifier trained on HSA was also not possible (AUC $= 0.47$), while an AUC score of 0.68 was obtained using CEL. All in all, cross-organismic EG predictions in eukaryotes were not as successful as it was in bacteria.

4   Conclusion

We performed prediction of EGs in the three domains of life. The proposed machine learning based predictor applies information-theoretic measures to the DNA sequences of the genes and use them as features along with other commonly used non-information-theoretic features. The predictive powers of five feature sets, namely, mutual information, conditional mutual information, entropy, Markov, and features related to stop codon usage, length, and GC content were analyzed. A Random Forest classifier was used and performance evaluations were carried out considering both intra- and cross-organism predictions. Since the features were exclusively derived from the sequences, identification of EGs is possible in newly sequenced or under-studied organisms.

Applied in bacteria, our proposed method yielded a very good prediction performance. The prediction accuracy is better than most existing predictors which rely only on sequence information and it is as good as the methods using network topology, homology, and gene-expression in addition to sequence-based features. Intra-organism prediction capabilities were demonstrated in *B. subtilis* (AUC = 0.90), *E. coli* (AUC = 0.86), and *M. pulmonis* (AUC = 0.82). A cross-organism prediction was performed using models trained by using *B. subtilis* and *E. coli* genes and to identify the EGs of the 14 bacteria. Both models yielded a similar accuracy, an average AUC score of around 0.8 (Fig. 4). In a leave-one-out validation scheme, a model was trained on 14 bacteria and tested using the remaining bacterium. The obtained results, average AUC score 0.81, were better than in earlier publications [21,22].

In the archaeon *Methanococcus maripaludis*, an average AUC score of 0.77 was obtained. In eukaryotes, we studied the possible prediction of EGs in *Homo sapiens*, *Drosophila melanogaster*, *Mus musculus*, and *Caenorhabditis elegans*. In *H. sapiens*, the gene essentiality data is based on cancer cell lines. Hence, there are some genes whose essentiality is conditional, i.e., essential in one cell line and non-essential in another. Our model classified the human genes with an AUC score of 0.76, which is a decent performance but not as good as the method proposed by Guo et al. [26]. EGs of *D. melanogaster* and *C. elegans* were predicted with a very good accuracy, AUC scores of 0.87 and 0.85, respectively. However, in *M. musculus*, the prediction result was worse, AUC 0.66. We suspect that the reason for this is the reduced quality of the annotations in the data. Almost 50% of the 8881 investigated genes were EGs, which is inconsistent to the percentage of essential genes in other species. Cross-organism predictions among eukaryotes were also not as successful as they were between bacteria. Only *C. elegans* was predicted with a good accuracy using the other species.

To conclude, we demonstrated that information-theoretic features, which can be easily derived from the genetic sequences, allow the classification of EGs and NEGs in both prokaryotes and eukaryotes.

References

1. Koonin, E.V.: How many genes can make a cell: the minimal-gene-set concept 1. Annu. Rev. Genomics Hum. Genet. **1**(1), 99–116 (2000)
2. Itaya, M.: An estimation of minimal genome size required for life. FEBS Lett. **362**(3), 257–260 (1995)
3. Hutchison, C.A., Chuang, R.Y., Noskov, V.N., Assad-Garcia, N., Deerinck, T.J., Ellisman, M.H., Gill, J., Kannan, K., Karas, B.J., Ma, L., et al.: Design and synthesis of a minimal bacterial genome. Science **351**(6280), aad6253 (2016)

4. Chalker, A.F., Lunsford, R.D.: Rational identification of new antibacterial drug targets that are essential for viability using a genomics-based approach. Pharmacol. Ther. **95**(1), 1–20 (2002)
5. Lamichhane, G., Zignol, M., Blades, N.J., Geiman, D.E., Dougherty, A., Grosset, J., Broman, K.W., Bishai, W.R.: A postgenomic method for predicting essential genes at subsaturation levels of mutagenesis: application to Mycobacterium tuberculosis. Proc. Natl. Acad. Sci. **100**(12), 7213–7218 (2003)
6. Chen, L., Ge, X., Xu, P.: Identifying essential Streptococcus sanguinis genes using genome-wide deletion mutation. Gene Essentiality: Methods Protoc., 15–23 (2015)
7. Giaever, G., Chu, A.M., Ni, L., Connelly, C., Riles, L., Veronneau, S., Dow, S., Lucau-Danila, A., Anderson, K., Andre, B., et al.: Functional profiling of the Saccharomyces cerevisiae genome. Nature **418**(6896), 387–391 (2002)
8. Salama, N.R., Shepherd, B., Falkow, S.: Global transposon mutagenesis and essential gene analysis of Helicobacter pylori. J. Bacteriol. **186**(23), 7926–7935 (2004)
9. Cullen, L.M., Arndt, G.M.: Genome-wide screening for gene function using RNAi in mammalian cells. Immunol. Cell Biol. **83**(3), 217–223 (2005)
10. Blomen, V.A., Májek, P., Jae, L.T., Bigenzahn, J.W., Nieuwenhuis, J., Staring, J., Sacco, R., van Diemen, F.R., Olk, N., Stukalov, A., et al.: Gene essentiality and synthetic lethality in haploid human cells. Science **350**(6264), 1092–1096 (2015)
11. Hart, T., Chandrashekhar, M., Aregger, M., Steinhart, Z., Brown, K.R., MacLeod, G., Mis, M., Zimmermann, M., Fradet-Turcotte, A., Sun, S., et al.: High-resolution CRISPR screens reveal fitness genes and genotype-specific cancer liabilities. Cell **163**(6), 1515–1526 (2015)
12. Wang, T., Birsoy, K., Hughes, N.W., Krupczak, K.M., Post, Y., Wei, J.J., Lander, E.S., Sabatini, D.M.: Identification and characterization of essential genes in the human genome. Science **350**(6264), 1096–1101 (2015)
13. Mushegian, A.R., Koonin, E.V.: A minimal gene set for cellular life derived by comparison of complete bacterial genomes. Proc. Natl. Acad. Sci. **93**(19), 10268–10273 (1996)
14. Ning, L., Lin, H., Ding, H., Huang, J., Rao, N., Guo, F.: Predicting bacterial essential genes using only sequence composition information. Genet. Mol. Res. **13**, 4564–4572 (2014)
15. Song, K., Tong, T., Wu, F.: Predicting essential genes in prokaryotic genomes using a linear method: ZUPLS. Integr. Biol. **6**(4), 460–469 (2014)
16. Yu, Y., Yang, L., Liu, Z., Zhu, C.: Gene essentiality prediction based on fractal features and machine learning. Mol. BioSyst. **13**(3), 577–584 (2017)
17. Plaimas, K., Eils, R., König, R.: Identifying essential genes in bacterial metabolic networks with machine learning methods. BMC Syst. Biol. **4**(1), 1 (2010)
18. Acencio, M.L., Lemke, N.: Towards the prediction of essential genes by integration of network topology, cellular localization and biological process information. BMC Bioinf. **10**(1), 1 (2009)
19. Lu, Y., Deng, J., Rhodes, J.C., Lu, H., Lu, L.J.: Predicting essential genes for identifying potential drug targets in Aspergillus fumigatus. Comput. Biol. Chem. **50**, 29–40 (2014)
20. Cheng, J., Xu, Z., Wu, W., Zhao, L., Li, X., Liu, Y., Tao, S.: Training set selection for the prediction of essential genes. PLoS ONE **9**(1), e86805 (2014)
21. Palaniappan, K., Mukherjee, S.: Predicting essential genes across microbial genomes: a machine learning approach. In: 2011 10th International Conference on Machine Learning and Applications and Workshops (ICMLA), vol. 2, pp. 189–194. IEEE (2011)

22. Liu, X., Wang, B.J., Xu, L., Tang, H.L., Xu, G.Q.: Selection of key sequence-based features for prediction of essential genes in 31 diverse bacterial species. PLoS ONE **12**(3), e0174638 (2017)
23. Deng, J., Deng, L., Su, S., Zhang, M., Lin, X., Wei, L., Minai, A.A., Hassett, D.J., Lu, L.J.: Investigating the predictability of essential genes across distantly related organisms using an integrative approach. Nucleic Acids Res. **39**(3), 795–807 (2011)
24. Li, Y., Lv, Y., Li, X., Xiao, W., Li, C.: Sequence comparison and essential gene identification with new inter-nucleotide distance sequences. J. Theor. Biol. **418**, 84–93 (2017)
25. Wei, W., Ning, L.W., Ye, Y.N., Guo, F.B.: Geptop: a gene essentiality prediction tool for sequenced bacterial genomes based on orthology and phylogeny. PLoS ONE **8**(8), e72343 (2013)
26. Guo, F.B., Dong, C., Hua, H.L., Liu, S., Luo, H., Zhang, H.W., Jin, Y.T., Zhang, K.Y.: Accurate prediction of human essential genes using only nucleotide composition and association information. Bioinformatics **33**(12), 1758–1764 (2017)
27. Sharp, P.M., Li, W.H.: The Codon Adaptation Index-a measure of directional synonymous codon usage bias, and its potential applications. Nucleic Acids Res. **15**(3), 1281–1295 (1987)
28. Cheng, J., Wu, W., Zhang, Y., Li, X., Jiang, X., Wei, G., Tao, S.: A new computational strategy for predicting essential genes. BMC Genom. **14**(1), 910 (2013)
29. Chen, Y., Xu, D.: Understanding protein dispensability through machine-learning analysis of high-throughput data. Bioinformatics **21**(5), 575–581 (2005)
30. Seringhaus, M., Paccanaro, A., Borneman, A., Snyder, M., Gerstein, M.: Predicting essential genes in fungal genomes. Genome Res. **16**(9), 1126–1135 (2006)
31. Yuan, Y., Xu, Y., Xu, J., Ball, R.L., Liang, H.: Predicting the lethal phenotype of the knockout mouse by integrating comprehensive genomic data. Bioinformatics **28**(9), 1246–1252 (2012)
32. Lloyd, J.P., Seddon, A.E., Moghe, G.D., Simenc, M.C., Shiu, S.H.: Characteristics of plant essential genes allow for within-and between-species prediction of lethal mutant phenotypes. Plant Cell **27**(8), 2133–2147 (2015)
33. Guo, F.B., Ou, H.Y., Zhang, C.T.: ZCURVE: a new system for recognizing protein-coding genes in bacterial and archaeal genomes. Nucleic Acids Res. **31**(6), 1780–1789 (2003)
34. Nigatu, D., Henkel, W.: Prediction of essential genes based on machine learning and information theoretic features. In: Proceedings of BIOSTEC 2017 - BIOINFORMATICS, pp. 81–92 (2017)
35. Nigatu, D., Henkel, W., Sobetzko, P., Muskhelishvili, G.: Relationship between digital information and thermodynamic stability in bacterial genomes. EURASIP J. Bioinf. Syst. Biol. **2016**(1), 1 (2016)
36. Bauer, M., Schuster, S.M., Sayood, K.: The average mutual information profile as a genomic signature. BMC Bioinf. **9**(1), 1 (2008)
37. Date, S.V., Marcotte, E.M.: Discovery of uncharacterized cellular systems by genome-wide analysis of functional linkages. Nat. Biotechnol. **21**(9), 1055–1062 (2003)
38. Hagenauer, J., Dawy, Z., Göbel, B., Hanus, P., Mueller, J.: Genomic analysis using methods from information theory. In: Information Theory Workshop, pp. 55–59. IEEE (2004)
39. Luo, H., Lin, Y., Gao, F., Zhang, C.T., Zhang, R.: DEG 10, an update of the database of essential genes that includes both protein-coding genes and noncoding genomic elements. Nucleic Acids Res. **42**(D1), D574–D580 (2014)

40. Chen, W.H., Minguez, P., Lercher, M.J., Bork, P.: OGEE: an online gene essentiality database. Nucleic Acids Res. **40**(D1), D901–D906 (2011)
41. Cover, T.M., Thomas, J.A.: Elements of Information Theory. Wiley, Hoboken (2012)
42. Shannon, C.: A mathematical theory of communication. Bell System Technical Journal **27**, 379–423, 623–656 (1948). Mathematical Reviews (MathSciNet): MR10, 133e
43. SantaLucia, J.: A unified view of polymer, dumbbell, and oligonucleotide DNA nearest-neighbor thermodynamics. Proc. Natl. Acad. Sci. **95**(4), 1460–1465 (1998)
44. Kullback, S., Leibler, R.A.: On information and sufficiency. Ann. Math. Stat. **22**(1), 79–86 (1951)
45. Tong, H.: Determination of the order of a Markov chain by Akaike's information criterion. J. Appl. Probab. **12**, 488–497 (1975)
46. Katz, R.W.: On some criteria for estimating the order of a Markov chain. Technometrics **23**(3), 243–249 (1981)
47. Peres, Y., Shields, P.: Two new Markov order estimators. ArXiv Mathematics e-prints, June 2005
48. Dalevi, D., Dubhashi, D.: The Peres-Shields order estimator for fixed and variable length Markov models with applications to DNA sequence similarity. In: Casadio, R., Myers, G. (eds.) WABI 2005. LNCS, vol. 3692, pp. 291–302. Springer, Heidelberg (2005). https://doi.org/10.1007/11557067_24
49. Menéndez, M., Pardo, L., Pardo, M., Zografos, K.: Testing the order of Markov dependence in DNA sequences. Methodol. Comput. Appl. Probab. **13**(1), 59–74 (2011)
50. Papapetrou, M., Kugiumtzis, D.: Markov chain order estimation with conditional mutual information. Physica A: Stat. Mech. Appl. **392**(7), 1593–1601 (2013)
51. Papapetrou, M., Kugiumtzis, D.: Markov chain order estimation with parametric significance tests of conditional mutual information. Simul. Model. Pract. Theory **61**, 1–13 (2016)
52. Berthold, M.R., et al.: KNIME: the Konstanz information miner. In: Preisach, C., Burkhardt, H., Schmidt-Thieme, L., Decker, R. (eds.) GfKL 2007. Studies in Classification, Data Analysis, and Knowledge Organization. Springer, Heidelberg (2007). https://doi.org/10.1007/978-3-540-78246-9_38
53. Sarmiento, F., Mrázek, J., Whitman, W.B.: Genome-scale analysis of gene function in the hydrogenotrophic methanogenic archaeon Methanococcus maripaludis. Proc. Natl. Acad. Sci. **110**(12), 4726–4731 (2013)
54. Fraser, A.: Essential human genes. Cell Syst. **1**(6), 381–382 (2015)
55. Boone, C., Andrews, B.J.: The indispensable genome. Science **350**(6264), 1028–1029 (2015)
56. Dickinson, M.E., Flenniken, A.M., Ji, X., Teboul, L., Wong, M.D., White, J.K., Meehan, T.F., Weninger, W.J., Westerberg, H., Adissu, H., et al.: High-throughput discovery of novel developmental phenotypes. Nature **537**(7621), 508 (2016)

A Heuristic for the Live Parsimony Problem

Rogério Güths[1], Guilherme P. Telles[2], Maria Emilia M. T. Walter[3],
and Nalvo F. Almeida[1(✉)]

[1] School of Computing, Federal University of Mato Grosso do Sul,
Campo Grande, Brazil
`r.guths@ufms.br, nalvo@facom.ufms.br`
[2] Institute of Computing, University of Campinas, Campinas, Brazil
`gpt@ic.unicamp.br`
[3] Department of Computer Science, University of Brasilia, Brasilia, Brazil
`mariaemilia@unb.br`

Abstract. Live Phylogeny generalizes the phylogeny theory by admitting living ancestors among the taxonomic objects. This theory suits cases of fast-evolving species like virus, and phylogenies of non-biological objects like documents, images and database records. In character-based live phylogeny, the input is a matrix with n objects and m characters, such each position i,j keeps the state of character j for the object i. The output is a tree where the input objects are represented as leaves or internal nodes labeled with a string of m symbols, representing the state of the characters. The goal is to obtain a tree with the minimal number of state changes along the edges, considering all characters, called the most parsimonious tree. In this paper we analyze problems related to most parsimonious tree using Live Phylogeny. We propose an improvement to a previously presented branch-and-bound algorithm and also a new heuristic for the problem. We present the results of experiments with a set of 20 Zika virus genome sequences, comparing the performance of our heuristic.

Keywords: Phylogeny · Character state phylogeny · Live phylogeny
Parsimony · Algorithms

1 Introduction

Two main approaches for solving the problem of reconstructing the evolutionary history of taxonomic objects and their relations with common ancestors are present in the literature: distance-based and character-based.

In both cases a tree whose leaves represent the taxonomic objects and whose internal nodes represent hypothetical ancestors must be constructed. In distance-based methods the problem is to build a tree whose distances are equal to the distances in an input distance matrix. In character-based methods the problem

N. Peixoto et al. (Eds.): BIOSTEC 2017, CCIS 881, pp. 248–267, 2018.
https://doi.org/10.1007/978-3-319-94806-5_14

is to build a tree that reflects the changes of character states during evolution course, provided that the state of each character of the leaves are given as input.

Character-based phylogeny is the focus of this work. We investigate phylogeny reconstruction based on parsimony, where one tries to minimize the total number of character state changes along the edges of the tree [5,15]. There are two major problems related to parsimony: the *Large Parsimony Problem* (LPP), where a tree must be build and labels must be assigned to the nodes, and the *Small Parsimony Problem* (SPP), where the tree is given as input and the task is assigning labels to the nodes. The later is easier to solve.

An extended theory, called *Live Phylogeny*, was defined in [16]. Live phylogeny generalizes traditional phylogeny by admitting the presence of living ancestors among the input objects, called *live internal nodes*. Live phylogeny suits well for sets of fast-evolving objects, like viruses [2,8], and may be used to model the relationship of non-biological ones, such as documents, images or relational database entries [3,13]. Figure 1 shows a phylogenetic tree with two live internal nodes.

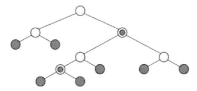

Fig. 1. Live phylogeny with two live internal nodes. Internal nodes are depicted with double lines.

In a previous work [9] we introduced new versions of the large and of the small parsimony problems called them *Large Live Parsimony Problem* (LLPP) and *Small Live Parsimony Problem* (SLPP), and showed that LLPP is NP-complete. These new problems generalize their traditional counterparts allowing the existence of live internal nodes in the trees. We started our exploration of live parsimony problems focusing on SLPP first, because it is easier and because it may useful to solve LLPP in the same fashion that SPP is used by many heuristics to solve LPP [17]. Also, while envisioning a branch-and-bound algorithm for the LLPP, the need for a solver of SLPP became clear.

This article extends our prior work [9] as follows:

- a detailed description of the original branch-and-bound is provided, including examples and a proof that it covers the search space,
- an improvement on the original branch-and-bound is introduced, based on the selection of choices leading to live internal nodes,
- a constructive heuristic for LLPP is proposed, and
- alternative topologies for a set of Zika virus strains are given.

The text is organized as follows. Section 2 introduces the parsimony problems. Section 3 presents solutions of SPP. Section 4 is devoted to the solution of SLPP. Section 5 presents a branch-and-bound for LLPP and introduces an improvement. A constructive heuristic for LLPP is presented in Sect. 6. Section 7 presents our experiments and introduces new topologies for a set of Zika virus strains. Finally, Sect. 8 brings our concluding remarks.

2   Parsimony Problems

The *Large Parsimony Problem* (LPP) takes n objects as input, each one labeled by a string of m symbols $s_1 \ldots s_m$ where s_j represents the state of character j, and a symmetric score function $\delta(a, b)$ that expresses the cost of changing any character from state a to state b. Each state of a character is a symbol from a set $\mathcal{S}$, with $|\mathcal{S}| = k$. The output is a binary rooted tree T where the leaves are the input objects, and each internal node v is labeled with a string of m symbols $v_1 \ldots v_m$, having symbol v_j representing the state of character j, such that $d(v, w) = \sum_{j=1}^{m} \delta(v_j, w_j)$ and $S(T) = \sum_{(v,w) \in T} d(v, w)$ is minimum. The distance $d(v, w)$ between adjacent nodes v, w expresses the cost of changes that occurred between them. The minimum score of a phylogeny is called *minimum parsimony score*. This problem has been proved NP-hard [7].

If the tree topology is given, the problem is easier. This version is called *Small Parsimony Problem* (SPP) and consists in labeling the internal nodes minimizing the total score [11].

3   Small Parsimony Problems

Two aspects involving the parsimony problems must be considered. The first one is the relationship among characters. We consider that each character is used as an independent hypothesis of evolution, and then SPP (and all the other problems in this article) can be solved separately for each character.

The second aspect is related to the score function used to account for character state changes in the evolution model. We will analyze two types of score function: general and binary. In the binary case, $\delta(a, b) = 1$ if $a \neq b$ or $\delta(a, b) = 0$ otherwise. In the general case, $\delta(a, b) \mapsto \mathbb{R}$.

3.1   SPP Using a General Score Function

SPP was solved by Sankoff [14] using dynamic programming. Let $s_t(v)$ be the minimum parsimony score of a subtree rooted at node v labeled with state t. Recall that the problem is being solved for a single character. Thus, $s_t(v)$ can be easily calculated as [9]:

$$s_t(v) = \min_{i \in \mathcal{S}}\{s_i(u) + \delta(i, t)\} + \min_{j \in \mathcal{S}}\{s_j(w) + \delta(j, t)\}, \tag{1}$$

where u and w are the children of v.

The initialization for the algorithm consists in setting, for each leaf v and each state t, $s_t(v) = 0$ if v is labeled with t, or $s_t(v) = \infty$ otherwise. At each step, after computing $s_t(u)$ and $s_t(w)$ for every state t, $s_t(v)$ may be calculated also for every state t. At the end of the algorithm, the minimum parsimony score is given by $\min_{t \in \mathcal{S}} s_t(\text{root})$.

As in any dynamic programming algorithm, an additional backtracking step is necessary in order to reconstruct an optimal assignment of labels. This is done by tracking the choices made at nodes. The whole algorithm takes $O(nk^2)$ time.

3.2   SPP Using a Binary Score Function

Even before Sankoff [14], Fitch [6] solved SPP for a binary score function using a similar approach. Fitch's Algorithm uses an auxiliary structure S_v, the set of possible values for label v. The algorithm has three steps and takes $O(nk)$ time.

Fitch's Algorithm firstly initializes S_v for all leaves. If v is a leaf labeled with t, $S_v = \{t\}$. Secondly, it does a post-order traversal on the tree to calculate S_v for the internal nodes. If v is a internal node with u and w as children, S_v can be calculated as follows [9]:

$$S_v = \begin{cases} S_u \cup S_w \text{ if } S_u \cap S_w = \emptyset, \\ S_u \cap S_w \text{ if } S_u \cap S_w \neq \emptyset. \end{cases} \tag{2}$$

Finally, it does a pre-order tree traversal labeling the nodes. The root is labeled with any element in S_{root}. Then, every node w with parent v is labeled as follows [9]:

$$label(w) = \begin{cases} label(v) & \text{if } label(v) \in S_w, \\ \text{any element of } S_w & \text{if } label(v) \notin S_w. \end{cases} \tag{3}$$

It is important to notice that Eq. 3 works even if w is a leaf, since S_w contains only one element.

4   Solutions for the Small Live Parsimony Problem

In this section we describe solutions for SLPP for binary and general functions, based on Sankoff's and Fitch's solutions. These solutions were originally defined in [9].

For both types of score function, we basically need to change how internal nodes representing objects, named *live internal nodes*, are dealt with. Like a leaf, a live internal node has its label already defined by the input and it cannot be changed.

4.1   SLPP Using a General Score Function

The modified version of Sankoff's algorithm preserves the original initialization, but now it is necessary to deal with live internal nodes. The algorithm starts by assigning, for each leaf v and each live internal node, zero to $s_t(v)$ if v is labeled with t, or ∞ otherwise. Figure 2 shows an example of the initialization, taking the score function δ showed in Table 1. Gray rectangles show the values of $s_A(v)$, $s_C(v)$, $s_G(v)$, $s_T(v)$ for each leaf or live internal node v.

Table 1. Function δ used in the examples, with characters from $\mathcal{S} =\{$A, C, G, T$\}$ [9].

δ	A	C	G	T
A	0	2	1	2
C	2	0	2	1
G	1	2	0	2
T	2	1	2	0

At each step, let v be an internal node with children u and w. If v is not live, then Eq. 1 is used as in SPP. Otherwise, let $\bar{t}$ be the state already defined for v. Since label $\bar{t}$ of v cannot be changed, the algorithm does not change any $s_t(v), t \neq \bar{t}$, previously defined as ∞, but instead calculates only $s_{\bar{t}}(v)$ using Eq. 1.

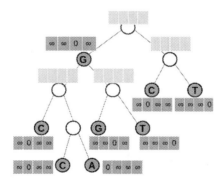

Fig. 2. First step of the algorithm for SLPP: evaluation of $s_t(v)$ for leaves and live internal nodes in a tree with one live internal node [9].

Although the label of v does not change, $s_{\bar{t}}(v)$ needs to be calculated in order to make sure that the minimum parsimony score for the subtree rooted by v is correctly computed, provided that $\bar{t}$ is the label of v. We can see this calculation in Fig. 3. The arrow shows the direction of calculation (from leaves to root).

Recovering the best choices and to label the nodes may be done exactly as before, since if the root is a live internal node with label $\bar{t}$ then $s_t(root) = \infty$ for each $t \neq \bar{t}$, and $s_{\bar{t}}(root) \neq \infty$. Thus, as in Sankoff's algorithm, the minimum parsimony score is given by $\min_{t \in \mathcal{S}} s_t(root)$.

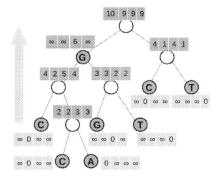

Fig. 3. Second step of the algorithm for SLPP: evaluation of $s_t(v)$ for internal nodes in a tree with one live internal node [9].

We can see an example of this step in Fig. 4. In the figure, the large arrow shows the direction of labeling (from root to leaves) and small arrows show, at each internal node, the characters of children that minimizes operations in Eq. 1.

The algorithm correctness is as follows. Let T be a binary rooted tree with a labeling of all live internal nodes and leaves, and let $\delta(a, b)$ be the symmetric function defining the cost of changing any character from state a to state b. By induction on the height h of T, if $h = 0$ then T has only one labeled live internal node r. After initialization, $s_{\bar{t}}(r) = 0$, and $s_t(r) = \infty$ for each $t \neq \bar{t}$, where $\bar{t}$ is the label of r. The minimum possible value that can be reached by $s_{\bar{t}}(r)$ is zero.

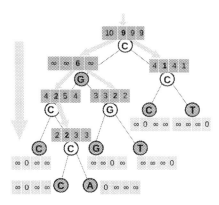

Fig. 4. Final labeling of nodes after the algorithm for SLPP on a tree with a single node [9].

As an induction hypothesis, assume that for each tree rooted by node r with height less than h, each state t is such that $s_t(r) = \infty$ or is the minimum parsimony, and there exists at least one t such that $s_t(r) \neq \infty$. Now, let T be a tree rooted by r with height $h > 0$. Let u, w be the children of r. For each state

t, $s_t(r)$ is calculated using Eq. 1. By induction hypothesis, there exists at least one state t_1 such that $s_{t_1}(u) \neq \infty$ and is minimum, and at least one state t_2 such that $s_{t_2}(w) \neq \infty$ and is minimum. The algorithm chooses, among all states t, one that minimizes $s_t(r)$. Then the modified Sankoff's Algorithm calculates the minimum parsimony score of T.

The running time is $O(nk^2)$ and the final labeling is optimal under the assumption that each live internal node label was previously chose.

4.2   SLPP with Binary Score Function

In order to solve SLPP efficiently with a binary score function, two modifications were made to Fitch's algorithm. In the initialization step the algorithm sets $S_v = \{t\}$ for each leaf and for each live internal node v labeled with t. Figure 5 shows the tree after this first step of the algorithm.

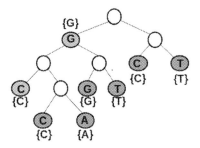

Fig. 5. First step of the algorithm for SLPP with binary score function: evaluating sets for leaves and live internal nodes on a tree with one live internal node [9].

During the post-order traversal of the tree we cannot apply Eq. 2 for live internal nodes because in SLPP they already have their corresponding sets with a single letter representing their labels. Figure 6 illustrates this step.

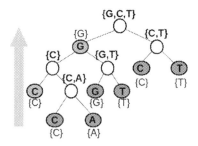

Fig. 6. Second step of algorithm for SLPP with binary score function: final evaluation of sets on a tree with one live internal node [9].

In the final step, the pre-order traversal is the same as in Fitch's Algorithm, since Eq. 3 works well for live internal nodes. Figure 7 shows the tree after the final step.

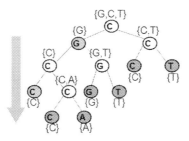

Fig. 7. Final step of algorithm for SLPP with binary score function: labeling the nodes of a tree with one live internal node.

The correctness of this algorithm follows easily from the traversals in the tree. In the top-down phase, if the label of a node was computed from the intersection of its children sets, then both children are labeled with the same state assigned to their father, resulting in cost zero for both edges. Otherwise, the label was computed from their union, and since the intersection of the children sets was empty, there is an edge of cost zero and the other edge has cost one, which is the minimum number of changes.

5   A Branch-and-bound for LLPP

In our previous work [9] we proposed a branch-and-bound to solve LLPP. In this section we will present it in more details with examples. We also introduce a refinement to the algorithm that keeps only live trees over branches.

Our branch-and-bound strategy for LLPP uses the same approach proposed by Hendy and Penny [10]. The idea basically consists in incrementally building the tree by inserting one species at a time and analyzing all possible edges where the new node can be included onto. Before completing the construction of the tree, the parsimony score is calculated by solving the SLPP and then comparing this parsimony score to the best score obtained so far. If the current score is greater than or equal to the current best, the tree under construction is discarded and the algorithm continues from the next possible alternative. This is the core of any branch-and-bound technique.

In order to allow species to be inserted into hypothetical internal nodes, turning them to live internal nodes, we need to make a change in the traditional strategy. Figure 8 illustrates two possibilities for the inclusion of node 4 (among others not shown). Figure 8(a) and (b) show the inclusion of node 4 as a leaf and as a live internal node, respectively.

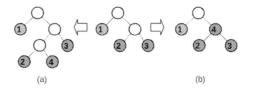

Fig. 8. Two possible inclusion scenarios for node 4 [9].

One of the premises of branch-and-bound is that all possible trees can be obtained and some of them are discarded by a good pruning strategy. With traditional phylogeny, as noted by [10], the order of inclusion of species does not matter. However, in live phylogeny some trees will not be generated depending on the previously defined order of inclusion of the nodes, as we can see in the example in Fig. 9, taking the order of inclusion $0, 1, 2, 3, 4$. Given the order $0, 1, 2, 3, 4$, at some point we will reach the central tree of Fig. 10. From this tree, all the possibilities are shown in the same figure. From any of them, it is impossible to obtain the tree showed in Fig. 9.

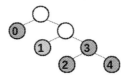

Fig. 9. A tree that cannot be reached when the order of species inclusion is $0, 1, 2, 3, 4$ [9].

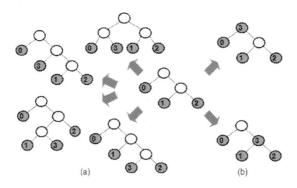

Fig. 10. A central tree after including nodes $0, 1, 2$, and the possible trees after including node 3.

In order to guarantee all that every possible tree is generated, the proposed solution shown in Algorithm 1 is generating all possible orders for including nodes and executing the previous strategy for each one. Obviously we need to pay an extra computational time, as we will see later.

Algorithm 1. Branch-and-bound for LLPP.

Require:

    (1) a set of n species $\{E_0, E_1, ..., E_{n-1}\}$,

    (2) a set of m characters $\{C_0, C_1, ..., C_{m-1}\}$.

Ensure:

    (1) tree T minimizing parsimony score.

1:   $best \leftarrow MaxNum; OS \leftarrow InitializeOS[n]$;

2: **while** $OS[0] < n$ {Not all OS tested} **do**

3:     $OC \leftarrow InitializeOC[n]$

4:     **while** $OC[1] = 0$ {Not all OC tested} **do**

5:        $i \leftarrow 0; Promising \leftarrow true$

6:        **while** $Promising = true$ and $i < n$ {T is promising incomplete tree} **do**

7:           TranverseTreeNumbering(T)

8:           **if** $OC[i] < 2(i-1)$ {Insert into edge} **then**

9:              $T \leftarrow InsertEdge(T, OS[i], OC[i])$

10:          **else**

11:             $T \leftarrow MakeLive(T, OC[i] - 2(i-1), OS[i])$

12:          **end if**

13:          $Promising \leftarrow TestParsimony(T, best)$ {T is promising}

14:          $i \leftarrow i + 1$

15:        **end while**

16:        **if** $i = n$ e $Promising = true$ {T is complete} **then**

17:           $best \leftarrow ParsimonyScore(T)$

18:           $bestTree \leftarrow T$

19:        **end if**

20:        $OC \leftarrow NextOC(OC, i)$ {Generate the next Order of Construction}

21:     **end while**

22:     $OS \leftarrow NextOS(OS)$ {Generate the next Order of Species}

23: **end while**

Algorithm 1 works with three nested loops: the outer loop generates all possible orders of inclusion of the species and stores them in a n-position array OS. The second loop generates all possible orders of construction of trees, controlling at which edge or node each species will be included (this order is stored in an n-position array OC). The inner loop repeats the following sequence of steps, controlled by i, to complete the tree or abandon the current construction:

- traverse the partial tree setting numbers for the edges and internal nodes.
- insert species $OS[i]$ breaking the edge $OC[i]$ or at the internal node indicated by $OC[i]$ (making it live).
- test whether the partial tree can generate an optimal solution. If it can't, interrupt the loop, indicating i as the position where the current search for the optimal tree failed and requesting the next OC position. If it can, we invoke the polynomial-time solution of SLPP to calculate the parsimony score of the partial tree and then test against the best score so far.

Except for the outer loop and of course for the possibility of creating live internal nodes, the algorithm works on the same way as the branch-and-bound proposed in [10].

Algorithm 1 uses an array OC to control tree construction. Given a partial tree T with $i-1$ species already inserted in it, the algorithm traverses T setting numbers for edges and also for internal nodes. $OC[i]$ indicates the position where the i-th species will be inserted. To deal with the inclusion of species as live internal nodes, we use values larger than the number of edges to flag during the construction order of the partial tree. For $i \geq 2$, OC has values larger than the number of edges in the partial tree, meaning that $OC[i] \geq 2(i-1)$. So, if $OC[i] < 2(i-1)$, then the i-th species will be inserted by breaking the edge numbered $OC[i]$, otherwise the species will be placed in the internal node indicated by $OC[i] - 2(i-1)$.

To illustrate the operation of arrays OC and OS consider, for example, species $0, 1, 2, 3, 4$ included in this order. Figure 11 presents the resulting trees when applying the construction orders 00105 (Fig. 11a) and 00123 (Fig. 11b). In these examples no live internal node was created because $OC[i] < 2(i-1), \forall i$.

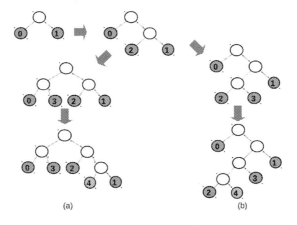

Fig. 11. Resulting trees when applying construction orders (a) 00105 and (b) 00123.

Figure 12 illustrates the construction of trees with live nodes for species $0, 1, 2, 3, 4$ inserted in this order and applying the construction orders 00152 and 00126. In the first order, species 3 is positioned in the internal node numbered 1 $(= 5 - 4 = OC[3] - 2(3-1))$. In the second order, the last species is positioned at the root (numbered 0).

To illustrate the branch, we will use the input matrix M shown in Fig. 13 with six species and two characters. By using the inclusion order $0, 1, \ldots, 5$ and construction order 000000, we obtain the tree shown in Fig. 14.

As another example, the central tree shown in Fig. 15 is obtained using the inclusion order of species $0, 1, 2, 3$ and construction order 001. The figure shows all possible inclusions of species 3.

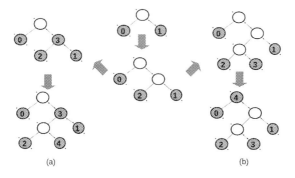

Fig. 12. Resulting trees when applying construction orders (a) 00152 and (b) 00126.

	1	2
0	A	A
1	T	T
2	C	G
3	A	C
4	G	A
5	C	T

Fig. 13. Input matrix M with species $0, 1, \ldots, 5$ and two characters 1 and 2 with states A, C, G and T [9].

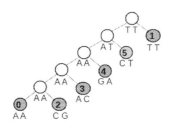

Fig. 14. Initial tree with score 7, obtained by inclusion order $0, 1, \ldots, 5$ and construction order 000000 [9].

Figure 16 shows a most parsimonious tree with minimal score for M obtained by the proposed branch-and-bound. Note that a most parsimonious tree obtained by branch-and-bound may be equal to the tree obtained by traditional branch-and-bound, or have the same score.

To see that all trees with $l \geq 0$ live internal nodes can be generated, consider T a tree with l live internal nodes. Because the traditional branch-and-bound is embedded in our Algorithm, all trees with $l = 0$ live internal nodes can be generated. Otherwise, if $l > 0$, it is sufficient to consider an order of species such that the l species that are live in T are the latest in the inclusion order of species. All construction orders are analyzed, in particular those orders that generate a partial tree T' equal to T, except for the labeling of the l live nodes.

Among those trees, the algorithm will process the one that promotes the l last species in the order to live internal nodes, exactly the same way that they are placed in T.

As pointed out by [10], the running time of traditional branch-and-bound for n species and m characters is $O(mn^n)$, although this time is not reached in most cases with biological sequence data. Because we included another external loop that generates all permutations of species, our branch-and-bound running time is now $O(n!mn^n)$.

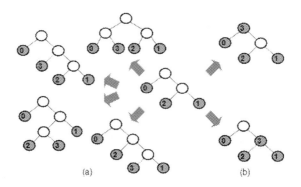

Fig. 15. Partial trees to be built and tested by the inclusion of species 3 [9]: (a) as a leaf and (b) as a live internal node.

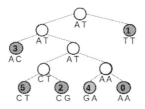

Fig. 16. Most parsimonious tree for M with score 6, obtained by branch-and-bound.

As expected, branch-and-bound may exhibit both acceptable and huge running times. For instance, two samples, one with 8 species and 10 characters and another with 9 species and 10 characters were solved by branch-and-bound in approximately 54 m and 20 h, respectively, on an Intel Core i5-4590 CPU at 3.30 GHz with 4 GB RAM.

An Improvement to the Branch-and-bound

If we want a most parsimonious tree with at least one live internal node, we may change Line 20 in the second loop of the branch-and-bound to generate construction orders with $l > 0$ live internal nodes. This is done by changing *NextOC*() in a such way that only construction orders with at least one live internal node are returned. Figure 17 shows a most parsimonious tree obtained by branch-and-bound with this restriction for matrix M (Fig. 13). Of course, there is no guarantee that the most parsimonious live phylogeny found using this approach will have the overall best parsimony score.

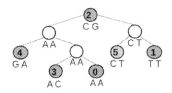

Fig. 17. Tree with live internal nodes and parsimony score 6.

An alternative change in the branch-and-bound it to allow keeping, at the same time, both the most parsimonious traditional phylogeny and the most parsimonious live phylogeny. To accomplish that, we just need to keep two additional variables, corresponding to *best* and *bestTree* (lines 17–18) for live phylogenies.

6 A Constructive Heuristic for LLPP

Because LLPP is NP-complete and the branch-and-bound is expensive, we propose a heuristic approach for LLPP. The constructive heuristic is based on the Sequential Addition presented by Felsenstein [5]. The idea is to construct the trees by adding one species at a time and testing for all possible places (edges or internal nodes), which one provides the largest score for a partial tree and proceeding only with the best one. All other possible trees are discarded.

We can add a Live Sequential Addition to this heuristic, that consists of, at each step, allowing and analyzing the inclusion of species also as live internal nodes. If the partial tree generated by the inclusion of the last species as live internal nodes is the best, then we proceed with this tree. So we can also construct trees with live internal nodes.

The main difference between this greedy strategy and the branch-and-bound presented at Sect. 5 consists in the fact that at this time we discard several branches, saving a lot of time. However, by doing this, we will probably not get the best parsimonious tree.

Considering the input matrix M shown in Figs. 13 and 18 shows the possible inclusions of species 2 after the tree obtained by the inclusion of species 0, 1. Note that the next step of the heuristic for the tree in Fig. 18 can be done from the right tree whose root node is live internal node. Continuing the execution of the heuristic using the inclusion order 012345, will generate the same tree shown in Fig. 17.

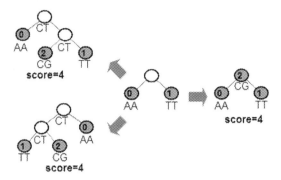

Fig. 18. Partial trees to be built and tested by the inclusion of species 2 by the Live Sequential Addition heuristic.

In fact, the execution of the heuristic allows the generation of trees with live internal nodes, but does not guarantee that the tree generated at the end has at least one live internal node. Then we will make one more addition to the heuristic. In each step, the best partial tree with live internal nodes obtained after the insertion of the i-th species will be stored in $TLive_i$.

Let's see how this will work. At each step T_1, the best tree with live internal node generated in the current step, will be stored temporarily. It will also temporarily store T_2, the best tree generated from $TLive_{i-1}$ by inserting E_i the i-th species. Note that since $TLive_{i-1}$ already has a live internal node, T_2 will have a live internal node not matter how inserting E_i. To finalize the step, we compare the parsimony score of T_1 and T_2 saving the lowest in $TLive_i$.

7   Experiments on a Set of Zika Virus Species

RNA viral genes have a high rate of mutations. Because of that, virus may evolve and at the same time co-exist [8]. A particular case is Zika virus. Outbreaks of Zika virus has been recently reported in Americas and in Africa. A huge importance has been given to Zika viruses because they have been associated with some pre-natal malformations, like microcephaly and other neurological diseases.

Lancioti and colleagues [12] proposed a phylogeny for 20 strains of Zika virus, shown in Table 2. Figure 19 shows the tree obtained by the authors.

In this section we propose an alternative topology for the 20 Zika virus strains shown in Table 2. The second column of the table presents clades proposed by the authors. The last two columns show the different numbering of the strains used in the trees in some of our tests.

Table 2. Twenty Zika virus strains described in [12].

Zika virus strain	Clade	Tests 1–2	Test 3
HQ234499 Malaysia 1966 P6-740	Asian	0	0
EU545988 Yap 2007	Asian		1
JN860885 Cambodia 2010 FSS13025	Asian	8	2
KF993678 Thailand 2013 PLCal_ZV	Asian		3
KU501215 Puerto Rico PRVABC59	Asian		4
KU501216 Guatemala 8375	Asian	6	5
KU501217 Guatemala 103344	Asian		6
KJ776791 French Polynesia H/PF/2013	Asian	4	7
KU321639 Brazil 2015 SPH2015	Asian	5	8
HQ234500 Nigeria 1968 IbH 30656	West African	1	9
KF383117 Senegal 1997 ArD128000	West African	3	10
HQ234501 Senegal 1984 ArD41519	West African		11
KF383116 Senegal 1968 ArD7117	West African		12
KF383118 Senegal 2001 ArD157995	East African		13
KF383119 Senegal 2001 ArD158084	East African		14
LC002520 Uganda 1947 MR766	East African	7	15
KF383115 Central African Republic ARB1362	East African	9	16
KF268949 Central African Republic 1980 ARB15076	East African		17
KF268948 Central African Republic 1979 ARB13565	East African	2	18
KF268950 Central African Republic 1976 ARB7701	East African		19

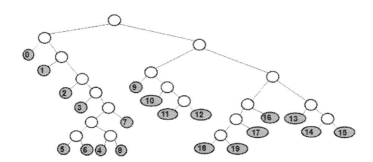

Fig. 19. Tree obtained for the 20 strains of Zika virus of Table 2 [12]. Node numbering follows the last column of the table.

Dataset

We used the 20 Zika virus strain genomic sequences, aligned using MUSCLE [4], resulting in 10,109 columns. After aligning, we used GBLOCKS [1] to remove non-informative characters, resulting in a shorter alignment with 2,169 columns.

7.1   Results

We run our heuristic taking as input the 20×2169 matrix (see Test 3 in this section). Three tests have been executed. In Test 1 we compared the branch-and-bound to the Live Sequential Addition heuristic. In Test 2 we compared the branch-and-bound in its plain and only with live phylogenies versions. Finally, in Test 3 we run our Live Sequential Addition heuristic using the whole input matrix.

The input matrix is large enough to make our branch-and-bound method computationally prohibitive. So, we built a set of 100 submatrices to be used in tests 1 and 2. These submatrices have been obtained by selecting 10 strains (with at least one representative strain of each clade shown in Table 2) and randomly picking 500 columns.

Test 1

This test evaluates the performance of the heuristic in searching a most parsimonious tree. In 50 cases out of the 100 10×500 submatrices, the heuristic worked very well, finding a tree with the same score as that one obtained by branch-and-bound, that is, the heuristic returned a most parsimonious tree. Overall, the heuristic obtained scores close to those of branch-and-bound ones, with average error of 0.19% and a maximum error of 2.07%.

It is interesting to note that in 24 cases the heuristic produced a tree containing at least one live internal node. In 9 of those, the tree returned by the heuristic was also most parsimonious.

Test 2

Comparing the standard branch-and-bound and the branch-and-bound that selects only live phylogenies, gives an idea on how close the scores of trees with live internal nodes are to the most parsimonious ones.

In 56 samples, the best tree with only one live node returned by branch-and-bound with only live phylogenies have the same parsimony score of the most parsimonious tree returned by standard branch-and-bound. The average difference was 0.13% and the maximum difference was 1.18%. Figure 20 shows the most parsimonious trees of a selected case.

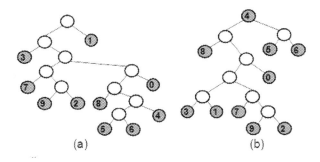

Fig. 20. Most parsimonious trees for a case. Figure 20(a) was built by branch-and-bound and Fig. 20(b) was built by branch-and-bound with only live phylogenies. Both have the same parsimony score 609.

Test 3

In Test 3 we used all 20 strains of Zika virus and all 2,169 columns on our heuristic. Figure 21 shows the resulting live phylogeny. The score of the tree obtained by Lanciotti and colleagues [12] is 3,233. Our heuristic obtained a score of 3,235, but with a live internal node. Note that all three clades suggested in [12] were preserved in our tree.

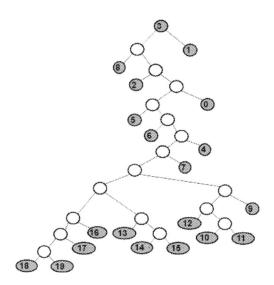

Fig. 21. Tree obtained by Sequential Addition heuristic for the 20 species of Zika virus.

8   Conclusion

In this article we extended the work presented in BIOSTEC'2017 [9], where we introduced the Large Live Parsimony and the Small Live Parsimony problems. These problems are an important step in the characterization of the problems in the family of Live Phylogeny.

As expected, the live small problem is easy, while the live large problem is hard. In this article we refined the branch-and-bound that was introduced earlier adding the possibility of constraining the trees to those that contain at least a live internal, broadening the possibilities of applying branch-and-bound to some instances of the problem, for instance to construct benchmarks to test future heuristics for LLPP.

In this article we also introduced a greedy heuristic for the large live problem, which was applied to datasets of Zika virus genomes. The results, when compared to those obtained by branch-and-bound, were good for these datasets.

The live parsimony problems still need further investigations. As mentioned in the introduction, they have a broad range of applications where there are typically large datasets to process. Better pruning and heuristics are probably welcome future research results.

Acknowledgments. RG and NFA thank Fundect grants TO141/2016 and TO 007/2015. NFA also thanks CNPq grants 305857/2013-4, 473221/2013-6 and CAPES grant 3377/2013. GPT acknowledges CNPq grant 310685/2015-0. MEMT thanks CNPq grant 308524/2015-2.

References

1. Cartresana, J.: Selection of conserved blocks from multiple alignments for their use in phylogenetic analysis. Mol. Biol. Evol. **17**, 540–552 (2000)
2. Castro-Nallar, E., Perez-Losada, M., Burton, G., Crandall, K.: The evolution of HIV: inferences using phylogenetics. Mol. Phylog. Evol. **62**, 777–792 (2012)
3. Cuadros, A.M., Paulovich, F.V., Minghim, R., Telles, G.P.: Point placement by phylogenetic trees and its application to visual analysis of document collections. In: Proceedings of the 2007 IEEE Symposium on Visual Analytics Science and Technology, pp. 99–106 (2007)
4. Edgar, R.C.: Muscle: multiple sequence alignment with high accuracy and high throughput. Nucleic Acids Res. **32**(5), 1792–1797 (2004)
5. Felsenstein, J.: Inferring Phylogenies. Sinauer Associates, Sunderland (2004)
6. Fitch, W.M.: Toward defining the course of evolution: minimum change for a specific tree topology. Syst. Zool. **20**, 406–416 (1971)
7. Goëffon, A., Richer, J., Hao, J.: Heuristic methods for phylogenetic reconstruction with maximum parsimony, pp. 579–597. Wiley (2011)
8. Gojobori, T., Moriyama, E.N., Kimura, M.: Molecular clock of viral evolution, and the neutral theory. P. Natl. Acad. Sci. **87**(24), 10015–10018 (1990)
9. Güths, R., Telles, G.P., Walter, M.E.M.T., Almeida, N.F.: A branch and bound for the large live parsimony problem. In: Proceedings of the 10th International Joint Conference on Biomedical Engineering Systems and Technologies (BIOSTEC 2017), pp. 184–189. SCITEPRESS - Science and Technology Publications, Lda (2017)

10. Hendy, M.D., Penny, D.: Branch and bound algorithms to determine minimal evolutionary trees. Math. Biosci. **59**(2), 277–290 (1982)
11. Jones, N.C., Pevzner, P.A., Pevzner, P.: An Introduction to Bioinformatics Algorithms, vol. 2004. MIT Press, Cambridge (2004)
12. Lanciotti, R., Lambert, A., Holodniy, M., Saavedra, S., Signor, L.: Phylogeny of Zika virus in western hemisphere, 2015. Emerg. Infect. Dis. **22**(5), 933–935 (2016)
13. Paiva, J., Florian, L., Pedrini, H., Telles, G., Minghim, R.: Improved similarity trees and their application to visual data classification. IEEE Trans. Vis. Comp. Graph. **17**(12), 2459–2468 (2011)
14. Sankoff, D.: Minimal mutation trees of sequences. SIAM J. Appl. Math. **28**(1), 35–42 (1975)
15. Setubal, J.C., Meidanis, J.: Introduction to Molecular Computational Biology, vol. 1997. PWS, Boston (1997)
16. Telles, G.P., Almeida, N.F., Minghim, R., Walter, M.E.M.T.: Live phylogeny. J. Comput. Biol. **20**(1), 30–37 (2013)
17. Yan, M., Bader, D.A.: Fast character optimization in parsimony phylogeny reconstruction. Technical report TR-CS-2003-53. University of New Mexico (2003)

Evaluating Runs of Homozygosity in Exome Sequencing Data - Utility in Disease Inheritance Model Selection and Variant Filtering

Jorge Oliveira[1,2]([⊠]), Rute Pereira[1], Rosário Santos[2], and Mário Sousa[1]

[1] Instituto de Ciências Biomédicas Abel Salazar (ICBAS),
Universidade do Porto, R. Jorge de Viterbo Ferreira nº 228, Porto, Portugal
`ruterpereira@gmail.com, msousa@icbas.up.pt`
[2] Centro de Genética Médica Dr. Jacinto Magalhães, Centro Hospitalar do Porto,
Praça Pedro Nunes nº 88, Porto, Portugal
`{jorge.oliveira, rosario.santos}@chporto.min-saude.pt`

Abstract. Runs of homozygosity (ROH) are regions consistently homozygous for genetic markers, which can occur throughout the human genome. Their size is dependent on the degree of shared parental ancestry, being longer in individuals descending from consanguineous marriages, or from inbred/isolated populations. Based on ROH existence, homozygosity mapping (HM) was developed as powerful tool for gene-discovery in human genetics. HM is based on the assumption that, through identity-by-descent, individuals affected by an autosomal recessive (AR) condition, are more likely to have homozygous markers surrounding the disease *locus*.

In this work, we reviewed some of the algorithms and bioinformatics tools available for HM and ROH detection, with special emphasis on those than can be applied to data from whole-exome sequencing (WES) data. Preliminary data is also shown demonstrating the relevance of performing ROH analysis, especially in sporadic cases. In this study, ROH from WES data of twelve unrelated patients was analyzed. Patients with AR diseases (n = 6) were subdivided into two groups: homozygous and compound heterozygous. ROH analysis was performed using the HomozygosityMapper software, varying the block length and collecting several parameters. Statistically significant differences between the two groups were identified for ROH total size and homozygosity score. The k-means clustering algorithm was then applied, where two clusters were identified, with statistically significant differences, corresponding to each predefined test group. Our results suggest that, in some cases, it may be possible to infer the most likely disease inheritance model from WES data alone, constituting a useful starting point for the subsequent variant filtering strategies.

Keywords: Whole-exome sequencing · Homozygosity mapping
Next-generation sequencing · Clinical genetics

J. Oliveira and R. Pereira—Equally contributing authors.

© Springer International Publishing AG, part of Springer Nature 2018
N. Peixoto et al. (Eds.): BIOSTEC 2017, CCIS 881, pp. 268–288, 2018.
https://doi.org/10.1007/978-3-319-94806-5_15

1 Introduction

Monogenic Mendelian diseases are a group of clinical entities caused by genetic defects present in a single *locus*, that mostly follows the inheritance laws originally proposed by Gregor Mendel [1]. They represent an opportunity to learn about gene functions and the pathophysiological mechanisms of diseases. The disease-causing gene may be in an autosome or in sex-chromosomes and of dominant or recessive nature. Individually these diseases are rare, which makes the genotype-phenotype association more complex than initially thought. But collectively they occur at a high incidence, with an estimated 7.9 million children being born annually with a serious birth defect of genetic origin [2]. Despite the extensive research being carried out in Mendelian diseases, only about 17% of genes have their function determined. According to the latest statistics available from Online Mendelian Inheritance in Man (OMIM, database initiated in 1997 by Prof. Victor A. McKusick, collecting data related with human genetic diseases) only 3810 genes have been listed as disease-causing (last accessed in 27/09/2017).

Over the last two decades, most of the Mendelian genes have been identified by linkage analysis studies, a strategy to map genes (i.e. find their location in chromosomes) that predispose to disease/traits. This method is based on the premise that the closer the two genes are on a chromosome, the lower is the likelihood of recombination between them and the more likely they are to be inherited together [3]. This linkage disequilibrium (LD) is thus defined as a non-random association between alleles at two or more *loci*. Besides a physical proximity, in LD the genes may be linked due to non-physical factors. Population subdivision, inbreeding events, changes in population size and the migration of individuals between populations affect LD throughout the genome. Besides mapping genetic diseases, linkage analysis and LD patterns throughout the genome have allowed scientists to understand the population history, the breeding system and the pattern of the geographic subdivision, as well as gene conversion, mutation and other forces that drive gene-frequency evolution [4].

In addition to gene mapping, another important technique in clinical genetics is Sanger Sequencing, a method of determining DNA sequence developed by Frederick Sanger and co-workers in 1975 [5], which is based on the selective incorporation of chain-terminating dideoxynucleotides during *in vitro* DNA synthesis mediated by the activity of a DNA polymerase. Sanger sequencing is considered the "gold standard" in genetic diseases diagnostics and also the first choice to confirm/validate sequence variants. Technological advances over the past decade led to the development of high-throughput sequencing platforms. The so-called "next generation sequencing" or, more accurately, massive parallel sequencing, transformed the sequencing strategies and boosted its capabilities and throughput, and was rapidly transposed both to research and to clinical diagnostic settings. With this new technology, the human genome can be completely sequenced within a short time span, allowing the simultaneous analysis of multiple genes and consequently the attainment of new important findings (see [6–8] for further reading).

Due to the extreme rarity of some Mendelian diseases, it is very difficult to find a sufficient number of individuals and affected families with exactly the same phenotype, which is usually a prerequisite for gene discovery. Population history and geographical events, such as genetic bottlenecks (i.e. a sharp reduction in the size of a population), and cultural factors such as marriage between close biological relatives (related as second cousins or closer), increases the probability of the offspring inheriting two deleterious copies of a recessive gene. These at-risk kindreds represent a particular context where the incidence of autosomal recessive disorders and its transmission to offspring is considerably higher [9]. Consanguinity is not evenly distributed worldwide. The global prevalence of consanguineous marriage is about 6,067 million. The communities of North Africa, Western and South Asia, particularly the highly religious transcontinental region of the middle-east, collectively account for 20–50% of all consanguineous marriages (http://consang.net/index.php/Summary). In 2013, 44 marriages between related individuals were reported in Portugal, which represents only 0. 1% of total marriages [10]. The affected offspring will have not only two identical copies of the ancestral allele, but the surrounding DNA segments will also be homozygous. Thus, the affected individual carries long stretches of DNA segments that are identical by descent (IBD), i.e. homozygous segments inherited from each parent. These homozygous DNA stretches are called 'runs of homozygosity' (ROH) (Fig. 1).

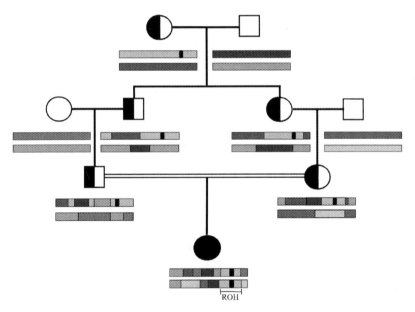

Fig. 1. Schematic representation of a small consanguineous pedigree and ROH with a pathogenic variant (black box).

The ROH length is dependent on the degree of shared parental ancestry and on the number of generations that share the DNA region. Therefore, longer ROH (measuring tens of Mb) can be identified in individuals from geographically isolated populations or belonging to ethnical groups with a higher consanguinity rate, due to cultural or religious reasons. In contrast, in larger and older populations with reduced consanguinity rates, ROH length is generally much shorter, as homozygous stretches have been broken down over successive generations by repeated recombination events during meiosis [11]. Nevertheless, there are small regions of our genome in which the recombination rates are considerably lower and thus IBD regions are always observed.

2   Homozygosity Mapping

Homozygosity mapping (HM, also known as autozygosity mapping), is a positional mapping strategy used for the first time by Lander and Bostein in 1987 [12]. This powerful technique for autosomal recessive disease mapping relies on the assumption that an affected individual inherits two identical alleles of a disease gene from a common ancestor. In cases of consanguinity or population bottlenecks, the IBD regions have longer ROH. Accordingly, to perform HM it is necessary to search for consistently homozygous regions in affected individuals from inbred families or from geographically confined populations. As autosomal recessive diseases can be extremely heterogeneous, HM is more robust when searching for a mutation segregating within a small, closed/consanguineous population. In these populations, each allele assumes a high frequency such that two individuals taken at random from the reproductive pool are likely to have alleles in common, hence likely to be carriers of the same disease-causing allele, and at risk of having clinically affected offspring [13, 14]. Detecting ROH requires the use of markers that both span the region in question and are sufficiently polymorphic to punctuate it as a distinct haplotype (i.e. a distinct profile for consecutive markers). Scanning for blocks of homozygosity initially resorted to microsatellite markers (stretches of short tandem repeats of 1–6 bases pairs) found throughout the human genome. However, although these are highly informative (polymorphic), polymerase chain reaction (PCR) reactions can be difficult to optimize and prone to artifacts. Microsatellites analysis has therefore been replaced by the analysis of single nucleotide polymorphisms (SNPs) [15]. SNPs are less informative, due to their lower heterozygosity scores but are much more abundant in the human genome (~ 1 per Kb) and allow the use of high-throughput assays, such array chips that allow the simultaneous calling of hundreds of thousands of SNPs [16–18].

3   Next-Generation Sequencing

During the last decade we have witnessed the development of new alternative strategies aiming to improve and eventually replace Sanger sequencing, those are collectively referred to next generation sequencing (NGS). Although initially developed to study the genome, they also allow the study of the transcriptome (RNA analysis, or RNA-seq) [19], the study of protein–DNA interactions (known as ChIP-Seq) [20], and the study of DNA patterns of methylation (or bisulfite-seq) [21]. NGS, enables sequencing of an entire human genome within a single day, being faster and more cost-effective than Sanger sequencing. Currently, at least four platforms are available for NGS: Illumina and Ion Torrent (2nd generation), PacBio and Oxford Nanopore Technologies (3rd generation). This number is expected to increase as technology improves and new equipment is being developed. Although these 2nd generation platforms are completely different, all follow a quite similar generic workflow. All start with library preparation, in which nucleic acids (study sample) are the template. It includes the random fragmentation of DNA, followed by *in vitro* ligation of platform-specific adaptors that allow the clonal amplification of the sequences by PCR. PCR products are spatially clustered, by different approaches depending on which can be recovered and arrayed. Finally, the sequencing process itself consists of alternating cycles of enzyme-driven biochemistry and signal-based data acquisition [8, 22].

As previously mentioned, NGS has enabled great advances in the study of genetic diseases and gene discovery [6, 23]. This holds true especially in genetically heterogeneous conditions where any one of several distinct genes, when mutated, may give rise to the same phenotype. As hereditary myopathies and primary ciliary dyskinesia (PCD), in which neither gene-by-gene Sanger sequencing nor linkage analysis are cost-effective or efficient approaches [24, 25]. Since nearly 85% of the known disease-causing variants are located in exonic regions or neighboring intronic sequences (donor or acceptor splice-sites) [26], whole-exome sequencing (WES) became a common application of NGS. WES includes all exonic regions of ~20,000 genes, performing a comprehensive analysis of the genome while still being manageable in terms of costs and amount of data generated. This approach is extremely useful for highly heterogeneous conditions and even for the identification of novel disease genes. Nevertheless, unveiling the genetic mechanism of a disease is not straightforward. Genetic and phenotypic heterogeneity, in which a disease can be caused or modulated by pathogenic variants in different genes, is not only confined to complex multigenic diseases but has also been recognized to occur in rare diseases. This, together with the enormous amount of novel variants of unknown clinical significance makes WES difficult to interpret and could lead to inconclusive results. But exome analysis has been shown to be a powerful tool, enabling the association of unlikely candidate genes with specific diseases. For instance, Gripp and collaborators identified truncating mutations in the last exon of the *NOTCH3* gene in patients with lateral meningocele syndrome (OMIM 130720, also known as Lehman syndrome) [27]. This gene was previously known to cause cerebral arteriopathy with subcortical infarcts and leukoencephalopathy 1 (CADASIL, OMIM 612954), a progressive disease with onset during adulthood, affecting the brain's small arterial vessels, and manifested by migraine, strokes, and white matter lesions, with subsequent dementia in some patients [28]. In spite of this usefulness, WES has still some limitations to that need addressing [29]. Firstly, there are intrinsic limitations, since some deleterious variations are located in non-coding regions and therefore not covered by WES. Sequencing errors are related to poor capture efficiency in difficult regions (such as GC-rich regions), mechanical and analytical errors, as well as misalignment of reads in repetitive regions, leading to erroneous results. These limitations make data analysis more difficult and impose the need to validate candidate causative variants by Sanger sequencing. Moreover, as a considerable number of variants are obtained (~35,000 to ~50,000 depending on the strategy), WES analysis requires the application of several filtering strategies, depending on the frequency of the disease, the predicted model of disease inheritance and the impact of the variants. This filtering step is critical as it will influence data analysis and final results outcome. For example, variants may be excluded for being synonymous; however, even though these are usually non-deleterious, numerous synonymous mutations have been implicated in human diseases [30], thus caution should be taken when dealing with this type of variants. In addition, during WES analysis a frequency filter is usually set to exclude variants with minor allele frequency above a certain threshold (above 1% in most cases). This threshold should be set according to the expected prevalence/incidence of the disease. Nonetheless, considering that in recessive disorders carriers do not show any signs of the disease, the frequency of damaging alleles in population variant databases can still be higher than the established threshold. This might lead to erroneous exclusion of these variants during filtering. To safeguard against some of these limitations, whole-genome sequencing (WGS) can be used instead of WES. Undoubtedly, WGS is more powerful and is able to detect all types of genomic variants [31, 32]; however, has the drawback of higher sequencing costs, informatics requirements, longer turnaround times, and more difficult and complex data analysis. This approach is therefore limited to gene discovery projects in large genome sequencing centers or service providers. For these reasons, the implementation of WGS in a routine diagnostic setting will be considerably more difficult than was that of WES, in the recent past.

4 Homozygosity Mapping Bioinformatics

4.1 Software for SNP-Array Data

Most of the disease-causing genes have been identified in the past by linkage analysis. This involves finding an association between the inheritance pattern of the phenotypic trait (usually a disease state) and a genetic marker, or a series of adjacent markers. Hence, genetic linkage analyses are useful to detect chromosomal regions containing disease genes, by examining patterns of inheritance in families [33]. Two main types of genetic linkage analysis are commonly used, namely model-based linkage analysis (or parametric analysis) and model-free linkage analysis (or non-parametric analysis). In parametric linkage analysis, it is assumed that models describing both the trait and marker loci are known. In contrast, in non-parametric methods some assumptions are made about the trait model, thus is more prone to errors [34]. For the analysis of simple Mendelian disorders with an extended pedigree, with a well-established mode of inheritance and where the family members are unambiguously clinically characterized as affected or unaffected, the parametric logarithm of odds (LOD) score method is one of the most popular statistical tool. It is based on an assessment of the recombination fraction, denoted by theta (θ), which is the probability of a recombination event between the two *loci* of interest and a function of distance. Two unlinked *loci* have a theoretical $\theta = 0.5$ (null hypothesis of no linkage) and the closer a pair of loci is, the lower is the recombination fraction, which favours the presence of linkage [35].

The LOD may be expressed as follows, (L denotes likelihood):

$$LOD = \log10(L(\theta)/L(\theta = 0.5)) \tag{1}$$

However, for complex traits with incomplete penetrance, phenocopies, multiple trait *loci* and possibly incorrectly specified dominance relationships, a precise genetic model cannot be specified, which makes LOD score analysis inadequate. Here, non-parametric linkage (NPL) analysis are commonly used [34].

As previously mentioned, two alleles can be identical by state (IBS), if they have the same DNA sequence, or identical by descent (IBD) if IBS alleles are derived from the same ancestral allele. A statistical test is performed to compare the observed degree of sharing to that expected when assuming that the marker and the trait are not linked. NPL analysis often examines IBD or IBS allele sharing in cases where siblings exhibit the same trait of interest [34].

Most of the genetic linkage analyses have been performed with the help of bioinformatic tools. The first generally available computer program for linkage analysis was LIPED [36]. It estimated the recombination fraction by calculating pedigree likelihoods for various assumed values of the recombination fraction, using only two-point parametric LOD scores and the Elston-Stewart algorithm [37]. Thereafter, several software solutions have been developed. Here we will briefly describe some of the most popular software used to perform gene mapping.

GENEHUNTER, developed by Kruglyak and co-workers is among the more frequently used software for parametric multipoint analysis of pedigrees, mainly because of its user-friendly interface and rapid operation. It was the first to calculate the exact multipoint linkage scores involving many markers, using the hidden Markov model (HMM) [38]. HMM is a probabilistic sequence model in which, given a sequence of units (e.g. DNA sequence), a probability distribution over possible sequences of labels is computed and the best label sequence is chosen [39]. This computer program is written in C language, usable in UNIX based systems through a command-line interface. It has a complete multipoint algorithm to determine the probability distribution over possible inheritance patterns at each point in the genome. The software then applies those concepts to define a unified multipoint framework for both parametric (the traditional LOD-score calculations) and non-parametric analysis [38]. However, it has the drawback of being limited to relatively small pedigrees (approximately 12 non-founders, i.e. individuals whose parents are in the pedigree) and not be feasible for large multigenerational pedigrees. Splitting pedigrees or discarding outlier individuals (trimming) is not a good option since this can result in a greater loss of information or invalidate the heterogeneity of the LOD score [40].

SIMWALK2 is another statistical tool, first described by Sobel and Lange to perform haplotype, parametric linkage, non-parametric linkage, IBD and mistyping analyses on a pedigree [41]. It uses Markov chain Monte Carlo (MCMC): an algorithm that is used to characterize a particular distribution without the knowledge about all of the distribution's mathematical properties, just by sampling values out of the distribution at random. The MCMC method can be employed to draw samples from distributions even when all that is known about the distribution is how to calculate the density for different samples [42]. SIMWALK2 applies the MCMC method to simulate annealing algorithms to perform multipoint analyses. In contrast to GENEHUNTER, it can handle up to 258 individuals as well as a considerable number of markers, although at cost of taking a longer processing time [43].

MERLIN is another software available for mapping genes by linkage [44]. It is written in C++ language and carries out single point and multipoint analyses of pedigree data, including IBD calculations, non-parametric and variance component linkage analyses and information content mapping. Compared with GENEHUNTER, it shows high computational speed and fewer memory constraints because it provides a swap file support to handle very large numbers of markers, thereby, making it more suited to very dense genetic maps. Moreover, it can detect genotyping errors in routine analysis to improve power, and simulates routines to estimate p-values. MERLIN can estimate haplotypes by finding the most likely path of gene flow or by sampling paths of gene flow at all markers jointly. It can also list all possible nonrecombinant haplotypes within short regions. MERLIN does not calculate parametric LOD scores, which are available in GENEHUNTER and ALLEGRO, but is the fastest for NPL, error checking and haplotyping analysis [45]. Finally, MERLIN can execute gene-dropping simulations for estimating empirical significance levels. Gene dropping simulation is a computer simulation in which founder genotypes are first simulated according to population allele frequencies. The genes are "dropped" down the pedigree by simulating gene-flow according to Mendel's laws. Finally, the phenotypes are simulated from the genotypes according to the penetrance. Simulated phenotypes are then compared to the observed, and outcomes inconsistent with the observed phenotypes are discarded. The result is a random sample of genotypes given the observed phenotypes [46].

ALLEGRO is similar to GENEHUNTER; it also uses an HMM to calculate multipoint parametric LOD scores, NPL scores and allele-sharing LOD scores, reconstruction of haplotypes, estimated recombination count between markers, and entropy information, but it is about 20–100 times faster [47]. In contrast to GENEHUNTER, for NPL analysis (which gives a p-value computed by comparing the observed NPL score with its complete data distribution), besides providing this value, ALLEGROcalculates an additional p-value by comparing the observed allele-sharing LOD score with its complete data distribution. This value increases the accuracy of the results.

4.2 Software for WES Data

Recent studies have clearly demonstrated the power and the effectiveness of applying HM to WES data, to identify causative genes for Mendelian disorders [48]. Krawitz and co-workers in 2010, developed a statistical model that allowed to infer IBD regions from the exome sequencing data of an affected child of a non-consanguineous couple, in which the disease followed the autosomal recessive inheritance mode [49]. In non-consanguineous families, the affected children do not share two equal haplotypes inherited from a single common ancestor, at the disease *locus,* but inherit identical maternal and paternal haplotypes in a region surrounding the disease gene, which is not necessarily from the same ancestor (IBD = 2). They used an algorithm based on an HMM, to identify chromosomal regions with IBD = 2 in the presence of sequencing data, to find the causative gene [49]. Another pioneering work from Becker et al., studied four patients from consanguineous families, extracting genotypes of all dbSNP130-annotated SNPs from the exome sequencing data, and using these 299,494 genotypes as markers for genome-wide identification of homozygous regions. From the analysis of these regions, the authors were able to identify a single homozygous truncating pathogenic variant [50].

The combination of exome sequencing with HM is so powerful to unveil the cause of autosomal-recessive disorders, special in consanguineous families, that finding the mutated gene might only require a single affected individual. The HM allows narrowing down the target data sets and the examination at the base-pair level, in order to enable the identification of candidate causative variants. This approach would start by mapping reads from exome sequencing against a reference genome (human hg19 in our examples). Data from whole-genome and RNA sequencing approaches can also be used. This step is usually performed through a bioinformatic pipeline that generates SAM/BAM (Sequence/Binary Alignment Map) and, at the end, variant call format (VCF) files. These files are then used as input for the HM analysis tools. The position and zygosity of resulted sequence variants can be used to retrieve/infer ROH regions. Longer ROH are indicative of homozygous regions. Table 1 lists some of the available tools to perform this analysis, supported by different algorithms.

The web-based tool HomozygosityMapper allows users to interactively analyses NGS data for HM and is freely available at http://www.homozygositymapper.org/ [51, 52]. It functions entirely on web-based software using the HTML interface, thus is user-friendly and does not require any local installation or specific data format [52]. It is independent of parameters such as family structure or allelic frequencies. The algorithm slides along an array of markers/SNPs (genotypes) inspecting zygosity and filling blocklength array. If the SNP is heterozygous the block length is 0, whereas if the SNP is homozygous it will determine the size of the homozygous block using the function DetectBlockEnd or until reaching the end of genotypes array.

Table 1. Main algorithms and bioinformatics tools used for ROH detection.

Algorithm	Software [Ref.]	UI	OS	Input data files	Range ROH size (Mb)
Sliding blocks	Homozygosity-Mapper [51, 52]	GUI	Unix/Linux web server[a]	VCF files + SNP genotypes	>1.5
	PLINK [53]	CLI & GUI	Unix/Linux, Mac OS, Windows	BED, PED, and FAM files	[0.5–1.5]; > 1.5
Sliding-window	GERMLINE [54]	CLI	Unix/Linux	PED, MAP and Hapmap files	>1.5
	HomSI [55]	GUI	Unix/Linux, Mac OS, Windows	VCF files	>1.5
Heterogeneous hidden Markov model	H^3M^2 [56]	CLI	Unix/Linux	BAF profiles	<0.5; [0.5–1.5]; > 1.5
Frequentistic genotype assigment	Agile- Genotyper and VariantMapper [57]	GUI	Windows	SAM + tab-delimited text files	>1.5

[a]http://www.homozygositymapper.org; BAM- Binary Alignment Map; BED- Browser Extensible Data; CLI-command-line interface; GUI- graphical user interface; OS- operative system; Ref.- references; SAM-Sequence Alignment Map; SNP- Single Nucleotide Polymorphism; UI- user interface; VCF- Variant Call Format.

Through the use of this function, the algorithm determines the end of each homozygous block, ignoring single heterozygous genotypes with seven or more homozygous/unknown genotypes on either side. HomozygosityMapper calculates a "homozygosity score", and it is very robust against genotyping errors due to the permissivity of the `DetectBlockEnd` function as mentioned above. HomozygosityMapper is not intended to replace other linkage tools, such a GENEHUNTER, but, as it is much faster it may be used in combination therewith. The software can rapidly identify the possible disease regions and then subsequently generate LOD scores and haplotypes with conventional software. HomozygosityMapper is linked with GeneDistiller [58], which is a database that includes information from various data sources such as gene-phenotype associations, gene expression pattern, and protein-protein interactions, allowing researchers to easily search information for the genes within a candidate interval, for instance with a high homozygosity score [51, 52]. Therefore, the HomozygosityMapper can be used as an indicator of the type of inheritance pattern and/or be used as a filter for the analysis of NGS data.

PLINK [53], GERMLINE [54] and EXome-HOMozygosity [59] are examples in which a sliding-window algorithm is applied for WES-based ROH detection. In a sliding window analysis, the statistics are calculated for a small frame of the data. The window incrementally advances across the region of interest and, at each new position, the reported statistics are calculated. In this way, chromosomes are scanned by moving a window of a fixed size along their entire length and variation in genetic markers across the region of interest can be measured. In practical terms, a sliding window is a sub-list that runs over an underlying collection of data (Fig. 2). This type of analysis

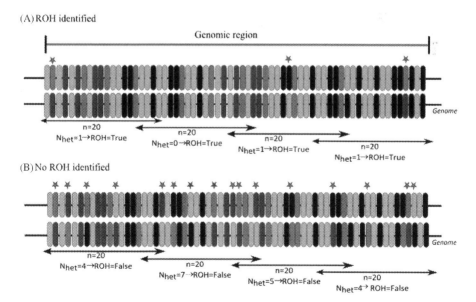

Fig. 2. Schematic representation of the sliding window algorithm. (A) Representation of genomic region that includes an ROH. (B) Representation of a genomic segment with no ROH. Stars represent heterozygous SNP.

allows investigation into the way patterns of variation change across a surveyed genomic segment [60].

PLINK is a user-friendly software tool, designed to facilitate the analysis of whole-genome data, with an efficient computationally routine analysis and new analyses that take advantage of whole-genome coverage [53]. It maps disease *loci* that contain multiple rare variants in a population-based linkage analysis, computes allele and genotypes frequencies, provides missing genotype rates, inbreeding, IBS and IBD statistics for individuals and pairs of individuals, detection of non-Mendelian transmission in family data, does sex checks based on X chromosome SNPs and tests non-random genotyping failure. The software's focus is the analysis of genotype/phenotype data, so there is no support for steps prior to this (e.g. study design and planning, generating genotype or copy number variation (CNV) calls from raw data). Very large whole-genome association studies (WGAS) data sets can be analyzed using standard hardware, and there are no fixed limits on the number of samples or SNPs [53]. The software uses a sliding-window algorithm to search for ROH along the genome. In this algorithm, the window moves forward from the 5′ to the 3′ extremity of a DNA sequence on a SNP-per-SNP basis. Each SNP is weighted as to whether looks 'homozygous' enough (yes/no) (i.e. allowing for a number of heterozygous or missed calls). Then, for each SNP, the proportion of 'homozygous' windows that overlap that position is calculated. If this proportion is higher than a defined threshold, the SNP is designated as being in a homozygous state. By default, PLINK consider a ROH only when containing at least 100 SNPs in a homozygous segment, and of total length $\geq$ 1000 kb, a ROH must have at least one SNP per 50 kb on average and the SNP-to-SNP distance is never greater than a user-specified threshold (default value = 1,000 kb) [62]. PLINK is the main WGAS analytic software that can run either as a stand-alone tool (from the command line or via shell scripting) or in conjunction with gPLINK, a Java-based graphical user interface. gPLINK also offers a simple project management framework to track PLINK analyses and facilitates integration with Haploview [61]. The combination of PLINK with gPLINK and Haploview offers users support for the subsequent visualization, annotation and storage of results.

GERMLINE is a tool designed for genome-wide discovery of IBD segments shared within large populations (by SNP arrays). It takes as input genotype or haplotype marker data for individuals (as well as an optional known pedigree) and generates a list of all pairwise segmental sharing [54]. Compared with similar tools, GERMLINE uses a novel hashing and extension algorithm, which is a linear-time algorithm (i.e. an algorithm in which plotting the runtime against the size of its input, a line is obtained) for identifying short identical genomic "slices" between pairs of individuals, and then extending the boundaries of these slices to discover long shared segments representative of IBD. For ROH detection, like the previous tool, it adopts a sliding-window algorithm that is flexible with respect to several parameters such as window size, minimum length of the ROH and tolerance for heterozygous mismatches. In contrast with PLINK, GERMLINE breaks up SNP stretches into non-overlapping windows of a user-specified length in terms of SNP, and only if several consecutive windows tagged as homozygous exceed a threshold in terms of physical or genetic distance is the region then labeled as homozygous [63]. GERMLINE is still significantly faster than similar IBD algorithms and compared to with PLINK has both a higher sensitivity and a overall lower false-positive rate. GERMLINE can identify shared segments of any specified length, as well as enable any number of mismatching markers.

EX-HOM (EXome HOMozygosity) demonstrated the possibility of exome sequencing to combine, in a single step, the identification of all the coding variants of a genome with the ability to perform homozygosity mapping as a way to limit candidate gene search to specific chromosomal regions [59]. EX-HOM authors used a sliding-window algorithm for WES based ROH detection by applying PLINK. This approach was developed specifically for when a single, small consanguineous family is available for mapping and identifying the genetic defect underlying a disease phenotype. As it uses WES data only, it was susceptible to the limitations which affect an exome sequencing approach, namely specific variants might have been missed due to low coverage or the lack of identification of large insertions or deletions, which would therefore have been missed. The efficiency of EX-HOM largely depends on the capacity to filter out all the variants which are not related to the disorder. It showed that regions >1 Mb in length overlap substantially with those identified as LOD score peaks by linkage analysis, leading to the conclusion that the EX-HOM approach can correctly identify disease-related long homozygous regions [59].

The three bioinformatic tools presented apply the sliding-window algorithm to identify ROH. This approach is efficient when working with longer ROH, as these may have few and unevenly spaced SNPs, whereas smaller and isolated ROH need a higher marker density. Thus, the sliding window algorithm is not as effective when used with short/medium ROH sizes. Magi et al. proposed a new tool, H^3M^2, that can detect small to longer-sized ROH [56]. The algorithm is based on a heterogeneous HMM, that incorporates distances between consecutive SNPs into transition probabilities matrix, to distinguish between the homozygosity and the heterozygosity states. Through this approach, the authors state that it can detect with high sensitivity and specificity ROH of every genomic sizes and being the main feature of the algorithm the heterogeneity, making it well-suited for WES data. To measure the homozygous/heterozygous genotype state of each SNP, this model uses B-allele frequency (BAF), which is defined as the ratio between B-allele counts (NB, the number of reads that match with the 1000 Genomes Project alternate allele at specific position) and the total number of reads mapped to that position (N, the depth of coverage) [56]. H^3M^2 showed better performances than GERMLINE and PLINK with the same dataset, it was less sensitive to parameter specification (which ensures that analysis results are not harshly affected by the user's chosen parameter configuration) and was considerably faster, namely in preparation of input genotype calls, as it only requires BAF profiles instead of NGS genotype calls [56].

Pippucci and co-workers tested H^3M^2, PLINK and GERMLINE and reported that all tools successfully identified the same 18 Mb homozygous region harboring the *CACNA2D2* gene, in which mutations were associated with epileptic encephalopathy. Although, higher accuracy was shown with H^3M^2 and PLINK [63]. Furthermore, H^3M^2 exhibited the highest accuracy in the detection of short and medium ROH, which highlights the applicability of WES-based HM in outbred individuals (i.e. non-consanguineous) [63].

AgileGenotyper/AgileVariantMapper [57] and HomSI [55] are two other examples of algorithms that can identify homozygous regions from an individual's exome sequence data. AgileGenotyper uses massive parallel sequencing reads to determine the genotypes at over 0.53 million known SNP identified by the 1000 Genomes Project, all located within exonic regions (also the flanking introns). Once the files imported into the software (in SAM format), it collates the sequence reads aligned to each exon and determines the read depth for each sequence variant at each known polymorphic position. It will then deduce the position's genotype, e.g. is called as heterozygous if 25% or more of the reads identify the minor variant base, and compares this to the possible genotypes as noted by the 1000 Genomes Project. If the genotype cannot be deduced or does not match the known genotypes, this are scored as "no-calls". The genotype data are exported as a single tab-delimited text file, which can then be analyzed by other programs such as AgileVariantMapper. AgileVariantMapper uses the total read depth and the read depth of the minor allele to determine the genotype at each position. These values can be interactively adjusted to determine the optimum values for defining the homozygous region [57].

In summary, all the presented methods have proven to be extremely valuable for the identification of ROH from WES data, with the possibility of performing HM mapping without resorting to SNP arrays. Still, although powerful, there is an error rate associated with this strategy that is difficult to estimate, since it is highly dependent on the exome metrics, sequencing platform and the bioinformatic tool used to infer ROH. Moreover, they have to take on the technical limitations of WES, namely the inadequate coverage of some exonic regions or sequencing errors which may be a source of false positive and/or false negative calls. Another issue is related with the incomplete annotation of the human genome, which can affect the accuracy of the mapping and annotation of variants; for instance, a deep intronic (pathogenic) variant, could indeed be the causative mutation in a non-annotated exon. With the improvement of NGS technologies, these limitations will be surpassed and this method will be even more powerful.

5   ROH Quantification in WES to Support Variant Filtering and Disease Inheritance Model Selection

Previously we presented HM data of two patients with distinct recessive conditions: a congenital neuromuscular disease (NMD) and PCD, caused by homozygous pathogenic variants identified by WES [64]. Although, only in one of the cases the disease-causing variant was located in a recognizable ROH, in both the overall HM data was compatible/suggestive with that of a homozygous autosomal recessive (AR) disease model.

With genetic conditions considered to be rare conditions, the patients are often found to represent sporadic, rather than having a family history. This means that, in a particular kindred, no other individuals with the same phenotype are found. In this context, variant filtering of WES data is more difficult, as the majority of disease models are still applicable. This scenario is even more complex when the WES is restricted to the patient (singleton), as is the case of adult patients where parental samples are not available for trio analysis. We postulate that ROH quantification could assist the choice of the suitable disease inheritance model. More specifically, if the

ROH regions are above a predetermined threshold value this would indicate that the homozygous AR model could contribute to identify the disease-causing variant. A lower ROH overall score, on the other hand, would indicate that this model is unsuitable for variant filtering (Fig. 3).

As a preliminary study, we analyzed ROH in WES data of twelve unrelated patients. In six cases the data was compatible with an autosomal recessive (AR) disease model and further six cases whose disease model (and disease-causing variants) are still unknown (UKN), used as test group. Among the AR disease model, we further sub-divide the patients in two groups: the first where the disease-causing variants were in homozygous state, thus we called this group "homozygous-AR" (n = 3, example in Fig. 4A); and the other group where the disease-causing variant was found in compound heterozygosity, known as "heterozygous-AR" (n = 3). To systemize this analysis, ROH were determined using HomozygosityMapper. In this software, we varied the block length (40, 60, 80, 100, 150, 200 and 250) and collected several parameters

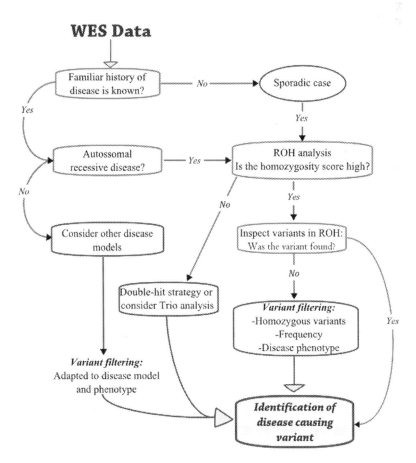

Fig. 3. Proposed workflow to identify disease-causing variants from WES data, with and without family history.

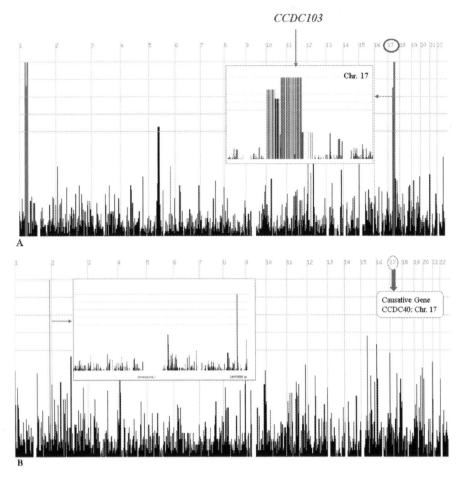

Fig. 4. Genome-wide homozygosity mapping using WES and the HomozygosityMapper software. The longest ROH are highlighted in red. (A) An example of a homozygous autosomal recessive case is shown, as previously presented in [64]. The patient has two long stretches of homozygous SNPs in chromosomes 1 and 17. The disease-causing gene is included in the second ROH (inserted blue box). (B) An example of a compound heterozygous autosomal recessive, longer stretches of homozygous SNP were not identified, just a small homozygous region in chromosome 1 is presented (inserted blue box). (Color figure online)

(highest homozygosity score, number of ROH, total size of ROH, average size of ROH, and the size of the largest ROH). With the generated data we could then evaluate how each parameter changed according to block length. A clear cut-off between the two groups (hom-AR and het-AR) for homozygosity score was identified (Fig. 5). In addition, for cases with longer ROH the block length of 80 was not sufficient and should be optimized (increased) to determine the highest score accurately (up to a value of 250 in the samples tested). It was interesting to note that scores above 60 were only detected in homozygous-AR cases (Fig. 5). We found statistically significant

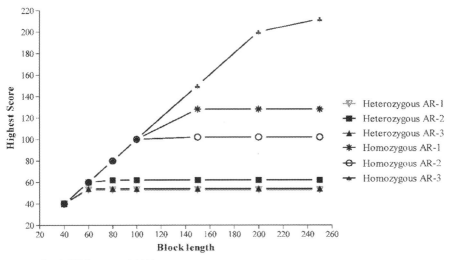

Kruskal-Wallis test: p=0,0146

Fig. 5. Correlation between highest homozygosity score and block length and comparison between heterozygous and homozygous autosomal recessive (AR) groups. Statistical analysis carried out with IBM SPSS statistics v.24; graphic in GraphPad Prism v.5. There is a clear cut-off between the two groups.

differences between the two groups using Kruskal–Wallis test (p = 0.0146). Further, we applied a Mann-Whitney U test, between homozygous-AR and heterozygous-AR groups which was found to be statistically significant, for the following parameters: highest score (Z = −3.302, p = 0.001), ROH average size (Z = −5.211, p = 0.000) and ROH largest size (Z = −3.429, p = 0.001). To further verify if the differences empirically observed in our cases could be statistically supported, we correlated the highest homozygosity score obtained in HomozygosityMapper with the total size in Mb of the respective ROH for each case. Next, we applied k-means clustering algorithm, a method of cluster analysis that allows the partition of n observations into k clusters, in which each observation is part of the cluster with the nearest mean.

Two different clusters were identified (Fig. 6). The first cluster corresponds to the heterozygous AR samples (k1) whose values seem to be more homogeneous compared with second cluster (k2, homozygous-AR) which has more dispersed data points. Kruskal-Wallis test demonstrated statistically significant differences between the two study groups ($\chi^{2(2)}$ = 6.2 and p = 0.044). No statistically significant differences were found between the UKN group and the other two (homozygous- and heterozygous AR), showing that it does not form a specific cluster. In the test group (unknown in Fig. 6), four samples are located in the vicinity of cluster k1 whereas the other two are nearer k2.

It should be noted that the number of cases analyzed are still very low, and these figures should be increased at least at 50 to 100 fold so that we can draw further conclusions. Nonetheless, we were able to show that, by computing the homozygosity highest score and ROH total size, it is possible to infer whether a homozygous or a heterozygous variant would be the cause of a particular disease.

The existence of longer stretches of homozygous SNP (ROH) may indeed provide a dual role: (i) indicate the pathogenic variant zygosity status (homozygous or heterozygous), and (ii) point towards the location of the disease-causing gene, since is likely to be located within these longer homozygous stretches. For instance, the case presented in Fig. 3A, represents a patient diagnosed with PCD; an AR genetic disorder that leads to anomalies in cilia/flagella structure, which results in chronic respiratory tract infections and in some patients, abnormalities in the position of internal organs (*situs inversus*), and/or infertility [65]. This case exemplifies how two longer ROH were identified, one in chromosome 1 and other on the 17, with the causative variant ultimately being found in the gene *CCDC103*, located in chromosome 17 [64].

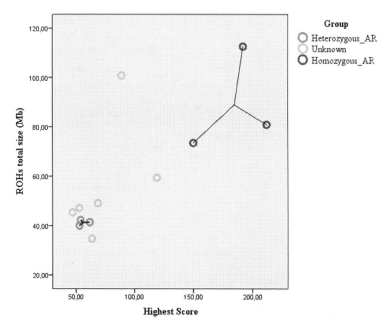

Fig. 6. Scatter plot presenting data analysis resorting tok-means clustering algorithm. Two clusters were identified for two groups: heterozygous AR (k1, green) and homozygous AR (k2, blue). Data analysis and plot performed with IBM SPSS statistics v.24. (Color figure online)

6   Conclusion

This work reviewed HM as an approach for gene discovery and the identification of disease-causing variants. The application of HM should be considered, not only in research but also in a routine clinical genetics setting, in cases where an autosomal recessive disease is suspected. The currently available algorithms and bioinformatic tools designed for ROH detection from array-SNP and WES data were also reviewed, highlighting their main features, advantages and limitations. Selection of appropriate algorithms should mainly consider the technology used to generate the data, but also specific features of the patient/family under study, such as genetic context, ROH average size and the number of relatives affected by the same condition. As depicted in Fig. 3, ROH analysis should be an option to include in the variant filtering strategies, in cases with familial AR transmission pattern or in sporadic cases.

As for identifying new associations between a gene and a particular phenotype, the presence of consanguinity in a specific kindred has its particularities; not only is the disease inheritance model self-evident (even in sporadic cases), but also concentrating the analysis of variants located in longer ROH regions reduces considerably the analytical burden. The term 'consanguineous' is somewhat ambiguous, as there are different levels, from the first to the 4th degree (e.g., first cousins). So the average percentage of DNA shared ranges from 50 to 12.5%. It should be noted that these percentages may influences the number and size of ROH. However, ROH analysis should not be confined to consanguineous cases as it may be found to be useful for cases with unknown parental consanguinity, especially if parents are from the same remote/confined village, where mutation founder effects or inbreeding events might be an issue.

This paper also shares some preliminary data that show how the analysis of ROH regions may also be extremely useful for variant filtering and for the selection of a disease inheritance model. More specifically, by correlating the highest homozygosity score and total size of ROH obtained with HomozygosityMapper two distinct clusters were obtained. If our assumption is correct, in the presence of a particular subject whose WES data clusters in k1 heterozygous variants, this should be verified first as a possible cause for the phenotype, corresponding to autosomal dominant (*de novo*) or compound heterozygous AR disease models. If the patient is a male, we cannot exclude an X-linked recessive inheritance, thus hemizygous variants should also be inspected. However, it should be noted that the number of cases analyzed is still limited, and further data needs to be collect and processed to verify these preliminary results.

In conclusion, the combination of WES and HM allow researchers to identify candidate *loci* and underlying genetic defect itself (at the nucleotide level) in a single step. Nonetheless, there are still several limitations and further bioinformatic developments are required. Considering the data presented, there are sensitivity issues that require addressing, especially if the genetic defect is located in a small ROH or if the pathogenic variant is *de novo* in an individual born to consanguineous parents. Finally, we consider that it would be useful to develop a tool that combines variant filtering and homozygosity mapping, which currently can only be performed individually.

Acknowledgements. The authors acknowledge support from: (i) Fundação para a Ciência e Tecnologia (FCT) [Grant ref.: PD/BD/105767/2014] (R.P.); (ii) Research grant attributed by "Fundo para a Investigação e Desenvolvimento do Centro Hospitalar do Porto" [Grant ref.: 336-13(196-DEFI/285-CES)] (J.O.). The work was also supported by the Institutions of the authors and in part by UMIB, which is funded by through FCT under the Pest-OE/SAU/UI0215/2014. The authors would like to thank the clinicians for patient referral.

References

1. Miko, I.: Gregor mendel and the principles of inheritance. Nat. Educ. **1**(1), 134 (2008)
2. Christianson, A., Howson, C.P., Modell, B.: Global report on birth defects: the hidden toll of dying and disabled children, New York (2006)
3. Lobo, I., Shaw, K.: Discovery and types of genetic linkage. Nat. Educ. **1**(1), 139 (2008)
4. Slatkin, M.: Linkage disequilibrium—understanding the evolutionary past and mapping the medical future. Nat. Rev. Genet. **9**(6), 477–485 (2008)
5. Sanger, F., Nicklen, S., Coulson, A.R.: DNA sequencing with chain-terminating inhibitors. PNAS **74**(12), 5463–5467 (1977)
6. Boycott, K.M., et al.: Rare-disease genetics in the era of next-generation sequencing: discovery to translation. Nat. Rev. Genet. **14**(10), 681–691 (2013)
7. Xia, J., et al.: NGS catalog: a database of next generation sequencing studies in humans. Hum. Mutat. **33**(6), E2341–E2355 (2012)
8. Koboldt, D.C., et al.: The next-generation sequencing revolution and its impact on genomics. Cell **155**(1), 27–38 (2013)
9. Bittles, A.H.: Consanguinity and its relevance to clinical genetics. Clin. Genet. **60**(2), 89–98 (2001)
10. Instituto Nacional de Estatística: Marriages (Between persons of the opposite sex - No.) by Place of registration (NUTS - 2002), Sex, Relationship or affinity between the spouses and Spouse previous marital status; Annual
11. McQuillan, R., et al.: Runs of homozygosity in European populations. Am. J. Hum. Genet. **83**(3), 359–372 (2008)
12. Lander, E.S., Botstein, D.: Homozygosity mapping: a way to map human recessive traits with the DNA of inbred children. Science **236**(4808), 1568–1570 (1987)
13. Alkuraya, F.S.: Autozygome decoded. Genet. Med. **12**(12), 765–771 (2010)
14. Goodship, J., et al.: Report autozygosity mapping of a Seckel syndrome locus to chromosome 3q22.1-q24. Am. J. Hum. Genet. **67**, 498–503 (2000)
15. Alkuraya, F.S.: Homozygosity mapping: one more tool in the clinical geneticist's toolbox. Genet. Med. **12**(4), 236–239 (2010)
16. Syvänen, A.-C.: Toward genome-wide SNP genotyping. Nat. Genet. **37**(6s), S5 (2005)
17. Gibbs, J.R., Singleton, A.: Application of genome-wide single nucleotide polymorphism typing: simple association and beyond. PLoS Genet. **2**(10), e150 (2006)
18. Evans, D.M., Cardon, L.R.: Guidelines for genotyping in genomewide linkage studies: single-nucleotide–polymorphism maps versus microsatellite maps. Am. J. Hum. Genet. **75**(4), 687–692 (2004)
19. Wang, Z., Gerstein, M., Snyder, M.: RNA-seq: a revolutionary tool for transcriptomics. Nat. Rev. Genet. **10**(1), 57–63 (2009)
20. Park, P.J.: ChIP-seq: advantages and challenges of a maturing technology. Nat. Rev. Genet. **10**(10), 669–680 (2009)
21. Li, Y., Tollefsbol, T.O.: DNA methylation detection: bisulfite genomic sequencing analysis. In: Tollefsbol, T. (ed.) Methods in Molecular Biology, vol. 791, pp. 11–21. Springer, Heidelberg (2011). https://doi.org/10.1007/978-1-61779-316-5_2
22. Mardis, E.R.: The impact of next-generation sequencing technology on genetics. Trends Genet. **24**(3), 133–141 (2008)
23. Ng, S.B., et al.: Exome sequencing identifies the cause of a mendelian disorder. Nat. Genet. **42**(1), 30–35 (2010)
24. Oliveira, J., et al.: New splicing mutation in the choline kinase beta (CHKB) gene causing a muscular dystrophy detected by whole-exome sequencing. J. Hum. Genet. **60**(6), 305 (2015)

25. Pereira, R., et al.: Mutation analysis in patients with total sperm immotility. J. Assist. Reprod. Genet. **32**(6), 893–902 (2015)
26. Antonarakis, S.E., Krawczak, M., Cooper, D.N.: Disease-causing mutations in the human genome. Eur. J. Pediatr. **159**(Suppl), S173–S178 (2000)
27. Gripp, K.W., et al.: Truncating mutations in the last exon of NOTCH3 cause lateral meningocele syndrome. Am. J. Med. Genet. Part A **167**(2), 271–281 (2015)
28. Norton, N., et al.: Genome-wide studies of copy number variation and exome sequencing identify rare variants in BAG3 as a cause of dilated cardiomyopathy. Am. J. Hum. Genet. **88**(3), 273–282 (2011)
29. Sirmaci, A., et al.: Challenges in whole exome sequencing: an example from hereditary deafness. PLoS ONE **7**(2), e32000 (2012)
30. Sauna, Z.E., Kimchi-Sarfaty, C.: Understanding the contribution of synonymous mutations to human disease. Nat. Rev. Genet. **12**(10), 683–691 (2011)
31. Meienberg, J., et al.: Clinical sequencing: is WGS the better WES? Hum. Genet. **135**(3), 359–362 (2016)
32. Belkadi, A., et al.: Whole-genome sequencing is more powerful than whole-exome sequencing for detecting exome variants. Hum. Genet. **135**, 359–362 (2016)
33. Xu, W., et al.: Model-free linkage analysis of a binary trait. Stat. Hum. Genet.: Methods Protoc. **850**, 317–345 (2012)
34. Bailey-Wilson, J.E.: Parametric and nonparametric linkage analysis. In: Encyclopedia of Life Sciences. Wiley, Chichester (2006)
35. Pulst, S.M., et al.: Genetic linkage analysis. Arch. Neurol. **56**(6), 667 (1999)
36. Ott, J.: Estimation of the recombination fraction in human pedigrees: efficient computation of the likelihood for human linkage studies. Am. J. Hum. Genet. **26**(5), 588 (1974)
37. Elston, R.C., Stewart, J.: A general model for the genetic analysis of pedigree data. Hum. Hereditary **21**, 523–542 (1971)
38. Kruglyak, L., et al.: Parametric and nonparametric linkage analysis: a unified multipoint approach. Am. J. Hum. Genet. **58**, 1347–1363 (1996)
39. Ghahramani, Z.: An introduction to hidden Markov models and Bayesian networks. Int. J. Pattern Recogn. Artif. Intell. **15**(1), 9–42 (2001)
40. Goedken, R., et al.: Drawbacks of GENEHUNTER for larger pedigrees: application to panic disorder. Am. J. Med. Genet. **96**(6), 781–783 (2000)
41. Sobel, E., Lange, K.: Descent graphs in pedigree analysis: applications to haplotyping, location scores, and marker-sharing statistics. Am. J. Hum. Genet. **58**(6), 1323–1337 (1996)
42. Geyer, C.: Introduction to Markov chain Monte Carlo. In: Brooks, S., et al. (eds.) Handbook of Markov Chain Monte Carlo, pp. 3–48. CRC Press, Boca Raton (2011)
43. Romero-Hidalgo, S., et al.: GENEHUNTER versus SimWalk2 in the context of an extended kindred and a qualitative trait locus. Genetica **123**(3), 235–244 (2005)
44. Abecasis, G.R., et al.: Merlin—rapid analysis of dense genetic maps using sparse gene flow trees. Nat. Genet. **30**(1), 97–101 (2002)
45. Dudbridge, F.: A survey of current software for linkage analysis. Hum. Genomics **1**(1), 63 (2003)
46. MacCluer, J.W., et al.: Pedigree analysis by computer simulation. Zoo Biol. **5**(2), 147–160 (1986)
47. Gudbjartsson, D.F., et al.: Allegro, a new computer program for multipoint linkage analysis. Nat. Genet. **25**(1), 12–13 (2000)
48. Alkuraya, F.S.: The application of next-generation sequencing in the autozygosity mapping of human recessive diseases. Hum. Genet. **132**(11), 1197–1211 (2013)

49. Krawitz, P.M., et al.: Identity-by-descent filtering of exome sequence data identifies PIGV mutations in hyperphosphatasia mental retardation syndrome. Nat. Genet. **42**(10), 827–829 (2010)
50. Becker, J., et al.: Exome sequencing identifies truncating mutations in human SERPINF1 in autosomal-recessive osteogenesis imperfecta. Am. J. Hum. Genet. **88**(3), 362–371 (2011)
51. Seelow, D., Schuelke, M.: HomozygosityMapper2012—bridging the gap between homozygosity mapping and deep sequencing. Nucleic Acids Res. **40**(W1), W516–W520 (2012)
52. Seelow, D., et al.: HomozygosityMapper—an interactive approach to homozygosity mapping. Nucleic Acids Res. **37**(Web Server issue), W593–W599 (2009)
53. Purcell, S., et al.: PLINK: a tool set for whole-genome association and population-based linkage analyses. Am. J. Hum. Genet. **81**(3), 559–575 (2007)
54. Gusev, A., et al.: Whole population, genome-wide mapping of hidden relatedness. Genome Res. **19**(2), 318–326 (2009)
55. Görmez, Z., et al.: HomSI: a homozygous stretch identifier from next-generation sequencing data. Bioinformatics **30**(3), 445–447 (2013)
56. Magi, A., et al.: H^3M^2: detection of runs of homozygosity from whole-exome sequencing data. Bioinformatics **30**(20), 2852–2859 (2014)
57. Carr, I.M., et al.: Autozygosity mapping with exome sequence data. Hum. Mutat. **34**(1), 50–56 (2013)
58. Seelow, D., et al.: GeneDistiller—distilling candidate genes from linkage intervals. PLoS ONE **3**(12), e3874 (2008)
59. Pippucci, T., et al.: EX-HOM (EXome HOMozygosity): a proof of principle. Hum. Hered. **72**(1), 45–53 (2011)
60. Tang, R., et al.: A variable-sized sliding-window approach for genetic association studies via principal component analysis. Ann. Hum. Genet. **73**(Pt 6), 631–637 (2009)
61. Barrett, J.C., et al.: Haploview: analysis and visualization of LD and haplotype maps. Bioinformatics **21**(2), 263–265 (2004)
62. Chang, C.: PLINK: whole genome data analysis toolset-identity by descent. https://www.cog-genomics.org/plink/1.9/ibd#homozyg
63. Pippucci, T., et al.: Detection of runs of homozygosity from whole exome sequencing data: state of the art and perspectives for clinical, population and epidemiological studies. Hum. Hered. **77**(1–4), 63–72 (2014)
64. Oliveira, J., et al.: Homozygosity mapping using whole-exome sequencing: a valuable approach for pathogenic variant identification in genetic diseases. In: Proceedings of the 10th International Joint Conference on Biomedical Engineering Systems and Technologies, BIOINFORMATICS, (BIOSTEC 2017), vol. 3, pp. 210–216 (2017)
65. Leigh, M.W., et al.: Clinical and genetic aspects of primary ciliary dyskinesia/Kartagener syndrome. Genet. Med.: Off. J. Am. Coll. Med. Genet. **11**(7), 473–487 (2009)

Virus Disassembly Pathways Predicted from Geometry and Configuration Energy

Claudio Alexandre Piedade, Marta Sousa Silva, Carlos Cordeiro, and António E. N. Ferreira[✉]

Laboratório de FTICR e Espectrometria de Massa Estrutural,
Centro de Química e Bioquímica, Departamento de Química e Bioquímica,
Faculdade de Ciências, Universidade de Lisboa, 1749-016 Lisbon, Portugal
claudioalexandrepiedade@gmail.com,
{mfsilva,cacordeiro,aeferreira}@fc.ul.pt

Abstract. Virus are supramolecular structures that are responsible for some of the most significant epidemics around the world. The disassembly of virus particles, a key event during viral infection is triggered by numerous intracellular factors. The investigation of the mechanisms of protein subunit loss during viral disassembly has generally been overlooked, in sharp contrast with the research on the assembly process of virus particles, which has been the focus of both experimental and theoretical studies. In this work, we address the problem of predicting the sequence of protein subunit removal from a viral capsid, by assuming that the order of subunit loss is mainly determined by each capsid's structural geometry and configuration energy. We modelled the early stages of virus disassembly in a sample of 51 icosahedral viruses of class $T = 1$, predicting the sequence of removal of up to five subunits. Due to the high symmetry of viral structures, we established the geometrical equivalence of subunit configurations of capsid fragments, decreasing the size of the search space. The energy of a given configuration was estimated by using heuristic functions of the number and types of inter-subunit contacts. We found a disassembly pathway common to a large group of viruses, consisting of the removal of a triangular trimer. Exceptions to this general pattern include the loss of a pentagon-shaped pentamer. These results point at specific subunit interactions as putative targets for novel antiviral drugs developed to interfere with the disassembly process.

Keywords: Virus capsid disassembly · Combinatorial geometry
Symmetry groups · Structural biology

1 Introduction

Viruses are intracellular parasites that replicate inside living cells by using its genetic and protein synthesis machinery to create new copies [1, 2]. Although they can infect several different organisms, from bacteria and fungi to algae, plants, insects and vertebrates, human viruses have deserved a special attention by researchers all over the world [3]. Since ancient times, viruses have coexisted and have evolved with humans (reviewed in [4]). Examples include several strains of herpes, measles and dengue viruses. More recent examples include the HIV and Ebola [4]. Viruses caused severe

© Springer International Publishing AG, part of Springer Nature 2018
N. Peixoto et al. (Eds.): BIOSTEC 2017, CCIS 881, pp. 289–301, 2018.
https://doi.org/10.1007/978-3-319-94806-5_16

epidemic outbreaks during human history, like the smallpox virus (also known as variola virus), causing the death of more than 400 thousand people in Europe each year in the 18th century [5], or the four influenza pandemics, responsible for over 4 million deaths all over the world [6].

Viral particles are composed by a nucleic acid (DNA or RNA, single or double stranded) and, in most cases, a protein-based supramolecular structure, the capsid, that protects the genetic material between the infection phase of the virus life cycle [1, 7, 8]. Round-shaped viruses have a fixed number of proteins surrounding the genetic material in an icosahedral symmetry [7, 8]. This geometrical feature was first described in 1962 by Caspar and Klug, who developed a scheme to classify the different levels of icosahedral symmetry by triangulating the icosahedron facets [7]. The Triangulation number (or T number) represents the number of equilateral triangles that compose a triangular face of the icosahedron [8].

The assembly of a complete viral capsid from its protein subunits has been addressed in many studies, both experimentally and theoretically (reviewed in [2, 9]). Viruses' capsid subunits are held together by non-covalent interactions such as electrostatic salt bridges, hydrophobic contacts and hydrogen bonds [10–12]. The combined effect of many of these interactions accounts for the stability of the virus capsid [13].

Virus assembly is spontaneous *in vitro* under close to physiological conditions [2] and the resulting capsids are stable for a long period of time. Many of the theoretical models of capsid assembly agree on the prediction that three bound protomers, pentamers of trimers and capsids that have just a triangular icosahedron face missing are stable intermediate forms found during the formation of a complete capsid [10, 12, 14–17]). If capsid disassembly is just the reverse process of capsid assembly, these findings suggest that the same structures may be found during capsid disassembly.

In sharp contrast to the number of studies addressing the assembly process, there are very few experimental studies on the pathways of capsid disassembly. Furthermore, since it is expected that intermediates of this process are transient and very difficult to detect, theoretical models of capsid disassembly are also difficult to validate experimentally. Moreover, the assembly and disassembly pathways are, most likely, not entirely symmetric since some viruses undergo maturation steps after assembly completion, such as proteolysis, cross-linking or conformational changes [13], which are not expected to occur during disassembly. In an *in vitro* study of capsid disassembly using atomic force microscopy (AFM), Castellanos et al. observed the removal of a triangle of subunits (a face of the icosahedron) when force was applied on capsids of Minute Virus of Mice, followed sometimes by the loss of an adjacent triangle [18]. In other cases, a removal of a pentamer of triangles (15 proteins) was observed. These disassembly pathways follow the predictions of the assembly models [14–17]. Horton and Lewis stated that, when possible intermediates are surveyed, energy minimums appear every multiple of three subunits [19]. Ortega-Esteban et al. have shown, also by AFM, that the first step of disassembly of Human Adenoviruses, starting from both mature and immature capsids, is the loss of a pentagon of proteins [20].

In this work, we address the problem of predicting the sequence of subunit loss during the early steps of viral capsid disassembly, the "disassembly pathway", focusing on $T = 1$ icosahedral capsid structures. We assume that the main factors that determine these pathways are geometry and subunit interaction energy. Due to symmetry, many of the fragments obtained from removing protein subunits from a virus capsid are geometrically equivalent, if the remaining subunits remain in the same place with the same inter subunit interactions. To establish such equivalence, we applied rigorous geometrical and combinatorial considerations.

The work is meant as a contribution to overcome the lack of theoretical studies targeting the disassembly process, with the long-term goal of providing insights which may guide the development of antiviral drugs designed to interfere with the formation of intermediate fragments during this process.

2 Methods

2.1 Structures of Viral Capsids

Atomic coordinates of capsids of type $T = 1$, present in the database ViperDB (http://viperdb.scripps.edu, [21]), were obtained from the Protein Data Bank (PDB, http://www.rcsb.org/, [22]). The structures were divided into groups according to the criteria of similarity of the infection host and the genes coding for the capsid proteins. The list of the 51 structures and their division into 14 groups are presented in Table 1. In this study we included Human Adenovirus of penton-dodecahedron type (Pt-Dd, abbreviated in our work as HAPD). Despite these are mainly $T = 25$, the structures studied in this work were a stable capsid formed with the pentagons of the $T = 25$, forming a dodecahedron.

Table 1. Groups and PDB IDs of viral capsids analyzed in this work. Viruses marked with † are Parvoviruses (Family Parvoviridae).

Group	PDB IDs
Adeno-Associated Virus†	1LP3, 2G8G, 2QA0, 3J1Q, 3J4P, 3NTT, 3RA2, 3RA4, 3RA8, 3RA9, 3RAA, 3UX1, 4IOV, 4RSO, 5EGC
Avian Birnavirus	1WCD
Bombyx mori Densovirus†	3P0S
Bovine Parvovirus†	4QC8
Canine and Feline Panleukopenia Virus†	1C8D, 1C8E, 1C8G, 1C8H, 1FPV, 1IJS, 1P5W, 1P5Y, 2CAS, 4DPV, 1C8F
Galleria mellonella Densovirus†	1DNV
Hepatitis E Virus	2ZTN, 2ZZQ, 3HAG
Human Adenovirus (HAPD)	1X9T, 4AQQ, 4AR2
Human Parvovirus†	1S58
Penaeus stylirostris Densovirus†	3N7X
Porcine Circovirus	3JCI, 3R0R
Porcine Parvovirus†	1K3V
Rodent Protoparvovirus†	1MVM, 1Z14, 1Z1C, 2XGK, 4G0R, 4GBT
Satellite Tobacco Mosaic Virus	1A34, 4OQ8, 2BUK, 4BCU

2.2   Structure Representation and Equivalence

Virus capsid structures with $T = 1$ have 60 subunits and, although having icosahedral symmetry, are best described by a 60-face polyhedron, in which each triangular face of the icosahedron is divided into three deltoids. This is a Deltoidal Hexecontahedron.

Due to the high degree of symmetry of the Deltoidal Hexecontahedron, the number of different fragments obtained by removing n subunits from a capsid is not simply the combinations $\binom{60}{n}$, since many of these fragments are equivalent by symmetry operations. The exact number of non-equivalent structures can be obtained by applying the Burnside's Lemma [23] and is shown in Table 2 for up to $n = 6$.

Table 2. Number of different fragments obtained by removal of n subunits from a $T = 1$ viral capsid.

n	Number of geometrically non-equivalent fragments	$\binom{60}{n}$
1	1	60
2	37	1,770
3	577	34,220
4	8,236	487,635
5	91,030	5,461,512
6	835,476	50,063,860

If the predictions about capsid disassembly can be restricted to non-equivalent forms, as opposed to using all the possible capsid configurations, then the computational complexity of all the methods can be dramatically decreased. To perform an exhaustive search for the fragments that are geometrically equivalent we built up the group of permutations associated with the rotations of a Deltoidal Hexecontahedron. For that purpose, the faces were numbered as shown in Fig. 1, which is the standard numbering in the Protein Data Bank for $T = 1$ structures, and equivalence was established by the analysis of the transformations done on the numbering of the faces by the symmetry operators of the symmetry group I [24].

In this work, $\{i_1, i_2,..., i_n\}$ denotes the capsid fragment obtained from removing subunits $i_1, i_2,..., i_n$ from the complete capsid. Applying the different rotations on the symmetry axes of a Deltoidal Hexecontahedron, results in a permutation group. These permutations are also permutations of the faces of the Deltoidal Hexecontahedron or the vertices of its dual, the Rhombicosidodecahedron. The structures were represented as subgraphs of the graph depicted in Fig. 1 since, at any step of subunit removal, the generation of disconnected fragments could be assessed by graph-theoretic methods.

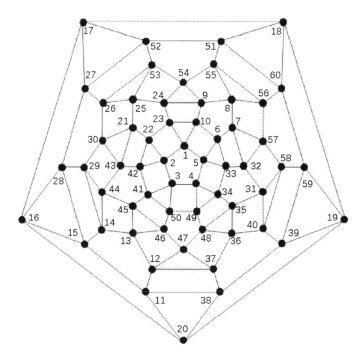

Fig. 1. Graph representation of the Deltoidal Hexecontahedron. Each vertex represents a subunit of the $T = 1$ virus capsid. Edges represent geometrical edges [25].

2.3 Energy Calculation

To calculate the energy of the full capsid and its disassembly products, the chemical interactions between protein subunits were considered (intra-protein contacts were ignored). These interactions are of three types: hydrogen bonds, salt bridges and hydrophobic contacts. The number of each type of interaction was calculated as follows: hydrogen bonds were counted if the positions of acceptor and donor's atoms, as indicated in Table 3, were found at a distance less than or equal to 4.0 Å [26]. A salt bridge bound was counted if a positively charged atom of an acidic amino acid (Asp or Glu) was found within 4.0 Å of a negatively charged atom of a basic amino acid (Arg or Lys), [27]. A hydrophobic interaction was counted when β-carbons of the residues Ala, Val, Leu, Ile, Met, Phe, Tyr and Trp, were found at the distance less than or equal to 7.0 Å [28].

Table 3. Donor and acceptor's atoms used to calculate the number of hydrogen bonds.

Donor	Arg (N_ε; $N_{\eta1}$; $N_{\eta2}$), Asn ($N_{\delta2}$), Cys (S_γ), Gln ($N_{\varepsilon2}$), His ($N_{\delta1}$; $N_{\varepsilon2}$), Lys (N_ζ), Ser (O_γ), Thr ($O_{\gamma1}$), Trp ($N_{\varepsilon1}$), Tyr (O_η)
Acceptor	Asn ($O_{\delta1}$), Asp ($O_{\delta1}$; $O_{\delta2}$), Gln ($O_{\varepsilon1}$), Glu ($O_{\varepsilon1}$; $O_{\varepsilon2}$), His ($N_{\delta1}$; $N_{\varepsilon2}$), Ser (O_γ), Thr ($O_{\gamma1}$), Tyr (O_η)

The energy of a complete capsid or a capsid fragment was calculated by three alternative heuristic measures, that are related to the number of hydrogen bonds (N_{HB}), salt bridges (N_{SB}) and hydrophobic contacts (N_{HC}) as follows:

$$E_I = N_{SB} + N_{HB} + N_{HC} \tag{1}$$

$$E_{II} = 20N_{SB} + N_{HB} + N_{HC} \tag{2}$$

$$E_{III} = 100N_{SB} + 10N_{HB} + N_{HC} \tag{3}$$

We proposed these three heuristic functions because of the complexity of using accurate energy functions for large macromolecular complexes. The three measures assign different weights for the three types of interactions. In Heuristic I (Eq. (1)), only the total number of interactions is considered, and the three types of bounds are equally weighted. Heuristic II (Eq. (2)) gives salt bridges 20 times more energy than hydrogen bonds, since they are usually stronger, with the hydrophobic contacts assumed to be energetically equivalent to hydrogen bonds. This assumption followed an entropy argument that solvation water is unbound when hiding hydrophobic amino acids in a hydrophobic contact, breaking hydrogen bonds between water and polar groups in amino acid residues [29]. Finally, in Heuristic III (Eq. (3)) increasing weights by powers of 10 were given to each type of interaction, in the known order of strength by contact type (salt bridges > hydrogen bonds > hydrophobic contacts), [29].

2.4   Generation of Equivalence Classes

Each possible capsid fragment corresponds to a configuration of the 60-subunit structure and was represented by a 60-element binary vector, where one (1) represents the absence and zero (0) the presence of each subunit, using the numbering scheme shown in Fig. 1. A list of binary vectors representing each equivalence class by one of its members was then obtained as follows: for each level of removing n subunits and for every possible combination of n indexes in the set of integers 1 to 60, a binary vector was generated with zeros in those index positions and ones elsewhere (subunit 1 was always considered as the first to be removed); the 60 permutations of the symmetry group I [24] were then applied to this vector; if any of the resulting vectors was not bitwise identical to any previously obtained vector it would be appended to the list. Thus, a set of non-geometrically identical vectors representing capsid fragments that lost n subunits was obtained. By using their representation as a subgraph of Fig. 1 the presence of disconnected fragments was checked and, if found, the largest fragment was retained and the search for non-redundant forms was also applied to this fragment. Finally, each fragment's energy was calculated by each of the three heuristic functions.

2.5   Optimal Path for Disassembly

For all the possible non-equivalent configurations resulting from the removal of n proteins, a directed graph was constructed with all the possible paths to reach each configuration from the intact virus capsid ($n = 0$). Nodes in this graph associate binary vectors representing the configuration of a capsid fragment with a list of numbers that enumerate all the possible fragments (with $n - 1$ subunits removed) from which the fragment may have originated, also following the numbering scheme shown in Fig. 1. Edges in this graph were assigned a transition energy weight, $E_{i \to j}$, based on the variation of the average heuristic energy per protein, as indicated by Eq. 4. In this equation, E_i represents the energy of fragment i and $m_i = 60 - n_i$ is the number of proteins in that fragment.

$$E_{i \to j} = E_j/m_j - E_i/m_i \qquad (4)$$

The Bellman-Ford algorithm [30] was then used on this graph to calculate the shortest path from the complete capsid to every possible configuration, recording the five shortest paths. The energy of a path is simply the sum of the transition energies of the edges in the path.

2.6   Implementation and Code Availability

All methods were implemented in Python 2.7 using scientific computing modules of this language. The graph theoretic algorithms are available in the Python bindings of package *igraph* [31]. All the analysis code is available on GitHub repository https://github.com/CAPiedade/Virus-Disassembly.

3   Results and Discussion

The final fragments resulting from the minimal energy paths of disassembly for the 51 capsid structures and n from 2 to 5 are shown in Table 4 assuming Heuristic I for energy calculations. It can be readily observed that most Parvoviruses (marked with a †) follow the same sequence of disassembly: {1} → {1, 10} → {1, 10, 23} → {1, 2, 10, 23} → {1, 2, 10, 22, 23}. Fragment {1, 10, 23} represents the loss of proteins forming a triangle on the capsid structure (Fig. 2A). This triangle is just one face of the Icosahedron from which the Deltoidal Hexecontahedron is derived (three adjacent deltoids).

In the mechanical removal of proteins by AFM applied on the Minute Mice Virus (on our work represented by the group of the Rodent Protoparvovirus) it was observed that the disassembly process tends to start by the loss of one of those triangular blocks, followed by the removal of another adjacent triangle [18]. Furthermore, the theoretical studies of Rapaport et al. revealed the existence of long-lived transient structures with just one last triangle of proteins missing to form the complete capsid [16, 17]. The same pattern for models of capsid assembly was showed by Reddy et al. using both individual proteins and trimers [14], suggesting that the path for disassembly also follows the triangle removal.

Going two more steps further in the disassembly of Parvoviruses, most of them end up with fragment {1, 2, 10, 22, 23} for $n = 5$ (Table 4). This fragment results from the removal of a trapezium-like shape group of subunits, centered on the triangle {1, 10, 23}, (Fig. 2C). Supposing this trend continues, it is not hard to see that there is a

Table 4. Capsid groups and final configurations for minimal energy paths after the removal of n subunits. Energy was computed by Heuristic I (Eq. 1). Viruses marked with † are Parvoviruses (Family Parvoviridae).

Group	PDB IDs	n			
		2	3	4	5
Adeno-Associated Virus†	1LP, 2G8G, 2QA0, 3J1Q, 3J4P, 3NTT, 3RA2, 3RA4, 3RA8, 3RA9, 3RAA, 3UX1, 4IOV, 4RSO, 5EGC	{1,10}	{1,10,23}	{1,2,10,23}	{1,2,10,22,23}
Avian Birnavirus	1WCD	{1,10}	{1,10,23}	{1,2,10,23}	{1,2,10,22,23}
Bombyx mori Densovirus†	3P0S	{1,2}	{1,10,23}	{1,2,10,23}	{1,2,10,22,23}
Bovine Parvovirus†	4QC8	{1,10}	{1,10,23}	{1,2,10,23}	{1,2,10,22,23}
Canine and Feline Panleukopenia Virus†	1C8D, 1C8E, 1C8G, 1C8H, 1FPV, 1IJS, 1P5W, 1P5Y, 2CAS, 4DPV,	{1,10}	{1,10,23}	{1,2,10,23}	{1,2,10,22,23}
	1C8F			{1,10,23,34}	
Galleria mellonella Densovirus†	1DNV	{1,2}	{1,10,23}	{1,2,10,23}	{1,2,10,22,23}
Hepatitis E Virus	2ZTN, 2ZZQ	{1,6}	{1,2,23}	{1,2,6,23}	{1,2,6,10,23}
	3HAG			{1,2,10,23}	
Human Adenovirus (HAPD)	1X9T, 4AQQ, 4AR2	{1,2}	{1,2,3}	{1,2,3,4}	{1,2,3,4,5}
Human Parvovirus†	1S58	{1,10}	{1,10,23}	{1,2,10,23}	{1,2,10,22,23}
Penaeus stylirostris Densovirus†	3N7X	{1,2}	{1,2,23}	{1,2,22,23}	{1,2,6,10,23}
Porcine Circovirus	3JCI	{1,10}	{1,10,23}	{1,2,10,23}	{1,2,10,22,23} {1,2,10,23,42}
	3R0R				{1,2,10,23,42}
Porcine Parvovirus†	1K3V	{1,10}	{1,10,23}	{1,2,10,23}	{1,2,10,22,23}
Rodent Protoparvovirus†	1MVM, 1Z14, 1Z1C, 2XGK, 4G0R 4GBT	{1,10}	{1,10,23}	{1,2,10,23}	{1,2,10,22,23}
Satellite Tobacco Mosaic Virus	1A34, 4OQ8	{1,6}	{1,2,23}	{1,2,6,23}	{1,2,6,10,23}
	2BUK, 4BCU		{1,2,6}	{1,2,6,24}	{1,2,6,10,24}

chance of removing the proteins around the five-fold axis. These could be the follow-up steps of the disassembly of these capsids, potentially resulting in the loss of 15 proteins such as {1, 2, 3, 4, 5, 6, 10, 22, 23, 33, 34, 41, 42, 49, 50}.

Castellanos et al.'s results [18] confirm the predictions of Reddy et al. [14], since the lowest energy configuration, just before the complete capsid, is missing a pentamer of triangles (corresponding to such 15-protein), inclusively for Parvoviruses [15].

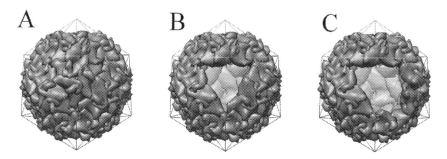

Fig. 2. Disassembly stages of Human Parvovirus with PDB ID 1S58. **A:** complete capsid, **B:** fragment {1, 10, 23}, **C:** fragment {1, 2, 10, 22, 23}.

The removal of four proteins can occur with more than one possibilities. Most Parvoviruses lose subunits {1, 2, 10, 23}. However, the structure 1C8F of Canine and Feline Panleukopenia virus is stabilized by the removal of the configuration {1, 10, 23, 34}, maintaining the triangular breach already formed (Table 4). Densoviruses, which belong to the Parvoviridae family, follow the main trend, except for the loss of two proteins, where configuration {1, 2} is favored, and in the case of *Penaeus stylirostris* Densovirus which follows the pathway {1} → {1, 2} → {1, 2, 23} → {1, 2, 22, 23} → {1, 2, 6, 10, 23}, (Table 4). Avian Birnavirus follow the same path as the majority of Parvovirus, as do Porcine Circoviruses, except when it comes to losing five subunits, in which case the latter family settles on configurations {1, 2, 10, 23, 42} or {1, 2, 10, 22, 23}, (Table 4).

Hepatitis E Virus capsids loses proteins in the order {1} → {1, 6} → {1, 2, 23} → {1, 2, 6, 23} → {1, 2, 6, 10, 23} or, alternatively, {1} → {1, 6} → {1, 2, 23} → {1, 2, 10, 23} → {1, 2, 6, 10, 23}, (Table 4). Although distinguishable from the Parvovirus, Hepatitis E Virus loses a pentamer that forms a triangular hole on the capsid structure.

HAPD follows the disassembly path {1} → {1, 2} → {1, 2, 3} → {1, 2, 3, 4} → {1, 2, 3, 4, 5}, an exception to all the others (Table 4). Human Adenovirus is the only group undergoing the loss of the subunits around the five-fold axis, the pentamer {1, 2, 3, 4, 5}, (Fig. 3B).

On Fig. 3 we can observe the structure of an HAPD, which is formed by very condensed clusters of pentagons, having very few contacts with the 2-fold and 3-fold proteins. The distance between the pentagonal clusters on the full capsid structure might make it easier for this set of subunits to be removed, in opposition to creating a bigger gap by removing, for example, proteins {1, 2, 10, 22, 23}. Our results are supported by those of Ortega-Esteban et al. which showed, through AFM, a loss of a pentagon-shaped pentamer of proteins for Human Adenoviruses [20].

Satellite Mosaic Tobacco Virus disassembly can be separated into two distinct groups, in which the structures 1A34 and 4OQ8 follow the pathway {1} → {1, 6} → {1, 2, 23} → {1, 2, 6, 23} → {1, 2, 6, 10, 23}, whereas structures 2BUK and 4BCU follow the pathway {1} → {1, 6} → {1, 2, 6} → {1, 2, 6, 24} → {1, 2, 6, 10, 24}. The first two structures were inferred from crystallized viruses with RNA still

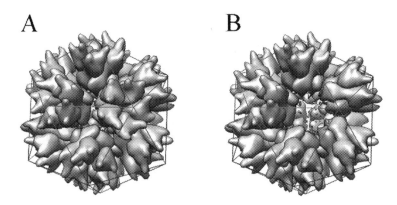

Fig. 3. Disassembly stages of Human Adenovirus (HAPD) with PDB ID 4AQQ. **A:** complete capsid (the highlighted proteins are the subunits around the five-fold axis), **B:** fragment {1, 2, 3, 4, 5}.

attached to the virus capsid while the latter structures were not. Since nucleic acids can assist the assembly of viral capsids [2], we can speculate that, although not accounted for in our methods, the presence of these extra macromolecules will contribute to significantly different full-capsid or fragment configuration energies, which will influence the pathway of disassembly.

We also investigated the effect of considering the other two heuristic functions for the calculation of configuration energies (Eqs. 2 and 3). Results were very similar to Heuristic I, with a slightly higher degree of branching. In particular, the same general trend of the loss of {1, 10, 23} and five proteins was observed in all three heuristics. Detailed results can be found as supplementary tables in the code repository associated with this work (see Sect. 2.6).

4 Conclusions

The aims of this study were to investigate whether there was a prevalent disassembly pathway among all virus capsids and, if not, if there were any pathways specific to some virus families. It seems clear that the results are in line with the idea that, for many $T = 1$ viruses, the disassembly of the capsid proceeds through the loss of three adjacent proteins. Geometrically, these subunits form one of the triangular faces of the icosahedron from which the deltoidal hexecontahedron is derived. The capsid fragment thus obtained still preserves a very high degree of symmetry. Families that follow this pattern include some Parvoviruses (Adeno-Associated Virus, Bovine Parvovirus, Human Parvovirus, Porcine Parvovirus, Rodent Protoparvovirus, Canine and Feline Panleukopenia Virus), Avian Birnavirus, Hepatitis E Virus and Porcine Circovirus. If our predictions are correct, then we expect to observe in many more viral types the experimental results obtained by Castellanos et al. with Rodent Protoparvovirus [18]. We can speculate that once this type of structure is formed, a capsid is sufficiently disassembled to export the genetic material out of the virus.

Exceptions to the general pattern can be found among the Human Adenoviruses (HAPD) which have a very particular pathway of disassembly, allowing for the removal of a pentagons of subunits.

Our 60-subunit model of viral capsids (Deltoidal Hexecontahedron) and a combinatorial method of searching for geometrical equivalence based on symmetry and geometry is generally superior to models based on 20 subunits (Icosahedron) or 12 subunits (Dodecahedron). Although we reached results comparable to those reported in previous literature, we were also able to investigate cases such as the Human Adenoviruses (HAPD type), which do not lose triangular faces of the Icosahedron, but a pentagon of faces of the Deltoidal Hexecontahedron. Our method is quite sensitive, being able to detect different structures with or without the presence of a nucleic acid, such as in the Satellite Mosaic Tobacco Viruses.

Two improvements can be envisaged for this work: one is the increase of the set of viral structures studied, which could provide more significance to the conclusions about the prevalence of the patterns found, and the other is the extension of the study above the removal of five subunits, a follow-up step which would be of considerable more computational cost.

As a major insight of this work, the prevalence of the removal of the triangular trimer from a complete capsid suggests that it can be a viable target for interfering with virus disassembly process and the subsequent infection mechanism. Antiviral drugs can thus be designed to disrupt the interactions between these specific capsid proteins.

Acknowledgments. Work supported by project RECI/BBB-BEP/0104/2012 from Fundação para a Ciência e Tecnologia, Portugal. We also had support from the Portuguese Mass Spectrometry Network, integrated in the National Roadmap of Research Infrastructures of Strategic Relevance (ROTEIRO/0028/2013; LISBOA-01-0145-FEDER-022125). The funders had no role in study design, data collection and analysis, decision to publish, or preparation of the manuscript.

References

1. Poranen, M.M., Daugelavicius, R., Bamford, D.H.: Common principles in viral entry. Ann. Rev. Microbiol. **56**, 521–538 (2002)
2. Mateu, M.G.: Assembly, stability and dynamics of virus capsids. Arch. Biochem. Biophys. **531**(1–2), 65–79 (2013)
3. Strauss, J.H., Strauss, E.G.: Overview of viruses and virus infection, Chap. 1. In: Viruses and Human Disease, 2nd edn, pp. 1–33. Academic Press, London (2008)
4. Strauss, J.H., Strauss, E.G.: Emerging and reemerging viral diseases, Chap. 8. In: Viruses and Human Disease, 2nd edn, pp. 325–343. Academic Press, London (2008)
5. Babkin, I.V., Babkina, I.N.: The origin of the variola virus. Viruses **7**(3), 1100–1112 (2015)
6. Saunders-Hastings, P.R., Krewski, D.: Reviewing the history of pandemic influenza: understanding patterns of emergence and transmission. Pathogens **5**(4), 66 (2016)
7. Caspar, D.L., Klug, A.: Physical principles in the construction of regular viruses. In: Cold Spring Harbour Symposia on Quantitative Biology, vol. 27, pp. 1–24 (1962)

8. Prasad, B.V.V., Schmid, M.F.: Principles of virus structural organization. In: Rossmann, M., Rao, V. (eds.) Viral Molecular Machines. AEMB, vol. 726, pp. 17–47. Springer, Boston (2012)

9. Perlmutter, J.D., Hagan, M.F.: Mechanisms of virus assembly. Ann. Rev. Phys. Chem. **66**, 217–239 (2015)

10. Zlotnick, A.: To build a virus capsid. An equilibrium model of the self assembly of polyhedral protein complexes. J. Mol. Biol. **241**(1), 59–67 (1994)

11. Zlotnick, A.: Are weak protein-protein interactions the general rule in capsid assembly? Virology **315**(2), 269–274 (2003)

12. Zlotnick, A., Johnson, J.M., Wingfield, P.W., Stahl, S.J., Endres, D.: A theoretical model successfully identifies features of hepatitis B virus capsid assembly. Biochemistry **38**(44), 14644–14652 (1999)

13. Zlotnick, A., Stray, S.J.: How does your virus grow? Understanding and interfering with virus assembly. Trends Biotechnol. **21**(12), 536–542 (2003)

14. Reddy, V.S., Giesing, H.A., Morton, R.T., Kumar, A., Post, C.B., Brooks, C.L., Johnson, J. E.: Energetics of quasiequivalence: computational analysis of protein-protein interactions in icosahedral viruses. Biophys. J. **74**(1), 546–558 (1998)

15. Reddy, V.S., Johnson, J.E.: Structure-derived insights into virus assembly. Adv. Virus Res. **64**, 45–68 (2005)

16. Rapaport, D.C.: Role of reversibility in viral capsid growth: a paradigm for self-assembly. Phys. Rev. Lett. **101**(18), 186101 (2008)

17. Rapaport, D.C.: Modeling capsid self-assembly: design and analysis. Phys. Biol. **7**(4), 045001 (2010)

18. Castellanos, M., Perez, R., Carrillo, P.J., de Pablo, P.J., Mateu, M.G.: Mechanical disassembly of single virus particles reveals kinetic intermediates predicted by theory. Biophys. J. **102**(11), 2615–2624 (2012)

19. Horton, N., Lewis, M.: Calculation of the free energy of association for protein complexes. Protein Sci. **1**(1), 169–181 (1992)

20. Ortega-Esteban, A., Perez-Berna, A.J., Menendez-Conejero, R., Flint, S.J., San Martin, C., de Pablo, P.J.: Monitoring dynamics of human adenovirus disassembly induced by mechanical fatigue. Sci. Rep. **3**, 1434 (2013)

21. Carrillo-Tripp, M., Shepherd, C.M., Borelli, I.A., Venkataraman, S., Lander, G., Natarajan, P., Johnson, J.E., Brooks, C.L., Reddy, V.S.: VIPERdb2: an enhanced and web API enabled relational database for structural virology. Nucleic Acids Res. **37**(Database issue), D436–D442 (2009)

22. Berman, H.M., Westbrook, J., Feng, Z., Gilliland, G., Bhat, T.N., Weissig, H., Shindyalov, I. N., Bourne, P.E.: The protein data bank. Nucleic Acids Res. **28**(1), 235–242 (2000)

23. Burnside, W.: On the theory of groups of finite order. Proc. Lond. Math. Soc. **s2–7**, 1–7 (1909)

24. Vincent, A.: Molecular Symmetry and Group Theory: A Programmed Introduction to Chemical Applications, 2nd edn. Wiley, Chichester, New York (2001)

25. Piedade, C., Ferreira, A., Cordeiro, C.: How to disassemble a virus capsid - a computational approach. In: Proceedings of the 10th International Joint Conference on Biomedical Engineering Systems and Technologies, BIOSTEC 2017, pp. 217–222. SCITEPRESS, Porto (2017)

26. Jeffrey, G.A.: An Introduction to Hydrogen Bonding. Oxford University Press, Oxford (1997)

27. Kumar, S., Nussinov, R.: Relationship between ion pair geometries and electrostatic strengths in proteins. Biophys. J. **83**(3), 1595–1612 (2002)

28. Onofrio, A., Parisi, G., Punzi, G., Todisco, S., Di Noia, M.A., Bossis, F., Turi, A., De Grassi, A., Pierri, C.L.: Distance-dependent hydrophobic-hydrophobic contacts in protein folding simulations. Phys. Chem. Chem. Phys. **16**(35), 18907–18917 (2014)
29. Atkins, P.W., De Paula, J.: Physical Chemistry for the Life Sciences. Oxford University Press, Oxford (2006)
30. Cormen, T.H., Leiserson, C.E., Rivest, R.L., Stein, C.: Introduction to Algorithms, 2nd edn. The MIT Press, Cambridge (2002)
31. Csardi, G., Nepusz, T.: The igraph software package for complex network research. InterJ. Complex Syst. **1695**, 1–9 (2006)

Bio-inspired Systems and Signal Processing

Towards Swarm Intelligence of Alcoholics

Andrew Schumann[(✉)]

University of Information Technology and Management in Rzeszow,
Sucharskiego 2, 35-225 Rzeszow, Poland
andrew.schumann@gmail.com

Abstract. I distinguish the swarm behaviour from the social one. The swarm behaviour is carried out without symbolic interactions, but it is complex, as well. In this paper, I show that an addictive behaviour of humans can be considered a kind of swarm behaviour, also. The risk of predation is a main reason of reducing symbolic interactions in human group behaviours, but there are possible other reasons like addiction. An addiction increases roles of addictive stimuli (e.g. alcohol, morphine, cocaine, sexual intercourse, gambling, etc.) by their reinforcing and intrinsically rewarding and we start to deal with a swarm. I show that the lateral inhibition and lateral activation are two fundamental patterns in sensing and motoring of swarms. The point is that both patterns allow swarms to occupy several attractants and to avoid several repellents at once. The swarm behaviour of alcoholics follows the lateral inhibition and lateral activation, too. In order to formalize this intelligence, I appeal to modal logics K and its modification K'. The logic K is used to formalize preference relation in the case of lateral inhibition in distributing people to drink jointly and the logic K' is used to formalize preference relation in the case of lateral activation in distributing people to drink jointly.

1 Introduction

It is known that any swarm can be controlled by replacing stimuli: attractants and repellents [24], therefore we can design logic circuits based on topology of stimuli to build biological computers [2,25]. For swarms there are no symbolic meanings and the behaviour is completely determined by outer stimuli. In this paper, we will consider how the alcohol dependence syndrome impacts on the human behaviour.

We claim that alcohol-dependent humans embody a version of swarm intelligence [3] to optimize the alcohol-drinking behaviour. Our research is based on statistical data which we have collected due to the questionnaire of 107 people who have treated at the Private Health Unitary Enterprise "Iscelenie," Minsk, Belarus. The interviews were made by Vadim Fris, the Chief Psychiatrist of this centre. Their theoretical analysis was carried out by me.

In Sect. 2, a swarm behaviour is distinguished from a social one. In Sect. 3, lateral activation and lateral inhibition are regarded as two basic patterns in

© Springer International Publishing AG, part of Springer Nature 2018
N. Peixoto et al. (Eds.): BIOSTEC 2017, CCIS 881, pp. 305–327, 2018.
https://doi.org/10.1007/978-3-319-94806-5_17

sensing and motoring of swarms. In Sect. 4, some statistical data on 107 people addicted to alcohol and questioned by us are collected. In Sect. 5, a modal logic for simulating lateral activation and lateral inhibition effects in the swarm behaviour of alcoholics is introduced.

2   Social Behaviour and Swarm Behaviour

Usually, a social behaviour is understood as a synonymous to a collective animal behaviour. It is claimed that there are many forms of this behaviour from bacteria and insects to mammals including humans. So, bacteria and insects performing a collective behaviour are called *social*.

For example, a *prokaryote*, a one-cell organism that lacks a membrane-bound nucleus (karyon), can build colonies in a way of growing slime. These colonies are called 'biofilms'. Cells in biofilms are organized in dynamic networks and can transmit signals (the so-called quorum sensing) [6]. As a result, these bacteria are considered social. Social insects may be presented by ants – insects of the family *Formicidae*. Due to a division of labour, they construct a real society of their nest even with a pattern to make slaves. Also, *Synalpheus regalis* sp., a species of snapping shrimp that commonly live in the coral reefs, demonstrates a collective behaviour like ants. Among shrimps of the same colony there is one breeding female, as well, and a labour division of other members [7]. The ant-like organization of colony is observed among some mammals, too, e.g. among naked mole-rats (*Heterocephalus glaber* sp.). In one colony they have only one queen and one to three males to reproduce, while other members of the colony are just workers [11]. The same collective behaviour is typical for Damaraland blesmols (*Fukomys damarensis* sp.), another mammal species – they have one queen and many workers [10, 12].

All these patterns of ant-like collective behaviour (a brood care and a division of labour into reproductive and non-reproductive groups) are evaluated as a form of *eusociality*, the so-called highest level of organization of animal sociality [16]. Nevertheless, it is quite controversial if we can regard the ant-like collective behaviour as a social behaviour, indeed. We can do it if and only if we concentrate, first, on outer stimuli controlling individuals and, second, on 'social roles' ('worker', 'queen', etc.) of individuals as functions with some utilities for the group as such, i.e. if and only if we follow, first, *behaviourism* which represents any collective behaviour as a complex system that is managed by stimulating individuals (in particular by their reinforcement and punishment) [30] and, second, if and only if we share the ideas of *structural functionalism* which considers the whole society as a system of functions ('roles') of its constituent elements [19]. In case we accept both behaviourism and structural functionalism, we can state that a collective animal behaviour has the same basic patterns from 'social' bacteria and 'social' insects to humans whose sociality is evident for ourselves.

However, there are different approaches to sociality. One of the approaches, alternative to behaviourism and structural functionalism, is represented by *symbolic interactionism*. In this approach, a collective behaviour is social if in the process of interaction it involves a thought with a symbolic meaning that arises out of the interaction of agents [3]. In other words, social behaviour is impossible without material culture, e.g. without using some tools which always have symbolic meanings. Obviously, in this sense the collective behaviour of ants cannot be regarded as social. There are no tools and no symbolic meanings for the ants.

But not only humans perform social behaviour in the meaning of symbolic interactionism. It is known that wild bottlenose dolphins (*Tursiops* sp.) "apparently use marine sponges as foraging tools" [15] and this behaviour of them cannot be explained genetically or ecologically. This means that "sponging" is an example of an existing material culture in a marine mammal species and this culture is transmitted, presumably by mothers teaching the skills to their sons and daughters [15].

Also, chimpanzees involve tools in their behaviours: large and small sticks as well as large and small stones. In [34], the authors discover 39 different behaviour patterns of chimpanzees, including tool usage, grooming and courtship behaviours. It is a very interesting fact that some patterns of chimpanzees are habitual in some communities but are absent in others because of different traditions of chimpanzee material cultures [34]. Hence, we see that the collective behaviour of chimpanzees can be evaluated as social, as well.

So, within symbolic interactionism we cannot consider any complex collective behaviour, like the ant nest, as a social behaviour. The rest of complex behaviours can be called a *swarm behaviour*. Its examples are as follows: swarming of insects, flocking of birds, herding of quadrupeds, schooling of fish. In swarms, animals behave collectively, e.g. in schools or flocks each animal moves in the same direction as its neighbour, it remains close to its neighbours, it avoids collisions with its neighbours [33].

A group of people, such as pedestrians, can also exhibit a swarm behaviour like a flocking or schooling: humans prefer to avoid a person conditionally designated by them as a possible predator and if a substantial part of the group (not less than 5%) changes the direction, then the rest follows the new direction [8]. An ant-based algorithm can explain aircraft boarding behaviour [22]. Under the conditions of escape panic the majority of people perform a swarm behaviour, too [9]. The point is that a risk of predation is the main feature of swarming at all [1,18] and under these risk conditions (like a terrorist act) symbolic meanings for possible human interactions are promptly reduced. As a consequence, the social behaviour transforms into a swarm behaviour.

Thus, *we distinguish the swarm behaviour from the social one*. The first is fulfilled without symbolic interactions, but it is complex, as well, and has an appearance from a collective decision making. In this paper, we will show that an addictive behaviour of humans can be considered a kind of swarm behaviour, also. The risk of predation is a main reason of reducing symbolic interactions in human collective behaviours, but there are possible other reasons like addiction. An addiction increases roles of addictive stimuli (e.g. alcohol, morphine, cocaine, sexual intercourse, gambling, etc.) by their reinforcing and intrinsically rewarding.

3   Common Patterns of Swarm Behaviour

3.1   The Müller-Lyer Illusion

There are many optical illusions which show that there are different modalities in perceiving signals which change our picture of reality. Let us consider the Müller-Lyer illusion, see Fig. 1. Traditionally, this illusion was explained as a combination of two opposing factors: (i) *lateral inhibition* increasing contrast when two points are seen closer than the objective display would justify (Fig. 1(a)), and (ii) *lateral activation* decreasing contrast when two points are seen too far apart to be considered currently (Fig. 1(b)). The matter is that simple cells in primary visual cortex have small receptive fields and respond preferentially to oriented bars. Then neurons increase or decrease a receptive field of visual cortex as a whole according to concentrations of stimuli, see [20]. In case of increasing we see Fig. 1(a), in case of decreasing we see Fig. 1(b).

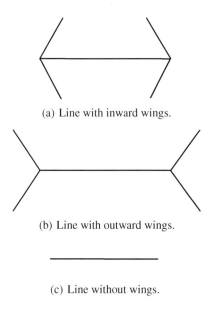

(a) Line with inward wings.

(b) Line with outward wings.

(c) Line without wings.

Fig. 1. The Müller-Lyer illusion. The lines of (a), (b), (c) are of the same length. Nevertheless, it seems to us that the line with the inward wings (i.e. (a)) is shorter than line (b), and the line with the outward wings (i.e. (b)) is longer than line (a).

Hence, perceiving the same line lengths is strongly biased by the neural-computation process in accordance with the stimulus distributions causing lateral inhibition or lateral activation. It is possible to show that the same patterns of perceiving signals can be detected at different levels of behaviours: from behaviours of unicellular organisms even to swarming, such as to group behaviours of ant nests. So, in [21] it was shown that the Müller-Lyer illusion

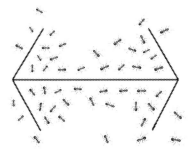

(a) Two points of highest concentrations of ants have a smaller distance than the distance between extremal points of the straight line.

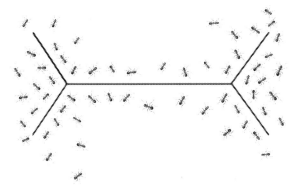

(b) Two points of highest concentrations of ants have a longer distance than the distance between extremal points of the straight line.

Fig. 2. An example from experiments performed in [21] to show that the Müller-Lyer illusion is detected in the swarm behaviour of ants. The authors of [21] located an attractant (honeydew solution of 50% w/w) on cardboard in the shape of the Müller-Lyer figure. The figure consisted of a 7.5-cm central shaft with two 3-cm wings pointing either inward or outward. As a result of this experiment proved statistically, the distribution of ants repeats the Müller-Lyer illusion. It means that the group sensing of ants repeats two patterns of perceiving performed by our neurons: (i) the first pattern is under condition of lateral inhibition (a); and (ii) the second pattern is under conditions of lateral activation (b).

holds for foraging ants, as well, see Fig. 2. It means that their swarm behaviour embodies lateral activation and lateral inhibition in the group perceptions of signals. The authors of [21] explain this phenomenon by that each swarm of ants has the following two main logistic tasks: (i) to build a global route system connecting the nest with food sources to monopolize all reachable food sources (it corresponds to the lateral activation, i.e. to the colony's ability to discover new food sources through exploration); (ii) to exploit effectively and efficiently each

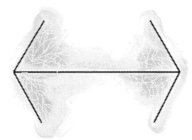

(a) Two points of highest concentrations of plasmodium have a smaller distance than the distance between extremal points of the straight line.

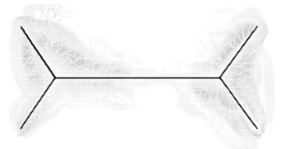

(b) Two points of highest concentrations of plasmodium have a longer distance than the distance between extremal points of the straight line.

Fig. 3. A possible experiment analogous to the experiment carried out in [21] to show that the Müller-Lyer illusion is detected in the swarm behaviour of *Physarum polycephalum*. We can locate an attractant (high nutrient concentration) in the shape of the Müller-Lyer figure. As a result, we can expect that the concentration of plasmodium repeats the Müller-Lyer illusion.

found food source (it corresponds to the lateral inhibition, i.e. to the colony's ability to concentrate on some food sources). And there is an economic balance which is analogous to the neurophysiological balance that generates the Müller-Lyer illusion [21]. In this analogy, each ant in a colony corresponds to a neuron or retinal cell and the behaviour of a swarm of ants corresponds to the behaviour of a neurological field.

The patterns of lateral activation and lateral inhibition in sensing and motoring can be detected even at the level of unicellular organisms, such as the slime mould, also called *Physarum polycephalum*. So, it is shown in [31] that Kanizsa illusory contours appear in the plasmodium pattern of *Physarum polycephalum*. We can show that the Müller-Lyer illusion holds for the plasmodium too, see Fig. 3. Indeed, we can observe (i) a lateral inhibition when there are two points of higher concentration of plasmodium with a distance that is shorter than the distance between two extremal points of the straight line (Fig. 3(a)), and (ii) a lateral activation when there are two points of higher concentration of plasmodium with a distance that is longer than the distance between two extremal points of the straight line (Fig. 3(b)).

Thus, some optical illusions, such as the Müller-Lyer illusion, are connected to combining lateral inhibition and lateral activation effects. Therefore, these illusions are repeated in the swarm behaviour of *Physarum polycephalum* and foraging ants.

3.2   Lateral Inhibition and Lateral Activation in Swarm Behaviour

Each animal behaviour can be stimulated by attractants ("pull") and repellents ("push"). For instance, in [17] there was proposed a combination of "pull" and "push" methods for managing populations of *German cockroach* (Dictyoptera: Blattellidae).

Different patterns in reacting to attractants and repellents are well visible on bacteria. In the absence of an attractant or repellent a bacterium such as *Salmonella typhimurium* has the following stages in its motions: (i) the stage of run (it swims in a smooth, straight line for several seconds); (ii) the stage of tumble (it thrashes around for a fraction of a second); (iii) the stage of twiddle (it changes its direction); (iv) the new stage of run (it again swims in a straight line, but in a new, randomly chosen direction), see [32]. Under conditions of sensing attractants or repellents, a bacterium has the same stages, but they lasted longer or shorter.

If there are different gradients of attractant, we face the following changes in the bacterium stages:

- if a concentration of attractant increases, cells tumble less frequently.
- if a concentration of attractant decreases, bacteria tumble more frequently.

Under conditions of different gradients of repellent, we see the following opposite reactions:

- if concentration of repellent increases, bacteria tumble more frequently.
- if concentration of repellent decreases, they tumble less frequently.

Some bacteria can be grouped into swarms. For example, *Myxococcus xanthus* is "a predatory surface-associated bacterium that moves in large multicellular groups and secretes digestive enzymes to destroy and consume other bacteria in the environment" [14]. Sometimes these multicellular groups form biofilms in which sessile bacteria secrete an extracellular matrix. Now, it is on open question how to define all the details for attracting and repelling bacterial swarms [14]. Nevertheless, there are some unicellular organisms, such as *Physarum polycephalum*, which have all the basic swarm patterns in their behaviour, but for them the mechanism of attracting and repelling is studied well.

Each bacterium can be attracted or repelled directly. But there are no bacteria which can occupy several attractants simultaneously or which can avoid several repellents at once. Only swarms can do it. And *Physarum polycephalum*

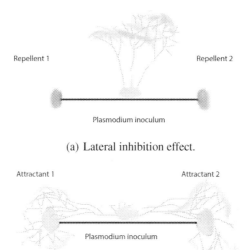

(a) Lateral inhibition effect.

(b) Lateral activation effect.

Fig. 4. The Müller-Lyer illusion can be detected in the following behaviour of plasmodium of *Physarum polycephalum*. Let an inoculum of plasmodium be located at the centre of a short line. Then the Müller-Lyer illusion holds if (i) at first we locate two repellents at two ends of the straight line respectively, (ii) then second we locate two attractants at both ends respectively. In the first case we observe a lateral inhibition. In the second case we observe a lateral activation. Hence, the distance between active zones is different for (a) and for (b), although the straight line is of the same length.

can do it, too. Let us consider an example of Fig. 4. On the one hand, the slime mould can react to both repellents (Fig. 4(a)) to run away from them. On the other hand, the slime mould can react to both attractants (Fig. 4(b)) to occupy them. As a consequence, we see a behavioural pattern of the Müller-Lyer illusion: (i) the distance between two extremal points of plasmodium distribution became shorter under condition of lateral inhibition in Fig. 4(a), and (ii) the distance between two extremal points of plasmodium distribution became longer under condition of lateral activation in Fig. 4(b). To compare, in the case of Fig. 3(a) the plasmodium behaves under conditions of informational noise, when there were too much attractants at a closer distance, to perform a lateral inhibition.

Hence, we can assume that lateral inhibition and lateral activation are important fundamental mechanisms which are combined for sensing and motoring in reactions of different swarms. So, swarms can have different biochemistries (different attractants and repellents), but algorithmically they realize the same patterns such as the Müller-Lyer illusion. In the next section, the alcoholic behaviour will be regarded as a new example of swarming with the same lateral inhibition and lateral activation in sensing and motoring of groups.

4   Statistical Data on Group Behaviours of Alcoholics

Vadim Fris and me have carried out a statistical research of group behaviour of 107 people addicted to alcohol who have been actually treated in the rehabilitation centre "Iscelenie," Minsk, Belarus. Vadim Fris is the Chief Psychiatrist of this centre. Some main characteristics of the sample for our survey are collected in Table 1. First, the majority of interviewees were men (82.2%). Second, most respondents were older than 41 (52.3%). Third, most respondents have a job at the moment (71%).

Table 1. Some general characteristics of people questioned by us.

	Quantity	Working	Jobless	Age less than 30	Age from 30 to 40	Age from 41 to 60
Women	19	15	4	1	8	10
Men	88	61	27	13	29	46

Table 2. The question whether the need for alcohol is satisfied.

	There are ever possibilities to drink as much as you want	There are no possibilities to drink as much as you want
Women	6	13
Men	28	60

Most interviewees (68.2%) claim that their need for alcohol is not satisfied properly, see Table 2. It means that logistics optimizing the drink behaviour is an actual trouble for them still.

Furthermore, most respondents (77.6%) buy alcohol at different places, see Table 3. It is correlated to their group behaviour. Joining different small groups for drinking or meeting the same small group at different places, they buy alcohol not at the same place. Some respondents live in the country, where there is only one store. This fact simplifies logistics for them.

Table 3. The question where they usually buy alcohol.

	There is the same place where you buy alcohol	There are different places where you buy alcohol
Women	4	15
Men	20	68

Some respondents (19.6%) prefer to drink alone, but sometimes they drink jointly. Others drink only in small groups (19.6%). So, the majority (60.8%) prefer to drink jointly, but sometimes they drink alone. See Table 4.

Table 4. The question whether they prefer to drink alone or jointly.

	You prefer to drink alone	You prefer to drink with somebody	You drink only with companions
Women	5	11	3
Men	16	54	18

Hence, we have detected that drinking is a form of group behaviour. The gender characteristics of these groups are collected in Table 5. Some women (42.1% off all women) drink in small groups consisting only of women and some men (44.3% of all men) drink in small groups consisting only of men. So, 56% of the respondents drink in mixed-gender groups. In the meanwhile, a sex/gender behaviour is mainly reduced in these groups.

Table 5. The question whether the group for drinking jointly consists of men or women.

	The community of your comrades who are your companions for drinking consists only of women	The community of your comrades who are your companions for drinking consists only of men	The community of your comrades who are your companions for drinking consists of both men and women
Women	8	0	11
Men	0	39	49

Joining small groups for drinking jointly supposes a kind of solidarity from participants. So, the companions can buy drinks if the interviewee has not enough money, see Table 6. For 68.4% of women and for 86.4% of men it is a common practice.

Table 6. The question whether the companions buy drinks for you sometimes.

	Your companions buy drinks sometimes to help you if you need	Your companions never buy drinks to help you if you need
Women	13	6
Men	76	12

On the other hand, joining small groups for drinking jointly has a requirement to help others; and 73.7% of women and 92% of men buy alcohol for others sometimes if their companions have not enough money currently, see Table 7.

Table 7. The question whether you buy drinks for your companions sometimes.

	You help your companions and sometimes you buy drinks for them if they need	You never help your companions to buy drinks if they need
Women	14	5
Men	81	7

According to our survey, all the respondents have affirmed that sometimes or always they drink in small groups from 3 to 7 people, but the same respondents can join different small groups in due course. The number of stable friends to drink commonly is from 2 to 5. The alcohol-addicted people distinguish their groups from relatives or colleagues and 63% of the respondents think that their family and job hinder them to drink safely.

Thus, these small groups from 3 to 7 people can be regarded as human swarms which help their members to drink safely and to logistically optimize the task to drink. 83.1% of all the respondents have responded that members of the group can pay for drinks if the respondent does not have money (Table 6); and 88.8% of all the respondents have claimed that they can buy alcohol for somebody from the group who does not have money (Table 7). So, we deal with a form of solidarity in helping to drink.

In the case of involving new members into groups the main reasons are as follows: they are neighbours or colleagues and they can help (it means, pay). Entering new groups is possible if a friend/acquaintance has invited to join them because it is more safe and interesting for the respondent to join the new group where there is his or her friend. Without an invitation it is impossible to enter the group.

Groups are very friendly and the only reason to expel somebody from the group is that (s)he quarrels (in particular, (s)he does not want to pay). 32% of respondents have noticed that it would be better to expel one member in their groups.

Only 28% of respondents have stated that in their groups there are leaders. They are men or women more than 40 years old. The leadership consists in a support of the group to drink together.

We have discovered that alcoholics form a *network consisting of several small groups*. And the task of optimizing common drinks is solved not by a small group, but by the whole network, i.e. by several groups whose members are interconnected. The point is that each small group of alcoholics appears and disappears under different conditions, but the network, these alcoholics belong to, is almost the same. We have studied that small groups of alcohol-addicted people are not stable and, by exchanging their members, *they can fuse or split in the optimization of drinking.* The same behavioural patterns are observed in the slime mould: fusing and splitting in front of attractants to optimize their occupation. Outer stimuli (attractants) for the slime mould are pieces of nutrients scattered before this organism. *Attractants for alcoholics are represented by places where they can drink in small groups safely*: flat or outside. 38% of the respondents prefer to drink at the same place and 62% at different places. The arguments in choosing the places are as follows: the short distance from the home, low price, quality of drinks.

To sum up, the alcohol-dependent people realize a version of swarm intelligence to optimize drinking in the way of fusing or splitting the groups under different conditions. In case the groups are splitting, we face a *lateral activation effect*; and in case the groups are fusing, we deal with a *lateral inhibition effect* of alcoholic networks. The lateral activation is observed in the following cases: (i) the behaviour is carried out under conditions of attractants rather than repellents; (ii) the behaviour is performed in relation to many well visible attractants simultaneously (there are many places where it is possible to drink safely). The lateral inhibition is examined in the following cases: (i) the behaviour is conducted under pressure or stress (there are more repellents than attractants); (ii) there are a few attractants for a choice or there is an information noise in choosing the attractants. For instance, some respondents have performed the swarm behaviour to drink jointly under stress recently (it means, they have fulfilled a lateral inhibition). Some other interviewees have performed the same behaviour under favourable conditions (it means, they have fulfilled a lateral activation). And both effects can be detected by answering the question by them why they choose this place to drink, see Table 8. We have proposed the following variants: (i) "pleasant company" (the most favourable condition); (ii) "comfortable atmosphere" (the less favourable condition); (iii) "closer to home" (the neutral condition); (iv) "no one interferes" (the less stress condition); (v) "easier to drink quickly" (the most stress condition). We do not know circumstances of drinking for the respondents currently, but according to the data, 43% of them have fulfilled a lateral activation recently, 40.1% of them fulfilled a lateral inhibition, see Table 8.

Table 8. The question why you choose this place to drink (jointly).

Why do you choose this place to drink?	Pleasant company	Comfortable atmosphere	Closer to home	No one interferes	Easier to drink quickly
Women	5	2	5	5	2
Men	29	10	13	22	14

Thus, small groups of alcoholics are considered by us as a kind of *human swarms*. These swarms build a network and within the same network alcoholics can freely move from one swarm to another. As a consequence, the swarms fuse or split.

5   Simulating Lateral Activation and Lateral Inhibition Performed by Alcoholics

As we have studied with Vadim Fris, the alcohol-addicted people prefer to drink in small groups from 3 to 7 persons. These groups are said to be *agents* of swarm intelligence in our formalization. Within this intelligence an appropriate network of alcoholics solves optimization tasks to drink. These swarm solutions are unconscious, but very effective. Each agent follows an unconscious collective decision-making mechanism that is decentralized and distributed among all members of the group. The same situation of distribution of intelligence is observed in any swarm.

The agents (swarms) are denoted by small letters $i, j, \ldots$ As well as all swarms, these agents can fuse and split to optimize a group occupation of attractants. Usually, there are many agents who communicate among themselves by exchanging people (their members), e.g. someone can be a member of agent i today and later became a member of agent j.

The places where agents $i, j, \ldots$ (appropriate small groups of humans addicted to alcohol) can drink safely are called *attractants* for swarm intelligence. They are denoted by $S, P, \ldots$

From the Müller-Lyer illusion we know that there are two different ways in occupying attractants by swarm agents: (i) with high concentration of people (lateral inhibition effect) at places of meeting and (ii) with low concentration of people (lateral activation effect) at places of meeting [13,28]. In the first case much less attractants are occupied. In the second case much more attractants are occupied. For instance, in snow winter there are less attractants (places to drink jointly and safely) and this causes a lateral inhibition effect in alcoholic swarming. In sunny summer there are more attractants (places to drink in a group) and this implies a lateral activation effect in alcoholic networking.

Lateral inhibition and lateral activation can be detected in any forms of swarm networking. For example, this mechanism is observed also in the true slime mould (plasmodium) of *Physarum polycephalum*. The plasmodium has the two distinct stages in responding to signals: (i) the sensory stage (perceiving signals) and (ii) the motor stage (action as responding). The effect of lateral activation in the plasmodium is to decrease contrast between attractants at the sensory stage and to split protoplasmic tubes towards two or more attractants at the motor stage (Fig. 4(b)). The effect of lateral inhibition is to increase contrast between attractants at the sensory stage and to fuse protoplasmic tubes towards one attractant at the motor stage or to increase contrast in front of repellents at the sensory stage and to fuse protoplasmic tubes just in one safe direction at the motor stage (Fig. 4(a)).

In human groups there are (i) the one sensory stage consisting in perceiving signals (as well as for the plasmodium) and the following two motor stages consisting in actions as responding: (ii) illocutionary stage and (iii) perlucotionary stage.

For the first time the well-known 20th-century philosopher John L. Austin has investigated speech acts as a way of coordination for human behaviour by a verbal communication as well as by a non-verbal communication (e.g. by gestures or mimics). His main philosophical claim that was accepted then by almost all later language philosophers has based on the idea that we coordinate our joint behaviour by *illocutionary acts* – some utterances which express our intentions and expectations to produce joint symbolic meanings for symbolic interactions: "I hereby declare," "I sentence you to ten years' imprisonment", "I promise to pay you back," "I pray to God", etc. These utterances can produce an effect on the hearer that is called a *perlocutionary act*. Hence, according to Austin, in order to commit a group behaviour, the humans should start with illocutionary acts (uttering illocutions) to coordinate their common symbolic meanings. As a result, their group behaviour appears as a kind of perlocutionary act grounded on previous illocutionary utterances.

Thus, the motor stage for the plasmodium is just a direct behaviour, while the motor stage for the humans starts from illocutionary acts to produce symbolic meanings for performing an interaction and then this stage is continued in perlocutionary acts (a direct coordinated behaviour of a human group).

Attractants S, P, ... are detected by alcoholics at the sensory stage. Then alcoholics perform illocutionary acts to share preference relations on detected attractants. Later they commit perlocutionary acts to occupy some detected attractants. A data point S is considered empty if and only if an appropriate attractant (the place denoted by S where it is possible to drink jointly) is not occupied by the group of alcohol-dependent people. Otherwise, it is not-empty. Let us define syllogistic strings of the form SP with the following interpretation: 'S and P are comparable positively', and with the following meaning: SP is true if and only if S and P are reachable for each other by members of the group i and both S and P are not empty, otherwise SP is false. Let $\mathcal{S}$ be a set of all true syllogistic strings.

Now we can construct an *illocutionary logic of alcohol-dependent people*. In this logic we deal with preference relations about detected attractants from $\mathcal{S}$.

5.1   Agents in Case of Lateral Inhibition

To formalize performative propositions used by alcoholics, let us construct an extension of modal logic **K**, please see [5] about **K**. This extension is to express preference relations of agents in case of lateral inhibition. Let 'A' and 'B' be metavariables ranging over syllogistic letters S, P, ... or over standard propositional compositions of syllogistic letters by means of conjunctions, disjunction, implication, negation. Let us introduce two modalities • and ◦ with the following meaning:

$$\bullet A \Rightarrow \circ A,$$

i.e. $\bullet A$ is modally stronger and $\circ A$ is modally weaker, e.g. $\bullet A$ means 'I like A' (or 'I desire A') and $\circ A$ means 'maybe A' (or 'it can be A'). So, the performative verb of • is stronger and the performative verb of ◦ is weaker with the same type of performativity (modality) to prefer A.

In our logic **K** for preference relations we have also only two axioms as in the standard **K** (the inference rules are the same also):

Necessitation Rule. If A is a theorem of **K**, then so is $\bullet A$.
Distribution Axiom. $\bullet(A \Rightarrow B) \Rightarrow (\bullet A \Rightarrow \bullet B)$.

The operator $\circ$ can be defined from $\bullet$ as follows:

$$\circ A := \bullet A,$$

where $\bullet$ are any performative verbs for expressing a preference relation with a strong modality: 'like', 'want', 'desire', etc.

Now let us add countable many new one-place sentential connectives $\bullet_{ki}$ to the language of **K**:

if A is a formula, then $\bullet_{ki} A$ is a formula, too.

These $\bullet_{ki} A$ are read as follows: "the k-th utterance of preference relation uttered by agent i to fulfil an illocutionary act". The weaker modality $\circ_{ki}$ is defined thus:

$$\circ_{ki} A := \neg \bullet_{ki} \neg A.$$

We assume that $\bullet_{ki}$ and $\circ_{ki}$ satisfy the necessity rule and distribution axiom as well.

Let us denote the new extension by $\mathbf{K}_i$.

Now let us define in $\mathbf{K}_i$ the four basic preference relations as atomic syllogistic propositions:
$k_i(S \preceq_{LI}^{good} P)$, $k_i(S \npreceq_{LI}^{bad} P)$, $k_i(S \preceq_{LI}^{bad} P)$, $k_i(S \npreceq_{LI}^{good})$. They are defined as follows.

$$k_i(S \preceq_{LI}^{good} P) := \bullet_{ki}(S \Rightarrow P) \tag{1}$$

The atomic proposition $k_i(S \preceq_{LI}^{good} P)$ means: "for agent i, alternative P is at least as good as alternative S by the k-th utterance" and it is defined under conditions of lateral inhibition. *In the model of alcohol-addicted swarms* it means: "for the grouping of alcohol-dependent people i, alternative P is at least as good as alternative S at the k-th utterance under conditions of lateral inhibition".

Let us define a model $\mathcal{M}$.

Semantic meaning of $k_i(S \preceq_{LI}^{good} P)$:

$\mathcal{M} \models k_i(S \preceq_{LI}^{good} P) :=$ at the utterance k uttered by i, there exists a data point $A \in \mathcal{M}$ such that $AS \in \mathcal{S}$ and for any $A \in \mathcal{M}$, if $AS \in \mathcal{S}$, then $AP \in \mathcal{S}$ and it is defined under conditions of lateral inhibition.

Semantic meaning of $k_i(S \preceq_{LI}^{good} P)$ *in alcohol-addicted swarms*: there is a group of alcoholics i at a place A such that places A and S are connected by exchanging of some members of i and for any place A, if A and S are connected by exchanging of some members of i, then A and P are connected by exchanging of some members of i.

$$k_i(S \npreceq_{LI}^{bad} P) := \circ_{ki}(S \wedge P) \tag{2}$$

The atomic proposition $k_i(S \npreceq_{LI}^{bad} P)$ means: "for agent i, alternative P is not at least as bad as alternative S by the k-th utterance" and it is defined under conditions of lateral inhibition. *In the model of alcohol-addicted swarms* it means: "for the grouping of alcohol-dependent people i, alternative P is not at least as bad as alternative S at the k-th utterance under conditions of lateral inhibition".

Semantic meaning of $k_i(S \not\preceq_{LI}^{bad} P)$:

$\mathcal{M} \models k_i(S \not\preceq_{LI}^{bad} P) :=$ at the utterance k uttered by i, there exists a data point $A \in \mathcal{M}$ such that both $AS \in \mathcal{S}$ and $AP \in \mathcal{S}$ and it is defined under conditions of lateral inhibition.

Semantic meaning of $k_i(S \not\preceq_{LI}^{bad} P)$ *in alcohol-addicted swarms*: there exists a group of alcoholics i at A such that A and S are connected by exchanging of some members of i and A and P are connected by exchanging of some members of i.

$$k_i(S \preceq_{LI}^{bad} P) := \bullet_{ki}(S \Rightarrow \neg P) \tag{3}$$

The atomic proposition $k_i(S \preceq_{LI}^{bad} P)$ means: "for agent i, alternative P is at least as bad as alternative S by the k-th utterance" and it is defined under conditions of lateral inhibition. *In the model of alcohol-addicted swarms*: "for the grouping of alcohol-dependent people i, alternative P is at least as bad as alternative S by the k-th utterance under conditions of lateral inhibition".

Semantic meaning of $k_i(S \preceq_{LI}^{bad} P)$:

$\mathcal{M} \models k_i(S \preceq_{LI}^{bad} P) :=$ at the utterance k uttered by i, for all data points $A \in \mathcal{M}$, AS is false or AP is false and it is defined under conditions of lateral inhibition.

Semantic meaning of $k_i(S \preceq_{LI}^{bad} P)$ *in alcohol-addicted swarms*: for all groups of alcoholics i at places A, A and S are not connected by exchanging of some members of i or A and P are not connected by exchanging of some members of i.

$$k_i(S \not\preceq_{LI}^{good} P) := \circ_{ki}(S \wedge \neg P) \tag{4}$$

The atomic proposition $k_i(S \not\preceq_{LI}^{good} P)$ means: "for agent i, alternative P is not at least as good as alternative S by the k-th utterance" and it is defined under conditions of lateral inhibition. *In the alcohol-addicted swarms*: "for the grouping of alcoholics i, alternative P is not at least as good as alternative S by the k-th utterance under conditions of lateral inhibition".

Semantic meaning of $k_i(S \not\preceq_{LI}^{good} P)$:

$\mathcal{M} \models k_i(S \not\preceq_{LI}^{good} P) :=$ at the utterance k uttered by i, for any data points $A \in \mathcal{M}$, AS is false or there exists $A \in \mathcal{M}$ such that $AS \in \mathcal{S}$ and AP is false and it is defined under conditions of lateral inhibition.

Semantic meaning of $k_i(S \not\preceq_{LI}^{good} P)$ *in alcohol-addicted swarms*: for all groups of alcoholics i at places A, A and S are not connected by exchanging of some members of i or there exists place A such that A and S are connected by exchanging of some members of i and A and P are not connected by exchanging of some members of i.

We can distinguish different swarms according to the acceptance of stronger or weaker modality:

Weak Agent. Agent i prefers $\circ_{ki}A$ instead of $\bullet_{ki}A$ iff $\bullet_{ki}A \Rightarrow \circ_{ki}A$.

Strong Agent. Agent i prefers $\bullet_{ki}A$ instead of $\circ_{ki}A$ iff $\bullet_{ki}A \Rightarrow \circ_{ki}A$.

An example of the weak agent: (s)he prefers not to like not-A instead of that to like A. An example of the strong agent: (s)he prefers to desire A instead of that to accept A.

Hence, in logic $\mathbf{K}_i$ we have the four kinds of atomic syllogistic propositions: $k_i(S \preceq_{LI}^{good} P)$, $k_i(S \npreceq_{LI}^{bad} P)$, $k_i(S \preceq_{LI}^{bad} P)$, $k_i(S \npreceq_{LI}^{good} P)$ for different k, i, S, and P. All other propositions of $\mathbf{K}_i$ are derivable by Boolean combinations of atomic propositions. Models for these combinations are defined conventionally:

$$\mathcal{M} \models \neg A \text{ iff } A \text{ is false in } \mathcal{M};$$
$$\mathcal{M} \models A \vee B \text{ iff } \mathcal{M} \models A \text{ or } \mathcal{M} \models B;$$
$$\mathcal{M} \models A \wedge B \text{ iff } \mathcal{M} \models A \text{ and } \mathcal{M} \models B;$$
$$\mathcal{M} \models A \Rightarrow B \text{ iff if } \mathcal{M} \models A, \text{ then } \mathcal{M} \models B.$$

Proposition 1. *Logic $\mathbf{K}_i$ is a conservative extension of $\mathbf{K}$.*   □

Proposition 2. *In $\mathbf{K}_i$, the conventional square of opposition holds, i.e. there are the following tautologies:*

$$k_i(S \preceq_{LI}^{good} P) \Rightarrow k_i(S \npreceq_{LI}^{bad} P);$$
$$k_i(S \preceq_{LI}^{bad} P) \Rightarrow k_i(S \npreceq_{LI}^{good} P);$$
$$\neg(k_i(S \preceq_{LI}^{good} P) \wedge k_i(S \preceq_{LI}^{bad} P));$$
$$k_i(S \npreceq_{LI}^{bad} P) \vee k_i(S \npreceq_{LI}^{good} P);$$
$$k_i(S \preceq_{LI}^{good} P) \vee k_i(S \npreceq_{LI}^{good} P);$$
$$\neg(k_i(S \preceq_{LI}^{good} P) \wedge k_i(S \npreceq_{LI}^{good} P));$$
$$k_i(S \preceq_{LI}^{bad} P) \vee k_i(S \npreceq_{LI}^{bad} P);$$
$$\neg(k_i(S \preceq_{LI}^{bad} P) \wedge k_i(S \npreceq_{LI}^{bad} P)).$$

Proof. It follows from (1)–(4).   □

The fusion of two swarms i and j for syllogistic propositions is defined in $\mathbf{K}_i$ in the way:

$$\frac{k_i(S_1 \preceq_{LI}^{good} P); \quad m_j(S_2 \preceq_{LI}^{good} P)}{(k \cup m)_{i \cup j}((S_1 \vee S_2) \preceq_{LI}^{good} P)}.$$

The splitting of one swarm $i \cup j$ is defined in $\mathbf{K}_i$ thus:

$$\frac{(k \cup m)_{i \cup j}(S \preceq_{LI}^{good} (P_1 \wedge P_2))}{k_i(S \preceq_{LI}^{good} P_1); \quad m_j(S \preceq_{LI}^{good} P_2)}.$$

Hence, the illocutionary logic $\mathbf{K}_i$ describes the preference relations of alcoholics towards attractants under the conditions of lateral inhibition.

5.2   Agents in Case of Lateral Activation

When the concentration of attractants (different places of grouping for common drinks) is high, the logic $\mathbf{K}$ for preference relations is unacceptable. Instead of $\mathbf{K}$ we will use its modification $\mathbf{K}'$ (with the same inference rules):

Necessitation Rule. If A is a theorem of $\mathbf{K}'$, then so is $\bullet A$.
Distribution Weak Axiom. $\bullet(A \wedge B) \Rightarrow (\bullet A \wedge \bullet B)$.

Now let us construct $\mathbf{K}'_i$ by adding countable one-place sentential connectives $\bullet_{ki}$ and $\circ_{ki}$ to the language of $\mathbf{K}'_i$ and then define the four basic preference relations $k_i(S \preceq_{LA}^{good} P)$, $k_i(S \npreceq_{LA}^{bad} P)$, $k_i(S \preceq_{LA}^{bad} P)$, $k_i(S \npreceq_{LA}^{good} P)$ in the following manner:

$$k_i(S \preceq_{LA}^{good} P) := \bullet_{ki}(S \wedge P). \tag{5}$$

The atomic proposition $k_i(S \preceq_{LA}^{good} P)$ means: "for agent i, alternative P is at least as good as alternative S by the k-th utterance" and it is defined under conditions of lateral activation. *In the model of alcohol-addicted swarms*: "for the group of alcoholics i, alternative P is at least as good as alternative S by the k-th utterance under conditions of lateral activation".

Let us define a model $\mathcal{M}'$.
Semantic meaning of $k_i(S \preceq_{LA}^{good} P)$:

$\mathcal{M}' \models k_i(S \preceq_{LA}^{good} P) :=$ there exists a data point $A \in \mathcal{M}'$ such that $AS \in \mathcal{S}$ and for any $A \in \mathcal{M}'$, $AS \in \mathcal{S}$ and $AP \in \mathcal{S}$ and it is defined under conditions of lateral activation.

Semantic meaning of $k_i(S \preceq_{LA}^{good} P)$ *in alcohol-addicted swarms*: there is a string AS and for any place A which is reachable for S and P by exchanging of members of i, there are strings AS and AP. This means that we have an occupation of the whole region where the places S and P are located.

$$k_i(S \npreceq_{LA}^{bad} P) := \bullet_{ki}(\neg S \wedge \neg P). \tag{6}$$

The atomic proposition $k_i(S \npreceq_{LA}^{bad} P)$ means: "for agent i, alternative P is not at least as bad as alternative S by the k-th utterance" and it is defined under conditions of lateral activation. *In the model of alcohol-addicted swarms*: "for the group of alcoholics i, alternative P is not at least as bad as alternative S by the k-th utterance under conditions of lateral activation".
Semantic meaning of $k_i(S \npreceq_{LA}^{bad} P)$:

$\mathcal{M}' \models k_i(S \npreceq_{LA}^{bad} P) :=$ for any data point $A \in \mathcal{M}'$, both AS is false and AP is false and it is defined under conditions of lateral activation.
Semantic meaning of $k_i(S \npreceq_{LA}^{bad} P)$ *in alcohol-addicted swarms*: for any place A which is reachable for S and P by exchanging of members of i, there are no strings AS and AP. This means that the group of alcoholics cannot reach S from P or P from S immediately.

$$k_i(S \preceq_{LA}^{bad} P) := \circ_{ki}(S \vee P). \tag{7}$$

The atomic proposition $k_i(S \preceq_{LA}^{bad} P)$ means: "for agent i, alternative P is at least as bad as alternative S by the k-th utterance" and it is defined under conditions of lateral activation. *In the model of alcohol-addicted swarms*: "for the group of alcoholics i, alternative P is at least as bad as alternative S by the k-th utterance under conditions of lateral activation".

Semantic meaning of $k_i(S \preceq_{LA}^{bad} P)$:

$\mathcal{M}' \models k_i(S \preceq_{LA}^{bad} P) :=$ there exists a data point $A \in \mathcal{M}'$ such that if AS is false, then $AP \in \mathcal{S}$ and it is defined under conditions of lateral activation.

Semantic meaning of $k_i(S \preceq_{LA}^{bad} P)$ *in alcohol-addicted swarms*: there exists a place A which is reachable for S and P by exchanging of members of i such that there is a string AS or there is a string AP. This means that the group of alcoholics i occupies S or P, but not the whole region where the places S and P are located.

$$k_i(S \npreceq_{LA}^{good} P) := \circ_{ki}(\neg S \vee \neg P). \tag{8}$$

The atomic proposition $k_i(S \npreceq_{LA}^{good} P)$ means: "for agent i, alternative P is not at least as good as alternative S by the k-th utterance" and it is defined under conditions of lateral activation. *In the model of alcohol-addicted swarms*: "for the group of alcoholics i, alternative P is not at least as good as alternative S by the k-th utterance under conditions of lateral activation".

Semantic meaning of $k_i(S \npreceq_{LA}^{good} P)$:

$\mathcal{M}' \models k_i(S \npreceq_{LA}^{good} P) :=$ for any data point $A \in \mathcal{M}'$, AS is false or there exists a data point $A \in \mathcal{M}'$ such that AS is false or AP is false and it is defined under conditions of lateral activation.

Semantic meaning of $k_i(S \npreceq_{LA}^{good} P)$ *in alcohol-addicted swarms*: for any place A which is reachable for S and P by exchanging of members of i there is no string AS or there exists a place A which is reachable for S and P by exchanging of members of i such that there is no string AS or there is no string AP. This means that the group of alcoholics i does not occupy S or there is a place which is not connected to S or P by exchanging of members of i.

Models for the Boolean combinations of atomic proposition of $\mathbf{K}'_i$ are defined thus:

$$\mathcal{M}' \models \neg A \text{ iff } A \text{ is false in } \mathcal{M}';$$
$$\mathcal{M}' \models A \vee B \text{ iff } \mathcal{M}' \models A \text{ or } \mathcal{M}' \models B;$$
$$\mathcal{M}' \models A \wedge B \text{ iff } \mathcal{M}' \models A \text{ and } \mathcal{M}' \models B;$$
$$\mathcal{M}' \models A \Rightarrow B \text{ iff if } \mathcal{M}' \models A, \text{ then } \mathcal{M}' \models B.$$

Proposition 3. *Logic $\mathbf{K}'_i$ is a conservative extension of $\mathbf{K}'$.* □

Proposition 4. *In $\mathbf{K}'_i$, the unconventional square of opposition holds, i.e. there are the following tautologies:*

$$k_i(S \preceq_{LA}^{good} P) \Rightarrow k_i(S \preceq_{LA}^{bad} P);$$
$$k_i(S \npreceq_{LA}^{bad} P) \Rightarrow k_i(S \npreceq_{LA}^{good} P);$$
$$\neg(k_i(S \preceq_{LA}^{good} P) \wedge k_i(S \npreceq_{LA}^{bad} P));$$
$$k_i(S \preceq_{LA}^{bad} P) \vee k_i(S \npreceq_{LA}^{good} P);$$
$$k_i(S \preceq_{LA}^{good} P) \vee k_i(S \npreceq_{LA}^{good} P);$$
$$\neg(k_i(S \preceq_{LA}^{good} P) \wedge k_i(S \npreceq_{LA}^{good} P));$$
$$k_i(S \preceq_{LA}^{bad} P) \vee k_i(S \npreceq_{LA}^{bad} P);$$
$$\neg(k_i(S \preceq_{LA}^{bad} P) \wedge k_i(S \npreceq_{LA}^{bad} P)).$$

Proof. It follows from (5)–(8). See [23].   □

Now, let us consider pairs $\bullet_{ki}A$ and $\bullet_{mi}A$, where different performative verbs $\bullet_{ki}$ and $\bullet_{mi}$ occur and these verbs belong to different groups of illocutions in expressing a preference relation, i.e. both cannot be simultaneously representatives, directives, declaratives, expressive, or comissives. For instance, 'believing' and 'knowing' are both representatives and 'ordering' and 'insisting' are both directives. Assume, 'believing' be denoted by $\bullet_{ki}$ and 'advising' by $\bullet_{mi}$. Notice that 'assuming' is modally weaker than 'believing', and 'advising' is modally weaker than 'insisting'. So, 'assuming' can be denoted by $\circ_{ki}$, and 'advising' can be denoted by $\circ_{mi}$, such that $\bullet_{ki}A \Rightarrow \circ_{ki}A$ and $\bullet_{mi}A \Rightarrow \circ_{mi}A$. The construction $\bullet_{ki}A \Rightarrow \bullet_{mi}\neg A$ (respectively, $\circ_{mi}A \Rightarrow \circ_{ki}\neg A$) fits the situation that a belief that A is ever stronger than some other illocutions (belonging to other illocution groups) related to not-A.

Let us distinguish different swarms according to the acceptance of stronger or weaker modality:

Meditative Agent. (i) agent i prefers $\bullet_{mi}\neg A$ instead of $\bullet_{ki}A$ iff $\bullet_{ki}A \Rightarrow \bullet_{mi}\neg A$; and (ii) agent i prefers $\circ_{ki}\neg A$ instead of $\circ_{mi}A$ iff $\circ_{mi}A \Rightarrow \circ_{ki}\neg A$.
Active Agent. (i) agent i prefers $\bullet_{ki}A$ instead of $\bullet_{mi}\neg A$ iff $\bullet_{ki}A \Rightarrow \bullet_{mi}\neg A$; (ii) and agent i prefers $\circ_{mi}A$ instead of $\circ_{ki}\neg A$ iff $\circ_{mi}A \Rightarrow \circ_{ki}\neg A$.

An example of the meditative agent: (s)he prefers to believe that not-A instead of that to order that A. An example of the active agent: (s)he prefers to insist that A instead of that to believe that not-A.

The fusion of two swarms i and j universal affirmative syllogistic propositions is defined in $\mathbf{K}'_i$ as follows:

$$\frac{k_i(S_1 \preceq_{LA}^{good} P);\quad m_j(S_2 \preceq_{LA}^{good} P)}{(k \cup m_{i\cup j}((S_1 \wedge S_2) \preceq_{LA}^{good} P)}.$$

The splitting of one swarm $i \cup j$ is defined in $\mathbf{K}'_i$:

$$\frac{(k \cup m)_{i\cup j}(S \preceq_{LA}^{good} (P_1 \wedge P_2))}{k_i(S \preceq_{LA}^{good} P_1);\quad m_j(S \preceq_{LA}^{good} P_2)}.$$

The illocutionary logic $\mathbf{K}'_i$ can express the preference relations of alcoholics in respect to attractants under the conditions of lateral activation.

6   Conclusions

I have shown that the lateral inhibition and lateral activation are two fundamental patterns in sensing and motoring of swarms. The point is that both patterns allow swarms to occupy several attractants and to avoid several repellents at once. Then I have shown that a habit of joint drinking of alcohol-addicted people in small groups can be considered a swarm behaviour controlled by outer stimuli (places to drink jointly). And this behaviour follows the lateral inhibition and lateral activation, also. As a result, the swarms of alcoholics can be managed by localization of safe places for meeting to drink jointly. Generally, the logic of lateral inhibition and lateral activation of groups of alcoholics has the same axioms as the logic of parasite propagation for *Schistosomatidae* sp. [26] as well as the same axioms as the logic of slime mould expansion [27]. The difference is that instead of syllogistics for *Schistosomatidae* sp. and for slime mould, where preference relations are simple and express only attractions by food, we say about performative actions (or verbs), which express a desire to drink together at a place. For simulating the swarm behaviour of alcoholics I propose two logics: the logic $\mathbf{K}_i$ to formalize a lateral inhibition in distributing people to drink jointly and the logic $\mathbf{K}_i'$ to formalize a lateral activation in distributing people to drink jointly.

Hence, we can state that some forms of human group behaviour are not social in fact. This unsocial behaviour can proceed as a human version of swarm behaviour. Many forms of human swarming have recently been studied – from crowds of people in escape panic [9] to aircraft boarding [22]. However, some stable patterns of interconnected people have never been analyzed as a swarm. I have proposed to consider a network of coordinated alcoholics as human swarming. The reasons are as follows: (i) their behaviour is controlled by replacing stimuli: attractants (places where they can drink jointly and safely) and repellents (some interruptions which can appear for drinking); this control is executed by the same algorithms as for standard swarms from social bacteria to eusocial mammals; (ii) the behaviour of alcoholics is collective and even cooperative, but it is subordinated to the only one uncontrolled intention, namely, how to drink; so, this motivation bears no symbolic meanings in the terms of symbolic interactionism [4] and, then, it cannot be evaluated as social.

Acknowledgement. The research was carried out by the support of FP7-ICT-2011-8. This paper is an extension of [29] presented at BIOSIGNALS, 2017, Porto, Portugal. I am thankful to Vadim Fris for helping in performing this research.

References

1. Abrahams, M., Colgan, P.: Risk of predation, hydrodynamic efficiency, and their influence on school structure. Environ. Biol. Fishes **13**(3), 195–202 (1985)
2. Adamatzky, A., Erokhin, V., Grube, M., Schubert, T., Schumann, A.: Physarum chip project: growing computers from slime mould. Int. J. Unconv. Comput. **8**(4), 319–323 (2012)
3. Beni, G., Wang, J.: Swarm intelligence in cellular robotic systems. In: Dario, P., Sandini, G., Aebischer, P. (eds.) Robots and Biological Systems: Towards a New Bionics. NATO ASI Series, pp. 703–712. Springer, Heidelberg (1993). https://doi.org/10.1007/978-3-642-58069-7_38
4. Blumer, H.: Symbolic Interactionism; Perspective and Method. Prentice-Hall, Englewood Cliffs (1969)
5. Bull, R.A., Segerberg, K.: Basic modal logic. In: The Handbook of Philosophical Logic, vol. 2, pp. 1–88. Kluwer (1984)

6. Costerton, J.W., Lewandowski, Z., Caldwell, D.E., Korber, D.R., et al.: Microbial biofilms. Annu. Rev. Microbiol. **49**, 711–745 (1995)
7. Duffy, J.E.: The ecology and evolution of eusociality in sponge-dwelling shrimp. In: Kikuchi, T. (ed.) Genes, Behavior, and Evolution in Social Insects, pp. 1–38. University of Hokkaido Press, Sapporo (2002)
8. Helbing, D., Keltsch, J., Molnar, P.: Modelling the evolution of human trail systems. Nature **388**, 47–50 (1997)
9. Helbing, D., Farkas, I., Vicsek, T.: Simulating dynamical features of escape panic. Nature **407**(6803), 487–490 (2000)
10. Jacobs, D.S., et al.: The colony structure and dominance hierarchy of the Damaraland mole-rat, Cryptomys damarensis (Rodentia: Bathyergidae) from Namibia. J. Zool. **224**(4), 553–576 (1991)
11. Jarvis, J.: Eusociality in a mammal: cooperative breeding in naked mole-rat colonies. Science **212**(4494), 571–573 (1981)
12. Jarvis, J.U.M., Bennett, N.C.: Eusociality has evolved independently in two genera of bathyergid mole-rats but occurs in no other subterranean mammal. Behav. Ecol. Sociobiol. **33**(4), 253–360 (1993)
13. Jones, J.D.: Towards lateral inhibition and collective perception in unorganised non-neural systems. In: Pancerz, K., Zaitseva, E. (eds.) Computational Intelligence, Medicine and Biology. SCI, vol. 600, pp. 103–122. Springer, Cham (2015). https://doi.org/10.1007/978-3-319-16844-9_6
14. Kearns, D.B.: A field guide to bacterial swarming motility. Nat. Rev. Microbiol. **8**(9), 634–644 (2010)
15. Krützen, M., Mann, J., Heithaus, M.R., Connor, R.C., Bejder, L., Sherwin, W.B.: Cultural transmission of tool use in bottlenose dolphins. PNAS **102**(25), 8939–8943 (2005)
16. Michener, C.D.: Comparative social behavior of bees. Annu. Rev. Entomol. **14**, 299–342 (1969)
17. Nalyanya, G., Moore, C.B., Schal, C.: Integration of repellents, attractants, and insecticides in a "push-pull" strategy for managing German cockroach (Dictyoptera: Blattellidae) populations. J. Med. Entomol. **37**(3), 427–434 (2000)
18. Olson, R.S., Hintze, A., Dyer, F.C., Knoester, D.B., Adami, C.: Predator confusion is sufficient to evolve swarming behaviour. J. R. Soc. Interface **10**(85), 20130305 (2013)
19. Parsons, T.: Social Systems and The Evolution of Action Theory. The Free Press, New York (1975)
20. Riesenhuber, M., Poggio, T.: Neural mechanisms of object recognition. Curr. Opin. Neurobiol. **12**(2), 162–168 (2002)
21. Sakiyama, T., Gunji, Y.-P.: The Müller-Lyer illusion in ant foraging. In: Hemmi, J.M. (ed.) PLoS ONE, vol. 8, no. 12, p. e81714 (2013)
22. Schadschneider, A., Klingsch, W., Klpfel, H., Kretz, T., Rogsch, C., Seyfried, A.: Evacuation dynamics: empirical results, modeling and applications. In: Meyers, R.A. (ed.) Encyclopedia of Complexity and Systems Science, pp. 3142–3176. Springer, Berlin (2009). https://doi.org/10.1007/978-0-387-30440-3_187
23. Schumann, A.: On two squares of opposition: the Leniewski's style formalization of synthetic propositions. Acta Analytica **28**, 71–93 (2013)
24. Schumann, A.: From swarm simulations to swarm intelligence. In: 9th EAI International Conference on Bio-inspired Information and Communications Technologies (formerly BIONETICS). ACM (2015)
25. Schumann, A., Pancerz, K., Szelc, A.: The swarm computing approach to business intelligence. Studia Humana **4**(3), 41–50 (2015)

26. Schumann, A., Akimova, L.: Syllogistic system for the propagation of parasites. The Case of *Schistosomatidae* (Trematoda: Digenea). Stud. Log. Gramm. Rhetor. **40**(1), 303–319 (2015)
27. Schumann, A.: Syllogistic versions of go games on physarum. In: Adamatzky, A. (ed.) Advances in Physarum Machines. ECC, vol. 21, pp. 651–685. Springer, Cham (2016). https://doi.org/10.1007/978-3-319-26662-6_30
28. Schumann, A., Woleński, J.: Two squares of oppositions and their applications in pairwise comparisons analysis. Fundamenta Informaticae **144**(3–4), 241–254 (2016)
29. Schumann, A., Fris, V.: Swarm intelligence among humans – the case of alcoholics. In: Proceedings of the 10th International Joint Conference on Biomedical Engineering Systems and Technologies, BIOSIGNALS, (BIOSTEC 2017), vol. 4. SCITEPRESS (2017)
30. Skinner, B.F.: About Behaviorism. Random House, Inc., New York (1976)
31. Tani, I., Yamachiyo, M., Shirakawa, T., Gunji, Y.-P.: Kanizsa illusory contours appearing in the plasmodium pattern of Physarum polycephalum. Front. Cellular Infect. Microbiol. **4**(10), 1–11 (2014)
32. Tsang, N., Macnab, R., Koshland, D.E.: Common mechanism for repellents and attractants in bacterial chemotaxis. Science **181**(4094), 60–63 (1973)
33. Viscido, S., Parrish, J., Grunbaum, D.: Individual behavior and emergent properties of fish schools: a comparison of observation and theory. Mar. Ecol. Prog. Ser. **273**, 239–249 (2004)
34. Whiten, A., Goodall, J., McGrew, W.C., Nishida, T., Reynolds, V., Sugiyama, Y., Tutin, C.E., Wrangham, R.W., Boesch, C.: Cultures in chimpanzees. Nature **399**(6737), 682–685 (1999)

Health Informatics

Technologies for Ageing in Place: A Systematic Review of Reviews and Meta-analyses

Luís Pereira[1], Ana Dias[2], Alexandra Queirós[3],
and Nelson Pacheco Rocha[4(✉)]

[1] Medtronic Portugal, Torres de Lisboa, Rua Tomás da Fonseca,
Torre E - 11º andar, 1600-209 Lisbon, Portugal
luis.pereira@medtronic.com
[2] Department of Economics, Management, Industrial Engineering and Tourism,
GOVCOP, University of Aveiro, Campo Universitário de Santiago,
3810-193 Aveiro, Portugal
anadias@ua.pt
[3] Health Sciences School, IEETA, University of Aveiro,
Campo Universitário de Santiago, 3810-193 Aveiro, Portugal
alexandra@ua.pt
[4] Department of Medical Sciences, IEETA, University of Aveiro,
Campo Universitário de Santiago, 3810-193 Aveiro, Portugal
npr@ua.pt

Abstract. Objectives - Assuming information technologies might help older adults in their residential environments (i.e. technologies for ageing in place), this study aims to identify: (i) the most relevant applications of technologies for ageing in place; (ii) the types of technologies for ageing in place; and (iii) the outcomes of technologies for ageing in place. Methods - A systematic review of reviews and meta-analyses was performed based on a search of the literature. Results - A total of 73 systematic reviews and meta-analyses were retrieved. These studies were classified in the following classes: (i) healthy lifestyles; (ii) loneliness and social isolation; (iii) home safety; and (iv) remote care of chronic conditions. Conclusion - The findings show the potential of technologies for ageing in place, but there is the need of additional evidence from randomized controlled trials and longitudinal studies with large sample sizes and robust evaluation methods.

Keywords: Technologies for ageing in place · Older adults · Chronic diseases

1 Introduction

The normal ageing process involves different types of alterations with repercussions on motor (e.g. less mobility), cognitive (e.g. attention capacity or short-term memory) or social (e.g. smaller social networks) capacities. These alterations influence perceived abilities, such as increasing difficulty of focusing on nearby objects or distinguishing them in poorly lit environments or even less ability to perform multitasking [1]. Consequently, diverse barriers tend to hamper the daily lives of older people, in particular about decision-making, problem-solving or day-to-day planning. On the other

© Springer International Publishing AG, part of Springer Nature 2018
N. Peixoto et al. (Eds.): BIOSTEC 2017, CCIS 881, pp. 331–353, 2018.
https://doi.org/10.1007/978-3-319-94806-5_18

hand, ageing is associated with many chronic diseases that influence the quality of older adults. All these circumstances have implications for the autonomy and independence of older adults and can lead to their institutionalization.

The concept of ageing in place [2] intents to satisfy the people's desire to stay in their own residential environments as they get older, despite possible declines in their physical and cognitive capacities. Ageing in significant places where many of the daily routines have taken place throughout life - such as neighbourhoods, churches, grocery stores, markets, cafes, libraries, recreational associations or gardens - allows a greater mediation of the alterations related to the ageing processes, and also the continuity of a (more or less) active lifestyle and, consequently, of contributions to the community.

Technological solutions emerge as potentially cost-effective to meet the needs of citizens and to promote the services' reorganization [3], which are the aims of concepts such as Medicine 2.0 [4], connected health [5], or holistic health [6, 7]. Moreover, many of the current health and social policies focus on providing products and services to compensate the declines of older adults, thus favouring the permanence in their homes. In this sense, ageing in place [2] reflects the idea that familiar environments provide a sense of belonging not only to the family, but also to the community, strongly related to the notion of identity, security, familiarity and autonomy, which are essential variables for a healthy ageing [8]. This perspective also enforces the role of information technologies, which may help older adults in their homes (i.e. technologies for ageing in place [9]) to overcome multiple impairments, and to allow them to live safely, independently, autonomously and comfortably, with the necessary support services to their changing needs [2, 10, 11].

There are several systematic reviews of reviews and meta-analyses related to technologies for ageing in place [12–15]. However, their studies focus on specific technologies (e.g. short message services [12]), or specific pathologies (e.g. congestive heart failure [13]). Therefore, the broad analysis of the study reported in the present article, which was partially presented in [16] (i.e. home monitoring of patients with chronic diseases), is useful to inform older adults, practitioners and researchers about the state of the art of technologies for ageing in place.

2   Methods

The systematic review of reviews and meta-analyses reported in this article aimed to systematize current evidence of technologies for ageing in place and was informed by the following research questions:

- RQ1: What are the most relevant applications of technologies for ageing in place?
- RQ2: What are the types of technologies for ageing in place?
- RQ3: What are the outcomes of technologies for ageing in place?

Since a large number of articles have been published, the study reported in this article was planned to include systematic reviews or meta-analyses only. Moreover, it followed the guidelines of the Preferred Reporting Items for Systematic Reviews and Meta-Analyses (PRISMA) [17].

The literature search was conducted using two general databases (i.e. Web of Science and Scopus) and two specific databases (i.e. PubMed, a medical sciences database, and IEEE Explorer, a technological database).

The database queries were prepared to include: (i) all the systematic reviews and meta-analyses where any of the keywords 'telecare', 'telehealth', 'telemedicine', 'homecare', 'telemonitoring', 'home monitoring', 'remote monitoring', ehealth', 'telerehabilitation', 'mobile health', 'mhealth' or 'assisted living' were presented in the title or abstract; and (ii) all the systematic reviews and meta-analyses where any the keywords 'technology-based', 'information technology', 'information and communication', 'internet-based', 'web-based', 'on-line', 'smartphones', 'mobile apps', 'mobile phone', 'monitoring devices' or 'consumer health information' were presented in the title or abstract together with any of the keywords 'healthcare', 'health care', 'patient', 'chronic disease', 'older' or 'elderly'.

The search was performed on 30 of April 2016 and intend to include systematic reviews and meta-analyses published during the preceding 10 years.

2.1   Inclusion and Exclusion Criteria

In terms of inclusion criteria, the study reported in the present article included systematic reviews and meta-analyses related to technological solutions that can be used to support older adults in their environments.

Moreover, the exclusion criteria were: (i) articles not published in English; (ii) articles reporting systematic reviews of reviews and meta-analyses; (iii) articles that target exclusively the formal and informal caregivers (i.e. studies that were clinicians focused or were intended primary to deal with the problems of caregivers rather than the patients); (iv) articles reporting applications that were designed to be used in an institutional environment and not in the domicile of older adults; and (v) articles that are not relevant for the objective of the study reported in this article.

2.2   Review Selection

After the removal of duplicates and articles not published in English, two authors independently reviewed all titles for relevance and assessed the abstracts of the retrieved articles against the inclusion and exclusion criteria. Afterwards, the same two authors assessed the full text of the articles according to the outlined inclusion and exclusion criteria. Any disagreement between the authors was discussed and resolved by consensus.

2.3   Data Extraction and Analysis

For every one of the selected articles, the following information was registered in a data sheet prepared by the authors: (i) authors, title and year of publication; (ii) scope of the review or meta-analysis; (iii) search strategy; (iv) inclusion and exclusion criteria; (v) data extraction procedure; (vi) quality assessment procedures used in the review; (vii) details of the research methods of the primary studies included in the review; (viii) total number of primary studies; (ix) total number of randomized clinical trials (RCT);

(x) total number of participants; (xi) technologies being reported; (xii) target chronic disease, when applicable; (xiii) primary outcomes; (xiv) secondary outcomes; (xv) evidence of the impact of the reported applications; (xvi) authors' interpretations; (xvii) conclusions; and (xviii) recommendations for the future.

Afterwards, the collected data was analysed to answer the research questions of the present study.

3   Results

Figure 1 presents the PRISMA flowchart of the systematic review of reviews and meta-analyses reported in the present paper.

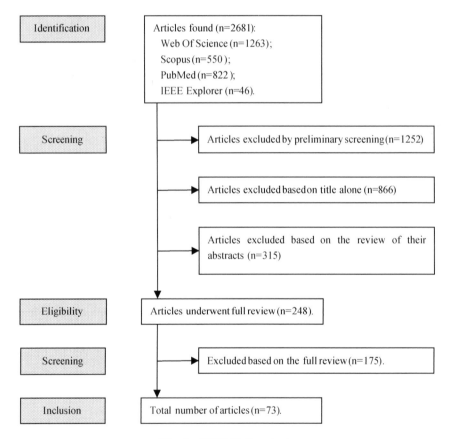

Fig. 1. PRISMA flowchart.

A total of 2681 articles were retrieved from the initial searches on Web of Science (1263 articles), Scopus (550 articles), PubMed (822 articles), and IEEE Explorer (46 articles). The initial screening yielded 1429 articles by removing the duplicates (1210 articles) or the articles without abstracts (42 articles). After exclusions based on title alone, 563 articles were retrieved. Additionally, 315 articles were eliminated based upon review of their abstracts.

The full texts of the 248 remaining articles were assessed and 175 articles were eliminated. Consequently, 73 articles [18–90] were included in this systematic review.

3.1 Characteristics of the Studies

Sixty eight of the 73 studies emanated from different journals, representing diverse fields and areas of research. Moreover, three studies were retrieved from the Cochrane library and two studies were published in conference proceedings. Most of the studies were published in clinical journals (n = 36) and the remainder studies published in journals were published in journals related to ehealth and medical informatics.

The journal in which studies were published most frequently was the Journal of Medical Internet Research (n = 13), followed by the Journal of Telemedicine and Telecare (n = 7).

The synthesis of the results was based on the process proposed by Ghapanchi and Aurum [91]. To classify the technologies for ageing in place being reported, the synthesis process involved extracting the terms and definitions used in the included articles to create a primary list of technologies and applications, and then this list was refined by further analyses.

Following this method, the authors identified technologies for ageing in place targeting:

- Healthy lifestyles.
- Loneliness and social isolation.
- Home safety.
- Remote care of chronic conditions.

A total of 20 articles were classified as promoting healthy lifestyles, one as targeting loneliness and social isolation, one as promoting home safety, and 51 as related to remote care of chronic conditions [16, 92, 93].

3.2 Healthy Lifestyles

Results of this study show that when dealing with healthy lifestyles the research is focused on health education, physical activity, nutrition and weight management. These results are consistent with the most common inappropriate behaviours affecting the industrialized countries' populations [95].

Health Education. Diverse range of media platforms (e.g. collaborative projects such as Wikipedia, content communities such as YouTube, social networking applications such as Facebook, or social worlds such as Second Life) are the foundations of the web 2.0 paradigm, also known as social media [94], which allows the creation and exchange of user generated content. One of the included systematic reviews or meta-analyses [51] evaluates the contribution of the social media for health communications to the general public, patients and health professionals about health issues. Although a significant percentage of the primary studies are exploratory or descriptive, the review concludes about several benefits of the social media, including: (i) increased interaction with others; (ii) more available, shared and tailored information; (ii) increasing accessibility and widening access to health information; (iv) peer support; and (v) potential influence of healthy policies. However, reliability, confidentiality and privacy are general concerns when using social media to communicate health issues and the quality and reliability of the exchanged information is quite diverse [51].

Information technologies also offer a medium to assist healthcare providers to meet educational-related responsibilities. One review [26] reports 25 RCT that evaluate the ability of interactive computer based education programs that can be viewed at home or during periodic clinic visits. Other eight systematic reviews reported the use of different technologies (e.g. social media or personal health records) for citizens' education [26, 41, 51, 69, 78, 90], covering a diverse population in terms of age, sex, education level, health status and healthcare intervention or disease state. The programs present significant variations in terms of features, implementations and integration strategies.

Physical Activity. Physical activity is one aspect of lifestyle changing that might be effective in reducing rates of hospital admission and reducing risk of mortality. Increasing physical activity to low or moderate levels can result in lower risk of mortality from all causes.

Eleven of the included systematic reviews and meta-analyses consider the promotion of physical activity among the behaviour change interventions analysed [27, 41, 44, 45, 48, 49, 56, 69, 80, 86, 89]. There are many applications that suggest a range of physical exercises, complemented with demo videos and the measurement of several outcomes.

When reported as an outcome, physical activity is being measured through validated questionnaires (e.g. the Short Questionnaire Assessing Health-enhancing - SQUASH, the Baecke Physical Activity Questionnaire, or the comprehensive evaluation of the Minnesota Leisure Time Physical Activity Questionnaire), and quantitative measures [65, 92]. Examples of quantitative measures are steps per day or minutes of weekly exercise [96] that can be performed by different types of devices [44, 97].

Technological applications appear to have positive effects on physical activity behaviours [27, 44, 48, 56, 80, 89], but the results are not consistent [27]. For instance, a review [44] reports that within the 14 RCT being analysed, six studies found that the intervention group had significant differences compared with the control group, four studies had mixed results, and another four had no significant differences between groups [92].

However, the retrieved studies are characterized by small sample sizes, heterogeneous effect sizes, and a lack of analysis of the cost-effectiveness of the interventions, especially in conjunction with clinical practice.

Nutrition and Weight Management. Nine of the included systematic reviews and meta-analyses [27, 34, 42, 62, 65, 68, 69, 79, 80] deal with nutrition and weight management. In terms of nutrition several studies reported nutrition applications able to capture dietary intake [42, 62] that can be divided into applications that allow controlling calories and keep food diary (e.g. applications that allow users to select food and portion size or applications that process food photograph taken by the users), and specific applications for food safety, namely considering people with allergies.

Overall, positive feedback was reported: the use of nutrition applications resulted in better self-monitoring adherence and changes in dietary intake when compared to conventional techniques (e.g. paper records).

Concerning weight management, remote interventions are being delivered using a wide range of technologies, including web-based applications and smartphone applications, or even more traditional methods, such as telephone calls [92]. The interventions might include [92]: (i) counselling or advice; (ii) self-directed or prescribed exercise; (iii) home based or facility based exercise; and (iv) written education or motivational support material, namely the promotion of knowledge using serious games [41].

In terms of outcomes, questionnaires such as the Food Frequency Questionnaire (FFQ) or the MEDFICTS score have been used [65, 92]. When compared to control groups, the majority of primary RCT studies of the included systematic reviews and meta-analyses pointed a significant net difference in weight between the intervention and control groups. This is valid for different types of technologies (e.g. web-based applications [42]), but is particularly evident when mobile applications are being used (e.g. periodic prompts of a smartphone applications [27, 80]).

Long-term, sustainable behaviour change and health benefits are not shown by the included systematic reviews and meta-analyses because of the lack of consistent follow-up data collection and reporting.

3.3   Loneliness and Social Isolation

Researchers report that the impact of social relationships on the risk of mortality is comparable with major, well-established risk factors such as smoking and alcohol consumption, and exceeds that of physical inactivity and obesity [98, 99].

One of the included systematic reviews and meta-analyses [87] analysed 26 primary studies (six primary studies were RCT) related to the use of technological solutions to surpass social isolation. The interventions in all but two primary studies were implemented in the regular living environments of the participants.

Most primary studies used some form web-based or mobile applications [92]. A minority of the studies were related to telephone befriending intervention, videogames and the use of a visual pet companion application that allowed the older adults to interact with an avatar in real time [87].

Technologies for ageing in place were consistently found to affect social support, social connectedness, and social isolation in general positively [92]. The results show that technological solutions can facilitate several mechanisms, including connecting to the outside world (e.g. family members, especially grandchildren, friends, former colleagues or new contacts of shared interests) and, mostly important, boosts self-confidence and empowerment which trigger positive feelings of the participants and their control over life and/or life satisfaction [87].

Although the potential impact of technologies for ageing in place might have in the promotion of social contacts, the included review [87] suggest more well-designed studies on the effect the interventions and the identification of how the training and implementation of such interventions should be tailored to maximize their effects.

3.4 Home Safety

Several types of technologies (e.g. personal alarms, home automation systems, video monitoring and smart technologies such as bed sensors, kitchen sensors, motion sensors or fall detection sensors) are being used to help older adults to overcome emergencies [59].

Older adults reported improved safety, independence and confidence, particularly when technologies with real time monitoring are connected to a response system [59]. However, there is still the lack of robust evidence. The results also show that applications aimed at predicting, monitoring and preventing should consider intrinsic factors related to older attitudes around control, independence and perceived requirements for safety [92].

3.5 Remote Care of Chronic Conditions

Concerning the use of technologies for ageing in place to optimize the care of patients with chronic conditions, several systematic reviews and meta-analyses deal with home monitoring of older adults with chronic diseases [16, 100, 101]. In addition, the promotion of the empowerment of older adults and their informal caregivers is also subject of a significant number of the studies [93]. The 51 retrieved systematic reviews and meta-analyses were classified accordingly the target chronic disease:

- Diabetes.
- Congestive heart failure.
- Chronic obstructive pulmonary disease.
- Hypertension.
- Mental health.
- Cancer.
- Other chronic conditions.

Diabetes. Of the retrieved articles, 19 dealt with home monitoring of patients with diabetes [18, 23, 24, 35–37, 40, 47, 52–54, 63, 64, 73, 75, 76, 82, 84, 85].

Furthermore, since self-management of diabetes requires patient adherence to best practice recommendations (e.g. glycaemia control, dietary management or physical activity) there has been an interest in increasing compliance of self-care applications: (i) self-management and care knowledge [35, 40, 47, 52, 54, 76, 88]; (ii) prescribed medication adherence [37, 72, 76]; and (iii) behaviour outcomes (e.g. diet and healthy eating or physical activity) [24, 35, 37, 40, 46, 47, 54, 72, 73, 76, 82, 85, 88].

A significant number of articles focuses both type 1 and type 2 diabetes [23, 24, 36, 47, 54, 63, 73, 75, 82, 84]. Other articles focus type 2 diabetes [18, 35, 37, 40, 75, 85]. Only one of the retrieved articles focuses exclusively on type 1 diabetes [64].

The articles of the diabetes domain include primary studies with high quality scientific evidence. All the retrieved articles targeting diabetes considered RCT primary studies and 11 of them considered RCT as one of the inclusion criteria [23, 24, 36, 37, 52–54, 63, 75, 84, 85]. On the other hand, aggregating all the primary studies it is evident that the number of the involved participants is relatively significant (e.g. one article reports the involvement of 3578 patients [52] and other reports the involvement of 3798 patients [75]).

In technological terms, several articles [35, 40, 47, 52–54, 75, 82, 84] refer web-based applications. In general, these applications allow synchronous (e.g. instant messaging or chat) and asynchronous (e.g. electronic mail or bulletin board) communications together with web pages to register clinical parameters (e.g. weight or blood pressure) and medication.

Besides web-based applications, there are other technological solutions reported in different articles:

- Computer-assisted applications integrating the management of clinical data with electronic practice guidelines, reminder systems, and feedback to the patients [18, 47].
- Smartphones (e.g. standalone smartphones or smartphones integrating specific devices such as glucometers for automatic glucose level upload) [36, 37, 40, 47, 52, 64, 73, 76, 84].
- Automatic patient data transmission by means of monitoring devices (e.g. devices to monitor vital signals or devices to monitor behaviour outcomes such as pedometers or accelerometers connected by wireless communications to monitor physical activity) [23].
- Video-conference [24, 47].
- Telephone calls [82].

The main outcome of most of the articles included in the diabetes domain is the control of glycaemia by using glycosylated haemoglobin (Hb1c) as a proxy. However, in all the studies, this aim is complemented with other health related outcomes (e.g. health related quality of life [24, 35, 53, 54], weight [35, 52, 73, 75], depression [52], blood pressure [24, 63, 73, 82], cholesterol level [35, 63], triglycemius level [63], or fluctuation index [35]), behaviour outcomes (e.g. physical activity) [18, 24, 35, 37, 54, 73, 82, 85], patient self-motivation [84], patient-clinician communication [84], medication adherence [42], and structural outcomes related to care coordination [23, 24].

Most of the articles of the diabetes domain report moderate to large significant reduction of Hb1c when compared with usual care [18, 23, 37, 40, 53, 63, 64, 73, 75, 76, 82, 84, 85]. However, several studies are not conclusive about the reduction of Hb1c [24, 35, 36, 52]. In particular, computer-based diabetes self-management interventions [52] and consultations supported by video-conference [24] appear to have a small beneficial effect on glycaemia control.

One article [47] reporting research gaps of the technological approaches identifies the need to improve the usability of the applications as well the need for more comprehensive solutions, including real-time feedback to the patients and integration with electronic health record systems.

Congestive Heart Failure. The number of RCT and non-RCT primary studies included in the nine articles dealing with congestive heart failure varies from nine to 42

[19–21, 25, 30, 39, 57, 58, 61]. Most of these systematic reviews (i.e. six systematic reviews [20, 25, 30, 39, 57, 61]) considered RCT as one of the inclusion criteria.

Concerning the supporting technologies, automatic patient data transmission by means of monitoring devices [19, 25, 30, 39, 61] is being used together with video-conference and standard telephone calls [20, 21, 57, 58] to allow the assessment of symptoms and vital signs, as well as the transmission of automatic alarms.

In terms of clinical outcomes, the main concerns are the impacts of home monitoring in heart failure-related hospitalizations and all-cause mortality [57] when compared with usual care. However, several secondary outcomes are also considered such as self-care behaviour (e.g. adherence to prescribed medication, daily weighing or adherence to exercise recommendations [39]).

According the reviewed articles, home monitoring has a positive effect on clinical outcomes of patients with congestive heart failure. Home monitoring reduces mortality when compared with usual care and it also helps to lower both the number of hospitalizations and the use of other healthcare services [25, 30, 57, 61].

However, there is a need for high-quality trials [20]. Additionally, Grustam and colleagues [58] state that evidence from the scientific literature related to home monitoring to support congestive heart failure patients is still insufficient. Also, more comprehensive economic analyses are needed to reach a sound conclusion. This means that further research is required in terms of comparisons of home monitoring with usual care of patients with congestive heart failure.

Chronic Obstructive Pulmonary Disease. All the four retrieved articles dealing with chronic obstructive pulmonary disease analyse RCT primary studies [29, 33, 79, 81]. In particular, three of them considered RCT as one of the inclusion criteria [29, 79, 81].

Home monitoring is supported by commercially available devices to measure and transmit different types of information (e.g. weight, temperature, blood pressure, oxygen saturation, spirometry parameters, symptoms, medication usage or steps in 6-min walking distance). In some cases, the automatic data acquisition is complemented by telephone interviews of clinical staff using questionnaires [29, 81], or by telephone or video-conference calls to provide feedback to the patients [79]. In this respect, one article also reports that telephone and videoconference calls when used to provide feedback are associated to improvements in the quality of life of patients with chronic obstructive pulmonary disease [79].

In what concerns the primary and secondary outcomes, three studies [29, 33, 81] compare home monitoring with usual care of patients with chronic obstructive pulmonary disease, considering mortality, admissions to hospital or other healthcare utilization as primary outcomes. Secondary outcomes include, among others, health related quality of life, patient satisfaction, physical capacity and dyspnea.

Home monitoring was found to reduce rates of hospitalization and emergency department visits, while the findings related to hospital bed days of care varied between studies [29, 81]. However, one study reports a greater mortality in a telephone-support group compared with usual care [29]. Additionally, there is evidence that home monitoring has a positive effect on physical capacity and dyspnea [79] and it is similar or better than usual care in terms of quality of life and patient satisfaction outcomes [85].

The evidence systematized by the articles related to chronic obstructive pulmonary disease does not allow drawing definite conclusions, as the studies are small. The benefits of home monitoring of patients with chronic obstructive pulmonary disease are not yet proven and further research is required before wide-scale implementation be supported.

Hypertension. Concerning patients with hypertension, one article systematizes the results of 12 RCT using devices with automated data transmission together with video-conference calls to monitor patients with hypertension [71]. The article reports improvements in the proportion of participants with controlled blood pressure compared to those who received usual care, but the authors conclude that more interventions are required and cost-effectiveness of the interventions should also be assessed [71].

A second article [32] related to the empowerment of patients with hypertension concludes that web-based or compute-computer based applications change the care knowledge and impact self-efficacy and self-care behaviours.

Mental Health. Concerning mental health, seven articles were retrieved [93]: (i) three articles report web-based applications [55, 72] and videoconference [31] to support people with psychosis; (ii) two articles analyse computer-based and web-based applications to support people with depression [28, 83]; (iii) one article is related to computer-based applications to support people with dementia [60]; and (iv) one article is focused on the interventions for people with insomnia [38].

Patients with psychosis seem to use the internet more frequently than control groups for the purposes of social networking, but participation varies across studies. Concerning the use of videoconference to treat people with psychosis, findings generally indicate that patient care via videoconference is equivalent to face-to-face therapy, but also offers numerous advantages such as reduction in the need for patients and professionals to travel [31]. However, the heterogeneity, poor quality and early stage of the reported research precludes any definite conclusions [55, 93].

In terms of patients with depression, a study [83] argues that there is evidence that supports the effectiveness of different treatments for depression and highlights participant satisfaction, but a second study [28] considers that there is insufficient scientific evidence regarding the effectiveness of computer-based cognitive behavioural therapy and self-help web-based applications in terms of the management of depression. Furthermore, there is a strong hypothesis that videoconference-based treatment obtains the same results as face-to-face therapy, and that self-help web-based applications could improve depression symptoms when traditional care is not available [28].

A study related to dementia analyses the usability and acceptability of the applications as well as the engagement, participation and enjoyment of the participation [60]. Benefits include the enjoyment derived by people with dementia from viewing reminiscing materials through various forms of multimedia, such as video and audio [60]. However, many of the systems described require technical expertise for setup or operation and may not be ready for independent use by family caregivers [60].

Finally, another study [38], considering the analysis of six RCT that involved 433 participants with insomnia problems, concludes that the overall adherence rate is satisfactory (78%) but there are very small to medium effects on the outcomes compared to control groups [93].

Cancer. To mitigate the undesirable side effects that can negatively affect the quality of life of patients with cancer, their empowerment is important [93]. The patients' empowerment can contribute to them being autonomous and respected, having knowledge, or psychosocial and behavioural skills, receiving support from community, family, and friends [74]. In this respect, technologies for ageing in place can support knowledge transmission, including electronic survivorship care plans, patient-to-patient and patient-to-caregiver communication, and electronic patient-reported outcomes [74].

The retrieved studies report that technologies for ageing in place (e.g. computer-based and web-based applications) were found to be effective in different health outcomes such as: (i) pain, depression and quality of life [66]; (ii) fatigue, depression, anxiety, and overall quality of life [77]; (iii) knowledge; (iv) satisfaction; and (v) other outcomes which were both directly and indirectly related to the healthcare interventions [22].

However, some of the primary studies included in the retrieved articles present only preliminary evaluations of the technological solutions being used [22] and the findings suggest that the application of technologies for ageing in place in cancer care is still at a very early stage [66].

Other Chronic Conditions. Finally, in terms of other chronic conditions, four articles were identified [93]: (i) one article considers that remote interventions, including the use of mobile applications designed for smartphones and tablets, appear to be well-accepted for the care of patients with asthma and increase self-care behaviours [50]; (ii) one article related to telerehabilitation for people with multiple sclerosis [67], including web-based applications and videoconference, highlights the lack of methodologically robust trials; (iii) one article shows the potential clinical benefits of dietary interventions based in mobile applications for chronic renal patients, although there is a need for additional robust trials [70]; and (iv) one article which aims was to analyse the impact of mobile applications targeting overweight or obese people concluded that when considering exclusively the use of mobile technologies (21 RCT) a significant reduction in weight (5–10%) was observed [43].

4   Discussion

The following subsections discuss the findings according to the different perspectives associated to the research questions formulated to inform the study reported in the present article.

4.1   Relevant Applications of Technologies for Ageing in Place

Concerning the relevant applications of technologies for ageing in place (i.e. the first research question), the study reported in this article identified 73 systematic reviews and meta-analyses that were classified into the following categories: (i) healthy lifestyles; (ii) loneliness and social isolation; (iii) home safety; and (iv) remote care of chronic conditions.

Since physical inactivity and obesity, together with smoking and alcohol consumption, are well-established risk factors with impact in health conditions and mortality, the promotion of healthy lifestyles assumes great importance [95]. In particular, several articles report the impact of health education and behaviour changing in terms of physical activity, nutrition and weight management.

One of the systematic reviews and meta-analyses target loneliness and social isolation and other target home safety. Loneliness and social exclusion are generally understood as dramatic consequences of the population ageing and the response to emergencies in terms of home safety is generally accepted as an important issue for older adults.

Concerning healthcare, according to the findings of the systematic review reported in this article, diabetes, congestive heart failure, chronic obstructive pulmonary disease and hypertension are the most relevant chronic diseases in terms of the use of technologies for ageing in place to support home monitoring. Type 1 and type 2 diabetes stand out from other chronic conditions with a total of 19 articles. In order of relevance, the second chronic condition was congestive heart failure (nine articles), which was followed by chronic obstructive pulmonary disease (four articles). Furthermore, one article reporting a systematic review related to home monitoring of patients with hypertension was also included in the present systematic review.

In terms of the empowerment of older adults and their informal caregivers, diabetes also stands out from other chronic conditions with a total of 15 articles. In order of relevance, seven articles are related to mental health and four articles are related to patients with cancer. Furthermore, five articles are related to one of the following chronic conditions: (i) hypertension; (ii) asthma; (iii) multiple sclerosis; (iv) renal chronic disease; and (v) obesity.

Diabetes requires constant monitoring of the glucose levels, congestive heart failure has a high rate of hospital readmission [102], and key aspects of the natural history of the chronic obstructive pulmonary disease are episodes of acute exacerbations [103]. On the other hand, self-management of diabetes requires patient adherence to best practice recommendations, engagement and participation [63], as well as efficient contacts between patients and clinical staff are essential when dealing with mental health conditions, and patients undergoing cancer treatment may experience many undesirable side effects that can negatively affect their quality of life. Therefore, the results of the systematic review reported in this article are in line with the current strong motivation for using technological solutions as a way to monitor older adults with chronic diseases at home and to promote an increasing compliance of self-care.

4.2   Types of Technologies for Ageing in Place

In terms of what technologies for ageing in place are being used to assist older adults (i.e. the second research question), the results show that there is a widespread use of general purpose information technologies (e.g. mobile communications, messaging, videoconference, social media, serious games, virtual reality or audio/video animations), and special purpose applications, including computer-based applications, web-based applications and smartphone applications.

Some technologies have gotten more attention than others. Particularly, mobile applications such as applications to deliver periodic prompts and reminders [27] were reported by a considerable number of articles. In this respect, the portability of smartphones enables users to have access 24 h a day, making possible the long-term management and reinforcement of health behaviours. This seems to promote the focus of the participants and their adherence to the programs.

Concerning home monitoring of patients with chronic diseases, the results show that the technological solutions being used include web-based applications, computer-based applications, smartphones applications, automatic patient data transmission by means of monitoring devices, video-conference and standard telephone calls. On the other hand, in terms of the empowerment of older adults and their informal caregivers, the technological solutions being used include computer-based applications, web-based applications, smartphone applications, videoconference, telephone calls and serious games.

Despite a high level of technological innovation and implementation, one of the findings is that telephone calls are still an important channel for the communication between patients and care providers.

Furthermore, it seems that important aspects are neglected during the technological developments, since there are reports of usability drawbacks as well as reports of the need for more comprehensive solutions, including provision of real-time feedback and the integration of the electronic health records systems being used by the care providers [47].

Therefore, the results show that not only disruptive technological solutions have a key role, since practical and robust solutions are required, which means that the integration and the interoperability of existing technologies assume a great importance [104].

4.3   Outcomes of Technologies for Ageing in Place

Concerning the third research question of the study reported in this article (i.e. what are the outcomes of technologies for ageing in place?) the analyses of the retrieved articles suggest that these outcomes depend on the specific applications.

Several systematic reviews and meta-analyses target behaviour changing, including health education, promotion of physical activity, and nutrition and weight management (i.e. healthy lifestyles). Knowledge gains, motivation, preventive behaviour, reduced education staff costs for low risk patients, level of physical activity, self-monitoring adherence, changes in dietary intake and weight management were the outcomes being considered by the studies targeting healthy lifestyles.

Two systematic reviews targeted loneliness and social isolation and home safety. In this respect, the outcomes being considered were social support, social connectedness, social isolation, safety, independence and confidence.

Concerning home monitoring of patients with chronic diseases, the results show that:

- In general, the systematic reviews and meta-analyses compare home monitoring with usual care and the primary outcomes depend on the type of the patients being considered (e.g. glycaemia control for patients with diabetes, patients' readmissions and mortality for patients with congestive heart failure and patients with chronic obstructive pulmonary disease, or blood pressure control of patients with hypertension).

- Secondary outcomes are quite diverse and include health related quality of life, weight, depression, blood pressure, behaviour change, self-management, care knowledge, medication adherence, patient-clinician communication, or structural outcomes related to care coordination.

Furthermore, in terms of technologies for ageing in place to promote the empowerment of patients with chronic conditions, the systematic reviews and meta-analyses compare the use of technological solutions with usual care and the outcomes depend on the type of the patients being considered, namely:

- Glycaemia control, health related quality of life or patient adherence to best practice recommendations, including care knowledge, behaviour outcomes (e.g. diet and healthy eating or physical activity) and adherence to prescribed medication, for patients with diabetes.
- Improvement of the symptoms, engagement and participation for patients suffering from mental health conditions.
- Knowledge, pain, depression, fatigue, anxiety, satisfaction and overall quality of life for patients with cancer.

Independently of the outcomes being measured, the retrieved articles show that the usage of technologies for ageing in place has positive effects with a moderate to large improvements in different outcomes when compared with conventional practices.

5 Conclusion

Considering the large number of articles reporting studies related to technologies for ageing in place, the authors decided to perform a systematic review of reviews and meta-analyses.

Although the authors tried to be as elaborate as possible in methodological terms to guarantee that the review selection and the data extraction were rigorous, it should be acknowledged that the study reported in this article has, however, some limitations that must be considered when interpreting the results. First, the search was not exhaustive because of the language restriction. Then, only the articles published in the scientific literature were included with a potential underestimation of the real number of works and researches related to this topic. Finally, it should be noted as the continuous evolution of the technology makes very difficult to provide an updated reporting of the evidence available.

However, it should also be pointed that the study reported in this article presents some strengths: (i) the methodological design was as elaborate as possible to guarantee that the review selection and the data extraction were rigorous; and (ii) the systematically collected evidence contributes to the understanding of the technologies for ageing in place to support older adults in their home environments.

The systematic reviews and meta-analyses being retrieved pointed out that technologies for ageing in place might facilitate immediate, intermediate and long-term health related outcomes in older adults.

One of the problems that emerge from the study reported in the present article is related to the outcomes being measured. Besides their diversity, it is important to refer that different measurement methods are being applied. This is an important difficulty when aggregating and analysing data from different trials, which is essential to achieve the statistical and clinical significance that is required to promote the adoption of new services.

On the other hand, it becomes increasingly important that the development technologies for ageing in place musts consider a variety of possible dangers to older adults.

One aspect to be considered is the risk of the reduction of the human relations, particularly between patients and healthcare providers. Therefore, technologies for ageing in place should not interfere on the quality of the human relations, which might require the implementation of specific training interventions for all the stakeholders.

These training programs are indispensable especially when it becomes evident that even highly educated people may experience difficulties in understanding instructions or other healthcare-related information. Therefore, there are significant problems in terms of health literacy that can be exacerbated when dealing with older adults. Moreover, health literacy is part of a complex issue known as 'digital divide', which is related to the existence of a gap between people who can effectively deal with information and communication tools and those who cannot [51] (e.g. difficulties in accessing specific services due to non-existent adequate communication infrastructures).

Finally, since technologies for ageing in place manage different types of personal information, including clinical data, there could be serious problems related to privacy of older adults. These problems might be exacerbated when using mobile technologies, such as mobile phones (e.g. when a smartphone is lost and the control or accesses is not performed).

Despite the potentially negative connotations, given the findings, technologies for ageing in place present an enormous potential and deserves further research. In particular, there is the need of additional scientific evidence from RCT and longitudinal studies with large sample sizes and robust methods.

Acknowledgments. This work was supported by Sistema de Incentivos à Investigação e Desenvolvimento Tecnológico (SI I&DT) of the Programa Portugal 2020, through Programa Operacional Competitividade e Internacionalização and/or Programa Operacional do Centro do FEDER - Fundo Europeu de Desenvolvimento Regional, under Social Cooperation for Integrated Assisted Living (SOCIAL), project number 017861.

References

1. Cota, T., Ishitani, L., Vieira, N.: Mobile game design for the elderly: a study with focus on the motivation to play. Comput. Hum. Behav. **51**, 96–105 (2015). https://doi.org/10.1016/j.chb.2015.04.026
2. Plaweck, H.: Aging in place: the role of housing and social supports. J. Gerontological Nurs. **18**, 53–54 (1990). https://doi.org/10.3928/0098-9134-19921001-14

3. Genet, N., Boerma, W.G., Kringos, D.S., Bouman, A., Francke, A.L., Fagerström, C., Melchiorre, M.G., Greco, C., Devillé, W.: Home care in Europe: a systematic literature review. BMC Health Serv. Res. **11**, 207 (2011). https://doi.org/10.1186/1472-6963-11-207
4. Eysenbach, G.: Medicine 2.0: social networking, collaboration, participation, apomediation, and openness. J. Med. Internet Res. **10**, e22 (2008). https://doi.org/10.2196/jmir.1030
5. Kvedar, J., Coye, M.J., Everett, W.: Connected health: a review of technologies and strategies to improve patient care with telemedicine and telehealth. Health Aff. **33**, 194–199 (2014). https://doi.org/10.1377/hlthaff.2013.0992
6. Koch, S.: Achieving holistic health for the individual through person-centered collaborative care supported by informatics. Healthc. Inform. Res. **19**, 3–8 (2013). https://doi.org/10.4258/hir.2013.19.1.3
7. Mori, A.R., Mazzeo, M., Mercurio, G., Verbicaro, R.: Holistic health: predicting our data future (from inter-operability among systems to co-operability among people). Int. J. Med. Inform. **82**, e14–28 (2013). https://doi.org/10.1016/j.ijmedinf.2012.09.003
8. Wiles, J.L., Leibing, A., Guberman, N., Reeve, J., Allen, R.E.S.: The meaning of "aging in place" to older people. Gerontologist **52**, 357–366 (2011). https://doi.org/10.1093/geront/gnr098
9. Connelly, K., Laghari, K.U.R., Mokhtari, M., Falk, T.H.: Approaches to understanding the impact of technologies for aging in place: a mini-review. Gerontology **60**, 282–288 (2014). https://doi.org/10.1159/000355644
10. Nutbeam, D.: Health promotion glossary. Health Promot. Int. **13**, 349–364 (1998). https://doi.org/10.1093/heapro/13.4.349
11. Walker, P.R.: Report from the World NGO Forum on Ageing and the United Nations Second World Assembly on Ageing. PsycEXTRA Dataset. https://doi.org/10.1037/e523502012-005
12. Househ, M.: The role of short messaging service in supporting the delivery of healthcare: an umbrella systematic review. Health Inform. J. **22**, 140–150 (2014). https://doi.org/10.1177/1460458214540908
13. Kitsiou, S., Paré, G., Jaana, M.: Effects of home telemonitoring interventions on patients with chronic heart failure: an overview of systematic reviews. J. Med. Internet Res. **17**, e63 (2015). https://doi.org/10.2196/jmir.4174
14. Mcbain, H., Shipley, M., Newman, S.: The impact of self-monitoring in chronic illness on healthcare utilisation: a systematic review of reviews. BMC Health Serv. Res. **15**, 565 (2015). https://doi.org/10.1186/s12913-015-1221-5
15. Slev, V.N., Mistiaen, P., Pasman, H.R.W., Leeuw, I.M.V.-D., Uden-Kraan, C.F.V., Francke, A.L.: Effects of eHealth for patients and informal caregivers confronted with cancer: a meta-review. Int. J. Med. Inform. **87**, 54–67 (2016). https://doi.org/10.1016/j.ijmedinf.2015.12.013
16. Queirós, A., Pereira, L., Dias, A., Rocha, N.P.: Technologies for ageing in place to support home monitoring of patients with chronic diseases. In: van den Broek, E.L., Fred, A., Gamboa, H., Vaz, M. (eds.) Proceedings of the 10th International Joint Conference on Biomedical Engineering Systems and Technologies - Volume 5: HEALTHINF, pp. 66–76. INSTICC, Porto (2017). https://doi.org/10.5220/0006140000660076
17. Moher, D., Liberati, A., Tetzlaff, J., Altman, D.G.: Preferred reporting items for systematic reviews and meta-analyses: the PRISMA statement. PLoS Med. **6**, e0000097 (2009). https://doi.org/10.1371/journal.pmed.1000097
18. Jackson, C.L., Bolen, S., Brancati, F.L., Batts-Turner, M.L., Gary, T.L.: A systematic review of interactive computer-assisted technology in diabetes care. J. Gen. Intern. Med. **21**, 105–110 (2006). https://doi.org/10.1007/s11606-006-0242-5

19. Martínez, A., Everss, E., Rojo-Álvarez, J.L., Figal, D.P., García-Alberola, A.: A systematic review of the literature on home monitoring for patients with heart failure. J. Telemedicine Telecare **12**, 234–241 (2006). https://doi.org/10.1258/135763306777889109

20. Chaudhry, S.I., Phillips, C.O., Stewart, S.S., Riegel, B., Mattera, J.A., Jerant, A.F., Krumholz, H.M.: Telemonitoring for patients with chronic heart failure: a systematic review. J. Card. Fail. **13**, 56–62 (2007). https://doi.org/10.1016/j.cardfail.2006.09.001

21. Clark, R.A., Inglis, S.C., Mcalister, F.A., Cleland, J.G.F., Stewart, S.: Telemonitoring or structured telephone support programmes for patients with chronic heart failure: systematic review and meta-analysis. BMJ **334**, 942 (2007). https://doi.org/10.1136/bmj.39156. 536968.55

22. Gysels, M., Higginson, I.J.: Interactive technologies and videotapes for patient education in cancer care: systematic review and meta-analysis of randomised trials. Support. Care Cancer **15**, 7–20 (2006). https://doi.org/10.1007/s00520-006-0112-z

23. Jaana, M., Paré, G.: Home telemonitoring of patients with diabetes: a systematic assessment of observed effects. J. Eval. Clin. Pract. **13**, 242–253 (2007). https://doi.org/10.1111/j. 1365-2753.2006.00686.x

24. Verhoeven, F., Gemert-Pijnen, L.V., Dijkstra, K., Nijland, N., Seydel, E., Steehouder, M.: The contribution of teleconsultation and videoconferencing to diabetes care: a systematic literature review. J. Med. Internet Res. **9**, e37 (2007). https://doi.org/10.2196/jmir.9.5.e37

25. Dang, S., Dimmick, S., Kelkar, G.: Evaluating the evidence base for the use of home telehealth remote monitoring in elderly with heart failure. Telemedicine e-Health **15**, 783–796 (2009). https://doi.org/10.1089/tmj.2009.0028

26. Fox, M.P.: A systematic review of the literature reporting on studies that examined the impact of interactive, computer-based patient education programs. Patient Educ. Couns. **77**, 6–13 (2009). https://doi.org/10.1016/j.pec.2009.02.011

27. Fry, J.P., Neff, R.A.: Periodic prompts and reminders in health promotion and health behavior interventions: systematic review. J. Med. Internet Res. **11**, e16 (2009). https://doi. org/10.2196/jmir.1138

28. García-Lizana, F., Muñoz-Mayorga, I.: Telemedicine for depression: a systematic review. Perspect. Psychiatr. Care **46**, 119–126 (2010). https://doi.org/10.1111/j.1744-6163.2010. 00247.x

29. Polisena, J., Tran, K., Cimon, K., Hutton, B., Mcgill, S., Palmer, K., Scott, R.E.: Home telehealth for chronic obstructive pulmonary disease: a systematic review and meta-analysis. J. Telemedicine Telecare **16**, 120–127 (2010). https://doi.org/10.1258/jtt.2009.090812

30. Polisena, J., Tran, K., Cimon, K., Hutton, B., Mcgill, S., Palmer, K., Scott, R.E.: Home telemonitoring for congestive heart failure: a systematic review and meta-analysis. J. Telemedicine Telecare **16**, 68–76 (2009). https://doi.org/10.1258/jtt.2009.090406

31. Sharp, I.R., Kobak, K.A., Osman, D.A.: The use of videoconferencing with patients with psychosis: a review of the literature. Ann. Gen. Psychiatry **10**, 14 (2011). https://doi.org/10. 1186/1744-859x-10-14

32. Saksena, A.: Computer-based education for patients with hypertension: a systematic review. Health Educ. J. **69**, 236–245 (2010). https://doi.org/10.1177/0017896910364889

33. Bolton, C.E., Waters, C.S., Peirce, S., Elwyn, G.: Insufficient evidence of benefit: a systematic review of home telemonitoring for COPD. J. Eval. Clin. Pract. **17**, 1216–1222 (2010). https://doi.org/10.1111/j.1365-2753.2010.01536.x

34. Kelders, S.M., Kok, R.N., Van Gemert-Pijnen, J.E.W.C.: Technology and adherence in web-based interventions for weight control. In: Haugtvedt, C., Stibe, A. (eds.) Proceedings of the 6th International Conference on Persuasive Technology: Persuasive Technology and Design: Enhancing Sustainability and Health - PERSUASIVE 2011, p. 3. ACM, Columbus (2011). https://doi.org/10.1145/2467803.2467806

35. Ramadas, A., Quek, K., Chan, C., Oldenburg, B.: Web-based interventions for the management of type 2 diabetes mellitus: a systematic review of recent evidence. Int. J. Med. Inform. **80**, 389–405 (2011). https://doi.org/10.1016/j.ijmedinf.2011.02.002

36. Baron, J., Mcbain, H., Newman, S.: The impact of mobile monitoring technologies on glycosylated hemoglobin in diabetes: a systematic review. J. Diab. Sci. Technol. **6**, 1185–1196 (2012). https://doi.org/10.1177/193229681200600524

37. Cassimatis, M., Kavanagh, D.J.: Effects of type 2 diabetes behavioural telehealth interventions on glycaemic control and adherence: a systematic review. J. Telemedicine Telecare **18**, 447–450 (2012). https://doi.org/10.1258/jtt.2012.gth105

38. Cheng, S.K., Dizon, J.: Computerised cognitive behavioural therapy for insomnia: a systematic review and meta-analysis. Psychother. Psychosom. **81**, 206–216 (2012). https://doi.org/10.1159/000335379

39. Ciere, Y., Cartwright, M., Newman, S.P.: A systematic review of the mediating role of knowledge, self-efficacy and self-care behaviour in telehealth patients with heart failure. J. Telemedicine Telecare **18**, 384–391 (2012). https://doi.org/10.1258/jtt.2012.111009

40. Frazetta, D., Willet, K., Fairchild, R.: A systematic review of smartphone application use for type 2 diabetic patients. Online J. Nurs. Inform. (OJNI) **16**(3) (2012)

41. Kennedy, C.M., Powell, J., Payne, T.H., Ainsworth, J., Boyd, A., Buchan, I.: Active assistance technology for health-related behavior change: an interdisciplinary review. J. Med. Internet Res. **14**, e80 (2012). https://doi.org/10.2196/jmir.1893

42. Lieffers, J.R.L., Hanning, R.M.: Dietary assessment and self-monitoring: with nutrition applications for mobile devices. Can. J. Diet. Pract. Res. **73**, e253–e260 (2012). https://doi.org/10.3148/73.3.2012.e253

43. Bacigalupo, R., Cudd, P., Littlewood, C., Bissell, P., Hawley, M.S., Woods, H.B.: Interventions employing mobile technology for overweight and obesity: an early systematic review of randomized controlled trials. Obes. Rev. **14**, 279–291 (2012). https://doi.org/10.1111/obr.12006

44. Blackman, K.C., Zoellner, J., Berrey, L.M., Alexander, R., Fanning, J., Hill, J.L., Estabrooks, P.A.: Assessing the internal and external validity of mobile health physical activity promotion interventions: a systematic literature review using the RE-AIM framework. J. Med. Internet Res. **15**, e224 (2013). https://doi.org/10.2196/jmir.2745

45. Buchholz, S.W., Wilbur, J., Ingram, D., Fogg, L.: Physical activity text messaging interventions in adults: a systematic review. Worldviews Evid.-Based Nurs. **10**, 163–173 (2013). https://doi.org/10.1111/wvn.12002

46. Connelly, J., Kirk, A., Masthoff, J., Macrury, S.: The use of technology to promote physical activity in type 2 diabetes management: a systematic review. Diabet. Med. **30**, 1420–1432 (2013). https://doi.org/10.1111/dme.12289

47. El-Gayar, O., Timsina, P., Nawar, N., Eid, W.: A systematic review of IT for diabetes self-management: are we there yet? Int. J. Med. Inform. **82**, 637–652 (2013). https://doi.org/10.1016/j.ijmedinf.2013.05.006

48. Foster, C., Richards, J., Thorogood, M., Hillsdon, M.: Remote and web 2.0 interventions for promoting physical activity. Cochrane Database Syst. Rev. (2013). https://doi.org/10.1002/14651858.cd010395.pub2

49. Geraedts, H., Zijlstra, A., Bulstra, S.K., Stevens, M., Zijlstra, W.: Effects of remote feedback in home-based physical activity interventions for older adults: a systematic review. Patient Educ. Couns. **91**, 14–24 (2013). https://doi.org/10.1016/j.pec.2012.10.018

50. Belisario, J.S.M., Huckvale, K., Greenfield, G., Car, J., Gunn, L.H.: Smartphone and tablet self management apps for asthma. Cochrane Database Syst. Rev. (2013). https://doi.org/10.1002/14651858.cd010013.pub2

51. Moorhead, S.A., Hazlett, D.E., Harrison, L., Carroll, J.K., Irwin, A., Hoving, C.: A new dimension of health care: systematic review of the uses, benefits, and limitations of social media for health communication. J. Med. Internet Res. **15**, e85 (2013). https://doi.org/10.2196/jmir.1933

52. Pal, K., Eastwood, S.V., Michie, S., Farmer, A.J., Barnard, M.L., Peacock, R., Murray, E.: Computer-based diabetes self-management interventions for adults with type 2 diabetes mellitus. Cochrane Database Syst. Rev. (2010). https://doi.org/10.1002/14651858. cd008776

53. Tao, D., Or, C.K.: Effects of self-management health information technology on glycaemic control for patients with diabetes: a meta-analysis of randomized controlled trials. J. Telemedicine Telecare **19**, 133–143 (2013). https://doi.org/10.1177/1357633x13479701

54. Vugt, M.V., Wit, M.D., Cleijne, W.H., Snoek, F.J.: Use of behavioral change techniques in web-based self-management programs for type 2 diabetes patients: systematic review. J. Med. Internet Res. **15**, e279 (2013). https://doi.org/10.2196/jmir.2800

55. Alvarez-Jimenez, M., Alcazar-Corcoles, M., González-Blanch, C., Bendall, S., Mcgorry, P., Gleeson, J.: Online, social media and mobile technologies for psychosis treatment: a systematic review on novel user-led interventions. Schizophr. Res. **156**, 96–106 (2014). https://doi.org/10.1016/j.schres.2014.03.021

56. Bort-Roig, J., Gilson, N.D., Puig-Ribera, A., Contreras, R.S., Trost, S.G.: Measuring and influencing physical activity with smartphone technology: a systematic review. Sports Med. **44**, 671–686 (2014). https://doi.org/10.1007/s40279-014-0142-5

57. Conway, A., Inglis, S.C., Clark, R.A.: Effective technologies for noninvasive remote monitoring in heart failure. Telemedicine e-Health **20**, 531–538 (2014). https://doi.org/10.1089/tmj.2013.0267

58. Grustam, A.S., Severens, J.L., Nijnatten, J.V., Koymans, R., Vrijhoef, H.J.M.: Cost-effectiveness of telehealth interventions for chronic heart failure patients: a literature review. Int. J. Technol. Assess. Health Care **30**, 59–68 (2014). https://doi.org/10.1017/s0266462313000779

59. Hawley-Hague, H., Boulton, E., Hall, A., Pfeiffer, K., Todd, C.: Older adults' perceptions of technologies aimed at falls prevention, detection or monitoring: a systematic review. Int. J. Med. Inform. **83**, 416–426 (2014). https://doi.org/10.1016/j.ijmedinf.2014.03.002

60. Lazar, A., Thompson, H., Demiris, G.: A systematic review of the use of technology for reminiscence therapy. Health Educ. Behav. **41**, 51S–61S (2014). https://doi.org/10.1177/1090198114537067

61. Nakamura, N., Koga, T., Iseki, H.: A meta-analysis of remote patient monitoring for chronic heart failure patients. J. Telemedicine Telecare **20**, 11–17 (2013). https://doi.org/10.1177/1357633x13517352

62. Ngo, J., Engelen, A., Molag, M., Roesle, J., García-Segovia, P., Serra-Majem, L.: A review of the use of information and communication technologies for dietary assessment. Br. J. Nutr. **101**, S102–S120 (2009). https://doi.org/10.1017/s0007114509990638

63. Or, C.K., Tao, D.: Does the use of consumer health information technology improve outcomes in the patient self-management of diabetes? A meta-analysis and narrative review of randomized controlled trials. Int. J. Med. Inform. **83**, 320–329 (2014). https://doi.org/10.1016/j.ijmedinf.2014.01.009

64. Peterson, A.: Improving type 1 diabetes management with mobile tools. J. Diab. Sci. Technol. **8**, 859–864 (2014). https://doi.org/10.1177/1932296814529885

65. Vegting, I., Schrijver, E., Otten, R., Nanayakkara, P.: Internet programs targeting multiple lifestyle interventions in primary and secondary care are not superior to usual care alone in improving cardiovascular risk profile: a systematic review. Eur. J. Intern. Med. **25**, 73–81 (2014). https://doi.org/10.1016/j.ejim.2013.08.008

66. Agboola, S.O., Ju, W., Elfiky, A., Kvedar, J.C., Jethwani, K.: The effect of technology-based interventions on pain, depression, and quality of life in patients with cancer: a systematic review of randomized controlled trials. J. Med. Internet Res. **17**, e65 (2015). https://doi.org/10.2196/jmir.4009

67. Amatya, B., Galea, M., Kesselring, J., Khan, F.: Effectiveness of telerehabilitation interventions in persons with multiple sclerosis: a systematic review. Multiple Sclerosis Relat. Disord. **4**, 358–369 (2015). https://doi.org/10.1016/j.msard.2015.06.011

68. Bardus, M., Smith, J.R., Samaha, L., Abraham, C.: Mobile phone and web 2.0 technologies for weight management: a systematic scoping review. J. Med. Internet Res. **17**, e259 (2015). https://doi.org/10.2196/jmir.5129

69. Bert, F., Giacometti, M., Gualano, M.R., Siliquini, R.: Smartphones and health promotion: a review of the evidence. J. Med. Syst. **38**, 9995 (2013). https://doi.org/10.1007/s10916-013-9995-7

70. Campbell, J., Porter, J.: Dietary mobile apps and their effect on nutritional indicators in chronic renal disease: a systematic review. Nephrology **20**, 744–751 (2015). https://doi.org/10.1111/nep.12500

71. Chandak, A., Joshi, A.: Self-management of hypertension using technology enabled interventions in primary care settings. Technol. Health Care **23**, 119–128 (2015). https://doi.org/10.3233/THC-140886

72. Farmer, A.J., Mcsharry, J., Rowbotham, S., Mcgowan, L., Ricci-Cabello, I., French, D.P.: Effects of interventions promoting monitoring of medication use and brief messaging on medication adherence for people with type 2 diabetes: a systematic review of randomized trials. Diab. Med. **33**, 565–579 (2015). https://doi.org/10.1111/dme.12987

73. Garabedian, L.F., Ross-Degnan, D., Wharam, J.F.: Mobile phone and smartphone technologies for diabetes care and self-management. Curr. Diab. Rep. **15**, 109 (2015). https://doi.org/10.1007/s11892-015-0680-8

74. Groen, W.G., Kuijpers, W., Oldenburg, H.S., Wouters, M.W., Aaronson, N.K., Harten, W. H.V.: Empowerment of cancer survivors through information technology: an integrative review. J. Med. Internet Res. **17**, e270 (2015). https://doi.org/10.2196/jmir.4818

75. Huang, Z., Tao, H., Meng, Q., Jing, L.: MANAGEMENT OF ENDOCRINE DISEASE: effects of telecare intervention on glycemic control in type 2 diabetes: a systematic review and meta-analysis of randomized controlled trials. Eur. J. Endocrinol. **172**, R93–R101 (2014). https://doi.org/10.1530/eje-14-0441

76. Hunt, C.W.: Technology and diabetes self-management: an integrative review. World J. Diab. **6**, 225 (2015). https://doi.org/10.4239/wjd.v6.i2.225

77. Kim, A.R., Park, H.A.: Web-based self-management support interventions for cancer survivors: a systematic review and meta-analyses. MedInfo (2015). https://doi.org/10.3233/978-1-61499-564-7-142

78. Laranjo, L., Arguel, A., Neves, A.L., Gallagher, A.M., Kaplan, R., Mortimer, N., Mendes, G.A., Lau, A.Y.S.: The influence of social networking sites on health behavior change: a systematic review and meta-analysis. J. Am. Med. Inform. Assoc. **22**, 243–256 (2014). https://doi.org/10.1136/amiajnl-2014-002841

79. Lundell, S., Holmner, Å., Rehn, B., Nyberg, A., Wadell, K.: Telehealthcare in COPD: a systematic review and meta-analysis on physical outcomes and dyspnea. Respir. Med. **109**, 11–26 (2015). https://doi.org/10.1016/j.rmed.2014.10.008

80. Mateo, G.F., Granado-Font, E., Ferré-Grau, C., Montaña-Carreras, X.: Mobile phone apps to promote weight loss and increase physical activity: a systematic review and meta-analysis. J. Med. Internet Res. **17**, e253 (2015). https://doi.org/10.2196/jmir.4836

81. Pedone, C., Lelli, D.: Systematic review of telemonitoring in COPD: an update. Pneumonol. Alergol. Pol. **83**, 476–484 (2015). https://doi.org/10.5603/piap.2015.0077

82. Riazi, H., Larijani, B., Langarizadeh, M., Shahmoradi, L.: Managing diabetes mellitus using information technology: a systematic review. J. Diab. Metab. Disord. **14**, 49 (2015). https://doi.org/10.1186/s40200-015-0174-x

83. Richards, D., Richardson, T.: Computer-based psychological treatments for depression: a systematic review and meta-analysis. Clin. Psychol. Rev. **32**, 329–342 (2012). https://doi.org/10.1016/j.cpr.2012.02.004

84. Tildesley, H.D., Po, M.D., Ross, S.A.: Internet blood glucose monitoring systems provide lasting glycemic benefit in type 1 and 2 diabetes. Med. Clin. North Am. **99**, 17–33 (2015). https://doi.org/10.1016/j.mcna.2014.08.019

85. Arambepola, C., Ricci-Cabello, I., Manikavasagam, P., Roberts, N., French, D.P., Farmer, A.: The impact of automated brief messages promoting lifestyle changes delivered via mobile devices to people with type 2 diabetes: a systematic literature review and meta-analysis of controlled trials. J. Med. Internet Res. **18**, e86 (2016). https://doi.org/10.2196/jmir.5425

86. Beishuizen, C.R., Stephan, B.C., Gool, W.A.V., Brayne, C., Peters, R.J., Andrieu, S., Kivipelto, M., Soininen, H., Busschers, W.B., Charante, E.P.M.V., Richard, E.: Web-based interventions targeting cardiovascular risk factors in middle-aged and older people: a systematic review and meta-analysis. J. Med. Internet Res. **18**, e55 (2016). https://doi.org/10.2196/jmir.5218

87. Chen, Y.-R.R., Schulz, P.J.: The effect of information communication technology interventions on reducing social isolation in the elderly: a systematic review. J. Med. Internet Res. **18**, 18 (2016). https://doi.org/10.2196/jmir.4596

88. Christensen, J., Valentiner, L.S., Petersen, R.J., Langberg, H.: The effect of game-based interventions in rehabilitation of diabetics: a systematic review and meta-analysis. Telemed. e-Health **22**, 789–797 (2016). https://doi.org/10.1089/tmj.2015.0165

89. Matthews, J., Win, K.T., Oinas-Kukkonen, H., Freeman, M.: Persuasive technology in mobile applications promoting physical activity: a systematic review. J. Med. Syst. **40**, 72 (2016). https://doi.org/10.1007/s10916-015-0425-x

90. Shingleton, R.M., Palfai, T.P.: Technology-delivered adaptations of motivational interviewing for health-related behaviors: a systematic review of the current research. Patient Educ. Couns. **99**, 17–35 (2016). https://doi.org/10.1016/j.pec.2015.08.005

91. Ghapanchi, A.H., Aurum, A.: Antecedents to IT personnels intentions to leave: a systematic literature review. J. Syst. Softw. **84**, 238–249 (2011). https://doi.org/10.1016/j.jss.2010.09.022

92. Queirós, A., Santos, M., Rocha, N.P., Cerqueira, M.: Technologies for ageing in place to support community-dwelling older adults. In: 2017 12th Iberian Conference on Information Systems and Technologies (CISTI) (2017). https://doi.org/10.23919/cisti.2017.7975990

93. Queirós, A., Pereira, L., Santos, M., Rocha, N.P.: Technologies for ageing in place to support the empowerment of patients with chronic diseases. In: Rocha, Á., Correia, A.M., Adeli, H., Reis, L.P., Costanzo, S. (eds.) WorldCIST 2017. AISC, vol. 570, pp. 795–804. Springer, Cham (2017). https://doi.org/10.1007/978-3-319-56538-5_80

94. Kaplan, A.M., Haenlein, M.: Users of the world, unite! The challenges and opportunities of social media. Bus. Horiz. **53**, 59–68 (2010). https://doi.org/10.1016/j.bushor.2009.09.003

95. Boggatz, T., Meinhart, C.M.: Health promotion among older adults in Austria: a qualitative study. J. Clin. Nurs. **26**, 1106–1118 (2017). https://doi.org/10.1111/jocn.13603

96. Southard, B.H., Southard, D.R., Nuckolls, J.: Clinical trial of an internet-based case management system for secondary prevention of heart disease. J. Cardiopulm. Rehabil. **23**, 341–348 (2003). https://doi.org/10.1097/00008483-200309000-00003

97. Consolvo, S., Klasnja, P., Mcdonald, D.W., Avrahami, D., Froehlich, J., Legrand, L., Libby, R., Mosher, K., Landay, J.A.: Flowers or a robot army? In: McCarthy, J., Scott, J., Woo, W. (eds) Proceedings of the 10th International Conference on Ubiquitous Computing - UbiComp 2008, pp. 54–63. ACM, Seoul (2008). https://doi.org/10.1145/1409635. 1409644

98. Dickens, A.P., Richards, S.H., Greaves, C.J., Campbell, J.L.: Interventions targeting social isolation in older people: a systematic review. BMC Public Health 11, 647 (2011). https://doi.org/10.1186/1471-2458-11-647

99. Holt-Lunstad, J., Smith, T., Layton, J.: Social relationships and mortality risk: a meta-analytic review. SciVee, e1000316 (2010). https://doi.org/10.4016/19865.01

100. Chronic Diseases and Associated Risk Factors in Australia. Australian Institute of Health and Welfare, Canberra (2006). ISBN 978-1-74024-619-4

101. Thrall, J.H.: Prevalence and costs of chronic disease in a health care system structured for treatment of acute illness. Radiology 235, 9–12 (2005). https://doi.org/10.1148/radiol. 2351041768

102. Bonow, R.O.: ACC/AHA clinical performance measures for adults with chronic heart failure: a report of the American College of Cardiology/American Heart Association task force on performance measures (writing committee to develop heart failure clinical performance measures): endorsed by the heart failure society of America. Circulation 112, 1853–1887 (2005). https://doi.org/10.1161/circulationaha.105.170072

103. Calvo, G.S., Gómez-Suárez, C., Soriano, J., Zamora, E., Gónzalez-Gamarra, A., González-Béjar, M., Jordán, A., Tadeo, E., Sebastián, A., Fernández, G., Ancochea, J.: A home telehealth program for patients with severe COPD: the PROMETE study. Respir. Med. 108, 453–462 (2014). https://doi.org/10.1016/j.rmed.2013.12.003

104. Queirós, A., Carvalho, S., Pavão, J., Da Rocha, N.P.: AAL information based services and care integration. In: Stacey, D., Solé-Casals, J., Fred, A., Gambo, H. (eds.) Proceedings of the 6th International Conference on Health Informatics - HEALTHINF 2013, pp. 403–406. INSTICC, Barcelona (2013). https://doi.org/10.5220/0004326004030406

A Model-Based Approach for Jump Analyses Regarding Strength and Balance
The Human as an Oscillating System

Sandra Hellmers[1(✉)], Sebastian Fudickar[1], Lena Dasenbrock[1],
Andrea Heinks[1], Jürgen M. Bauer[2], and Andreas Hein[1]

[1] Assistive Systems and Medical Technologies,
Carl von Ossietzky University Oldenburg, Oldenburg, Germany
sandra.hellmers@uni-oldenburg.de
[2] Chair of Geriatric Medicine, Heidelberg University,
Agaplesion Bethanien Hospital Heidelberg, Heidelberg, Germany

Abstract. To identify the functional decline as related to aging, geriatric assessments are an established instrument. Within such assessments, the functional ability is evaluated and consists of the three major components: strength, mobility, and balance. Counter movement jumps (CMJ) are well-suited to test these three essential elements of functional ability within a single assessment item. Since common balance measures have been shown to be significantly prone to algorithmic and technical variations, a robust alternative method is required. Thus, we introduce a model-based approach for balance and strength analyses, where the human lower extremities are modeled as an oscillating system during the phase of landing and recovery after a vertical jump. In the System and Control Technology, a transfer function of an oscillating system is described by a second-order delay element (PT2-element), which is characterized by the parameters natural frequency and damping. We analyze the jumps of 30 participants (70–87 years) regarding their jump phases and the mentioned parameters. A linear correlation between jump power and jump height, which are sensitive indicators of the muscle performance and the strength could be confirmed. While a correlation between jump power and spring constant could be observed, a significant relationship between the balance ability and natural frequency could not be identified.

1 Introduction

Geriatric assessments gain an increasing relevance with the ongoing age-related demographic shift. These assessments are well-established to identify early changes associated with functional and cognitive decline [1–3] and usually consist of several tests such as the Short Physical Performance Battery (SPPB) [4], the de Morton Mobility Index (DEMMI) [5] or the Frailty Criteria [6]. It is important to detect early changes in functional decline and to start interventions at

© Springer International Publishing AG, part of Springer Nature 2018
N. Peixoto et al. (Eds.): BIOSTEC 2017, CCIS 881, pp. 354–375, 2018.
https://doi.org/10.1007/978-3-319-94806-5_19

an early stage to slow or stop the progress of functional decline. Therefore, it is important to perform these assessments regularly. But, since these assessments require a lot of time and high personal efforts, they are often performed in irregular and long time intervals. In order to increase the density of assessments, the selection of tests can be reduced and optimized. The possibility of measuring all essential components of functional ability through a single test item instead of several tests leads to a minimized assessment. This reduces the time and effort by keeping the loss of information as low as possible. Another advantage of the reduced assessment items is that stress and potential fatigue for patients can be lowered since stress and fatigue hold the risk that assessment results lose significance [7].

The essential factors of functional ability are balance, strength and mobility [8,9], and are covered by various standardized assessments and tests (see Table 1). Most of these assessments consist of several assessment items. For example, the de Morton Mobility Index (DEMMI) consists of mobility tests (bed, chair), a walk test, and a static and dynamic balance test. The DEMMI can cover the parameters balance and mobility only in the combination of the assessment items. The Stair Climb Power Test is suitable for measuring mobility and strength [10], but the balance ability is not yet considered in this test. Consequently, among the common assessments, only the Counter Movement Jump (CMJ) is well-suited to test all three components, strength, balance, and mobility within a single item.

In detail, the CMJ allows measuring postural stability (balance) [11] via the time to stability (TTS) during the landing and stabilization phase and muscle performance of the lower extremities (strength) via muscle power ahead of jumps [12–15]. Furthermore, the ability of jumping requires an adequate mobility.

However, current CMJ-based balance measures (such as center of pressure COP and time to stabilization TTS) have been shown to be significantly prone to algorithmic and technical variations (Sect. 3.2) and the balance ability, as well as the strength, are evaluated in different phases of the jump (take-off and landing). Therefore, the results might not be related to each other. Thus, we present a new approach to measure postural stability and strength based on the natural frequencies and damping during the landing and recovery phase of CMJs and evaluate its practicability for 30 subjects with an age of 70 to 87 years. We already introduced this approach in [17]. But in contrast to our previous article, we show manual analyses instead of using the System Identification Toolbox of MATLAB in this article. This seems to lead to better results. Additionally, the strength is evaluated classically by the jump power and jump height.

Therefore, the remainder of this article is structured as follows: The biomechanics of a counter movement jump are described in Sect. 2. Related work is presented in Sect. 3. An introduction in the System and Control Technology fundamentals, as well as our model-based approach, follow in Sects. 4 and 5. The study design, the results, and the evaluation are described in Sects. 6 and 7, followed by a discussion and conclusion in Sects. 8 and 9.

Table 1. Selection of geriatric assessment tests, their classification regarding the components of physical fitness (− none, + significant, ++ highly significant), and test duration. The test durations are based on literature and estimated on own experiences (*) in a study with 250 participants [16].

Test	Balance	Strength	Mobility	Test duration
DEMMI	++	-	++	9 min
Static balance	++	-	-	
Dynamic balance	++	-	-	
Walk test	-	-	+	
Transition	-	-	++	
SPPB	++	++	+	15 min
Static balance	++	-	-	
Walk test	-	-	+	
Chair rise test	-	++	+	
Frailty criteria	-	++	+	10–17 min*
Grip strength	-	++	-	
Walk test	-	-	+	
Stair climb power test	-	++	++	2 min*
6 min walk test	-	+	++	6 min
Counter movement jump	++	++	(+)	5 min*

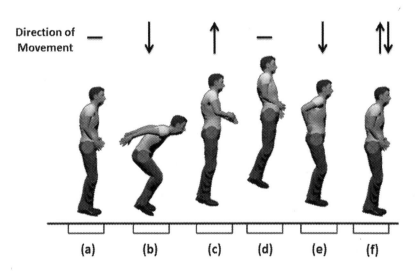

Fig. 1. Major phases of a counter movement jump: standing (a), preparation (b), take-off (c), flight (d), landing (e), and recovery (f). The orange marks indicate the participant's center of mass (COM) in each jump phase. Arrows mark the direction of the movement. This Figure is an extended version of Fig. 1 in [17]. (Color figure online)

2   Biomechanics of the Counter Movement Jump

Counter movement jumps (CMJs) are vertical jumps that are performed from standing. According to [18] they consist of the following phases (as shown in Fig. 1):

The directions of the movements are indicated by arrows. In the first phase (a) the participant is standing. Phase (b) is characterized by the preparation with a downward movement by the flexion of the knees and hips, followed by an immediate and impulsive extension of the knees and hips again to jump vertically up and take-off (c) and flight (d). When reaching the maximum height in the flight phase, the jumper stops for a short moment and then, falls downwards. At the end of the jump, a stage of landing (e) with the absorption of the forces of the impact, and a stage of recovery (f) of the balance can be identified, followed by a standing phase after compensation of the forces (a).

2.1   Technical Measurements via Force Plate and IMU

Jump analyses are typically supported by technology because subjective observations by health professionals are often insufficient, due to the fast and complex progress of a jump. Applied technologies for jump analyses are force platforms, contact mats or optical systems [19]. Inertial measurement units (IMUs) offer the possibility of a flexible, easy to use and low-cost measurement system since there is no need of a laboratory environment and IMUs are cheaper than the other mentioned technologies. Therefore, this article concentrates on technical jump measurements via force platform and IMUs and the comparison between these systems.

Force Platform: Force platforms measure the ground reaction force, which acts on the plate. Figure 2 shows the coordinate orientation and dimensions of the force platform used in our study. The main force, which acts perpendicular to the plate in the vertical direction is Fz. The force in the mediolateral direction is Fy and in the anterior-posterior direction Fx. The force platform in our study measures with a sample rate of 200 Hz. Jump parameters such as power and jump height are calculated automatically by the equations mentioned in Sect. 3.1.

Inertial Measurement Units: Inertial measurement units (IMU) often consist of accelerometers and gyroscopes. In this study, we used IMUs integrated into a hip-worn belt. The coordinate orientation of the IMU and the magnetometer are illustrated in Fig. 2. The acceleration in the vertical direction is called AccY, in mediolateral direction AccX and anterior-posterior direction AccZ. The same applies to the orientation of gyroscope and magnetometer. Additionally, the sensor unit includes a barometer which measures the air pressure and can give useful information about the height. Barometers with a high sensitivity can be used for jump height estimations. Since the barometer used in our study has a sensitivity of about 10 cm, the jump height is calculated based on the equation mentioned in Sect. 3.1.

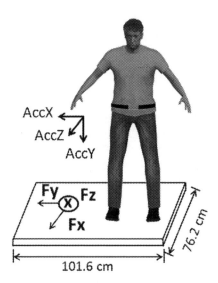

Fig. 2. Coordinate orientation of the force plate and the IMU integrated into a hip-worn belt. The force plate measures the force in the vertical (F_z), mediolateral (F_y), and anterior-posterior direction (F_x). The coordinate orientation of the triaxial sensors of the IMU is illustrated as well.

2.2 Comparison of Force Platform and IMU Measurements

Figure 3 compares the accelerometer measurements in vertical direction of a sequence of three counter movement jumps via IMU (red line) and force platform (blue line). There is an offset of $a = 9.81 \, \mathrm{m/s^2}$ in acceleration due to the gravity, which acts in vertical direction.

The advantages of IMUs in comparison to force plates are lower costs and their mobility, and flexibility. Besides these points, IMUs implicate also metrological advantages: Measurements during the flight phase are possible, which can't be measured by a force plate (no contact between jumper and platform during flight). Therefore, the quality and validity of a jump can be evaluated, since bending legs during flight is not allowed. In the case of bent legs, the flight time can be extended, and results for the jump height are distorted. For example, the third jump in Fig. 3 is a jump with bent legs, which can be identified by the strong positive peak during flight.

Although the counter movement jump is a vertical jump, movements in mediolateral and anterior-posterior direction can be also analyzed by the IMU. The calculation of jump power and jump height is possible with both systems, as well as detailed analyses of the specific jump phases.

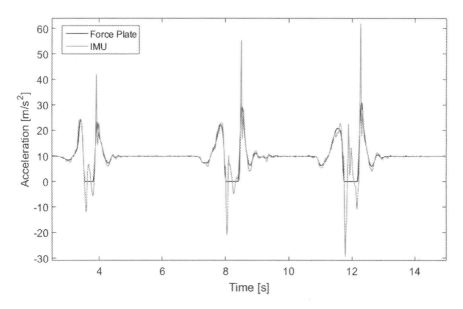

Fig. 3. Acceleration in vertical direction during a sequence of three counter movement jumps. In comparison to the measurement of the force plate (blue line), the IMU (red line) can also evaluate the flight phase of a jump. (Color figure online)

3   Related Work

3.1   Strength: Calculation of Jump Power and Jump Height

The Counter Movement Jump is an established test for strength evaluation of the lower extremities and can show an age-related decline in jump power [20]. According to [14,15] the parameters jump power and jump height seems to be significant indicators for muscle performance and strength and thus, for the functional ability. The jump power P can be calculated by the force acting on the plate during the take-off phase. According to Newton's second law, the force F is equal to the mass m of an object times its acceleration a.

$$F = m \cdot a \tag{1}$$

The power P is defined by the force F times the velocity v:

$$P = F \cdot v = ma \cdot v \tag{2}$$

The velocity v can be calculated by the integration of the acceleration a:

$$v = \int a \cdot dt \tag{3}$$

and the distance s of the center of mass (COM) from the neutral position by

$$s = \int v \cdot dt = \int \int a \cdot dt \tag{4}$$

The parameter jump height h can be estimated by the following equation, which is based on projectile motion equations:

$$h = (v_t \cdot t) - \frac{1}{2} \cdot g \cdot t^2, \tag{5}$$

where v_t is the vertical COM velocity at take-off, t is the time to peak flight and g the gravity. The height represents the maximum vertical coordinate of the COM trajectory following take-off of the jump.

3.2 Balance: TTS, DPSI

Besides measuring muscle strength, force platforms can be utilized to measure dynamic postural stability, which has been shown as related to balance and ankle stabilities. Therefore, functional deficits such as chronic functional ankle instability (FAI) can be indicated based on the recorded vertical, anterior-posterior or mediolateral reaction forces. These measures enable the calculation of time to stabilization (TTS) and variations over time of the center of pressure (COP), the range of motion (ROM), and the dynamic postural stability index (DPSI) as accepted measures for postural stability and FAI. The DPSI is at least as accurate and precise as TTS but provides a comprehensive measurement of dynamic postural stability that is sensitive to changes in 3 directions, since combining three stability indexes and considering as well the subject's weight for the vertical stability (see Eq. 6 [21]).

$$DPSI = \sqrt{\frac{\sum (0 - F_x)^2 + \sum (0 - F_y)^2 + \sum (m - F_z)^2}{n}}, \tag{6}$$

where F_x, F_y, F_z are the forces in anteroposterior (x), mediolateral (y) and vertical(z) direction, m the body weight, and n the number of data points.

Thus, the DPSI has been shown to be a reliable measure [21,22]. While COP and ROM have shown mixed correlations to functional ankle instabilities, TTS is a well-accepted measure to quantify performance. Typically, the force is considered in order to measure the TTS, as a measure of the ability to stabilize posture (which is applied within numerous studies). TTS typically ranges from 0 to 7 s. By investigating 20 TTS calculation methods (as identified via a structured literature review), Fransz et al. [23] have shown that all used threshold-based approaches based on the ground force and 90% can be described based on four aspects: (1) the input signal, (2) signal processing, (3) the stable state (threshold), and (4) the definition of when the (processed) signal is considered stable.

Wikstrom et al. identified a significant variability among TTS measurements due to differences between the TTS calculation methods used in various studies [24]. By evaluating the influence of parameter variations, Fransz et al. [23] have indicated that TTS measures produce non-standardized parameters if estimated via ground reaction forces. They indicated variations of the TTS of up to 56% for sample rate (100 to 1000 Hz), 37% for filter settings (no filter, 40, 15 or

10 Hz), 28–282% for trial lengths (20, 14, 10, 7, 5 and 3 s), as well as calculation methods. Thereby they clarified the difficulties to compare TTS results recorded among different systems based on the power measure.

While these analyses are performed based on single jump measurements for 25 healthy younger adults (20–53 years), its insights will apply due to the indicated computational differences and the drastic effect sizes. Consequently, alternative measures are desired, which are more robust regarding measurement-variations such as sample rates.

Ideally, these measures should be equally applicable to rather mobile measurement devices such as inertial measurement units (IMU), which will be increasingly applied due to their lower price and the higher grade of mobility [25–27].

4   System and Control Technology

According to Newton's third law of motion, a system reacts on a stimulation or force (input signal) by an opposite reaction or force (output signal). The prediction of a reaction of the system to an action is possible if the characteristics of the system are known. In the System and Control Technology the relation between an input F(s) and an output function Y(s), and therefore the system, can be described by a transfer function H(s) (see Fig. 4).

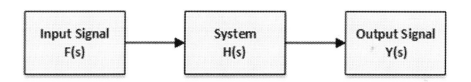

Fig. 4. Relation between input function F(s), the transfer function of a system H(s) and the output function Y(s).

Applying this concept on counter movement jumps, the input function is represented by the impact on the floor after a jump and defines the force which is acting on our system - the human. Consequently, the output function is the landing phase including the recovery and stabilization phase, which forms the reaction on the stimulation.

The mathematical relation between input and output function is given by:

$$Y(s) = H(s)F(s), \qquad (7)$$

where $Y(s)$ is the output function, $H(s)$ the transfer function and $F(s)$ the input function. If assuming, that the system is an oscillating system, the transfer function is described by a second-order delay element (PT2-element).

$$H(s) = \frac{Y(s)}{F(s)} = \frac{a}{cs^2 + bs + 1} \qquad (8)$$

Considering the general second-order system of an oscillator, $H(s)$ can be described by

$$H(s) = \frac{K\omega_0}{s^2 + 2D\omega_0 s + \omega_0^2}, \tag{9}$$

where ω_0 is the natural frequency, K the DC gain of the system and D the damping ratio. By comparison of Eq. 8 with 9, the relationship between the parameters b, c, and the physical parameters ω_0, and D can be found:

$$\omega_0 = \sqrt{\frac{1}{c}} \tag{10}$$

and

$$D = \frac{b\omega_0}{2}. \tag{11}$$

The natural frequency determines how fast the system oscillates during the response. The damping ratio determines how much the system oscillates as the response decays toward a steady state. Figure 5 shows an example to illustrate the damping D and the frequency ω_0. The damping can usually be characterized by an exponential function ($\sim e^{-x}$), which describes the exponential decay of the amplitude.

As we will see in the next section, these parameters might be an alternative possibility to characterize the balance ability, the muscle strength, and allow conclusions to postural stabilization and neuromuscular control.

5   Model-Based Approach

Current CMJ-based balance measures, such as COP and TTS, have been shown to be significantly prone to algorithmic and technical variations (see Sect. 3.2). Therefore, we propose the use of the oscillation behavior as an alternative approach to drawing conclusions about muscle strength, balance ability, postural stability, and neuromuscular control instead of using the DPSI, TTS, COP or ROM. The advantage of the model-based approach of the oscillation behavior (during the landing and recovery phase after a jump) over existing amplification-based methods might be its potentially lower dependability on sample rates, and trial lengths.

Our approach shall enable balance and strength analyses, which are more robust than present methods, independent of measurement setting, and applicable for different measuring devices.

In detail, we aim to model (as schematically illustrated in Fig. 6) the human's lower extremities as a spring that oscillates during the landing and recovery phase. This means that the spring is slack during free fall in the flight phase and will be compressed at the impact on the floor. After maximum compression, the spring depresses during the recovery and stabilization phase to the steady state in one or more oscillations.

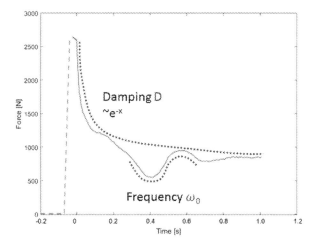

Fig. 5. The phase of landing after a jump: the natural frequency describes the oscillations per time and the damping the decay of oscillations, which can be mathematically described by an exponential function.

From a physical point of view, the spring (assumed as human's lower extremities) can be described by Hooke's law:

$$F = -kx,\tag{12}$$

with the force F, the displacement x and the spring constant k. The frequency can be estimated with

$$\omega_0 = \sqrt{k/m}.\tag{13}$$

This equation shows that the frequency correlates to the spring constant k.

In our model, the spring is characterized by the spring constant. Consequently, if comparing the spring with the muscles of the humans' lower extremities, the spring constant characterizes the stiffness of the muscles in a first approximation and is related to the damping. The natural frequency ω_0 of a system describes the dynamic quality and the ability how fast the system can react on a stimulation. Higher frequencies indicate a system of a higher quality since it reacts faster on a stimulation to compensate the force.

The damping ratio D characterizes the influence within or upon an oscillatory system that has the effect of reducing its oscillations and might also be a relevant parameter for the characterization of the balance ability, the postural stability, and strength. The damping ratio is given by the following equation:

$$D = \frac{c}{2\sqrt{mk}},\tag{14}$$

where c is the damping coefficient, k the spring constant and m the mass.

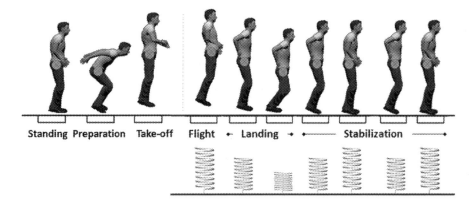

Fig. 6. Comparing of the human's lower extremities with a spring during the landing and stabilization phase of a jump: the spring is slack during the flight phase and will be compressed during the landing. After maximal compression, the spring depresses to steady state in one or more oscillations. This figure is an extended version of Fig. 5 in [17].

6   Study Design

We analyzed 30 participants aged 70–87 years (50% female, 50% male). Each participant performed three counter movement jumps in a sequence with a rest of one minute between the jumps to avoid signs of fatigue. Further characteristics of the study population are listed in Table 2. The group covers a typical range of age, body weight, and body height for the group of pre-frail elderlies.

The jumps were performed on the AMTI AccuPower force platform and with a sensor system integrated into a hip-worn sensor belt. The coordinate orientations of both systems are illustrated in Fig. 2. The sampling rate of the force platform is 200 Hz. The IMU consists of a triaxial accelerometer, gyroscope, and magnetometer measuring with a frequency of 100 Hz.

For standardization, we analyzed the second jump of each participant regarding the jump power, jump height, frequency in anterior-posterior, mediolateral and vertical direction, as well as the spring constant, which is defined by an acting force on the system and the resulting displacement due to this force (see

Table 2. Characteristics of our study population (n = 30) with the minimum (min), maximum (max), and mean-value (mean) as well as the standard deviation (SD) of age in years, body weight in kg and body height in cm.

n = 30	Min	Max	Mean	SD
age [years]	70	87	76.2	4.7
weight [kg]	51.6	104.6	73.9	14.2
height [cm]	145.8	188.7	166.2	11.2

Eq. 12). In contrast to [17] in which we made automatic analyzes of the parameters with the System Identification Toolbox of MATLAB, we decided to make a manual analyze in this article since this seems to lead to better results.

The test procedures were approved by the local ethics committee (ethical vote: Hannover Medical School No. 6948) and conducted in accordance with the Declaration of Helsinki.

7   Results

7.1   Analyses of Jump Phases

Understanding the specific jump phases and the related signals of our measurement systems is essential for the jump evaluation and parameter determination. Figure 7 shows exemplarily the force plate measurement of the counter movement jump of one participant. The blue line shows the acceleration, which was calculated from the measured force on the basis of Eq. 1. The velocity (red line) was calculated by the integration of the acceleration according to Eq. 3 and the center of mass (COM) displacement from neutral position (green line) by Eq. 4. We can clearly separate the phases mentioned in Sect. 2.

In detail: The jump starts from standing (a) with an almost constant acceleration a, velocity v, and COM-displacement s of about zero ($a = v = s = 0$). The transition from standing to the preparation phase (b) can be recognized by changes in the amplitudes of acceleration a and velocity v. In this phase, a downward movement can be observed (negative value of COM-displacement from neutral position) until the velocity amounts zero ($v = 0$). At this point (c) the movement direction changes in an upwards movement (positive values of velocity v). The Take-off with a maximum acceleration is marked by (d). In the flight phase (e) the acceleration amounts $a = -9.81 \, \mathrm{m/s^2}$, which equals the gravity because the plate doesn't measure anything when the participant is in the air and standing in a rest position is defined as $a = 0$. At (f) in the middle of the flight phase the velocity amounts zero again ($v = 0$) and the movement direction changes in a downwards movements after a standstill. The jumper falls downwards until he lands on the plate at point (g). The downward movement continues until (h). In phase (i) the jumper tries to compensate the forces in order to enter the phase of standing or resting (j) again.

The acceleration data of the IMUs can be analyzed in the same way. In comparison to the force plate data, further evaluation of the flight phase are possible.

Figure 8 shows the force measurement of the force plate during a jump. Each phase described in Fig. 7 can also be identified in this Figure. Regarding Eq. 1 the force is defined by $F = m \cdot a$ and thus, has a similar form than the acceleration. It is clear that the mean force acts perpendicular to the force plate in the vertical (z) direction. But there are also reaction forces in the mediolateral (y) and especially in the anterior-posterior (x) direction. In the anterior-posterior direction is a peak during the take-off phase pushing the feet off the ground, and during the landing while the toes and heels strike the ground and compensate the movements.

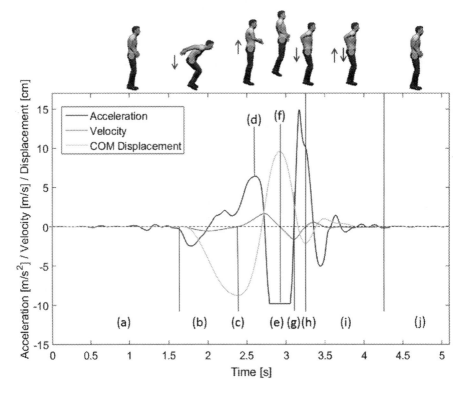

Fig. 7. Force plate measurement of a counter movement jump. The acceleration (blue), velocity (red) and COM-displacement (green) are shown over the time. The jump phases are standing (a), preparation (b) + (c), take-off (d), flight (e) + (f), landing and stabilization (g)–(i) and resting (j). (Color figure online)

7.2 Classical Strength Analyses

The maximum jump power and jump height are well-established parameters to characterize the muscle strength of the lower extremities [14,15]. The calculation of power and jump height are mentioned in Sect. 3.1. Figure 9 shows the jump power P in relation to the jump height h for our study participants. A linear relationship between these parameters can be recognized. The equation of the linear regression is

$$Jump\ Height = 0.0057 \cdot Jump\ Power + 0.064.$$

Therefore, the relationship between strength, jump power, and jump height is given by:

$$Strength \sim Jump\ Power \sim Jump\ Height$$

Table 3 lists the jump characteristics of our study population. It can be seen that we have a broad variety regarding the jump performance and therefore, observe strong as well as weak jumpers.

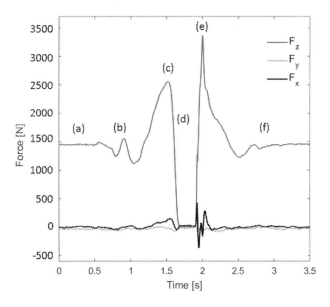

Fig. 8. Force per axes (x, y, z) over time during a counter movement jump. The major phases of the counter movement jump are marked in the graph: standing (a), preparation (b), take-off (c), flight (d), landing (e), and recovery (f). This Figure was already presented in [17].

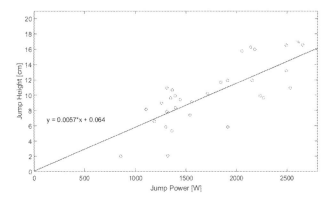

Fig. 9. Jump power P in relation to jump height h. It exists a linear relationship between these parameters.

Table 3. Jump characteristics of our study population with minimum (min), maximum (max), and mean-value (mean), as well as the standard deviation (SD).

n = 30	Min	Max	Mean	SD
Jump power [W]	855.9	2656.9	1723.1	494.5
Jump height [cm]	2.03	16.51	9.95	3.85

7.3   Analyses of the Oscillating Frequency

As already mentioned in Sect. 5 the frequency is an important parameter to characterize the dynamic quality of the system or rather the muscles of the lower extremities. Dynamic postural stability is the ability to maintain stability when transitioning from a dynamic to static state [28]. The ability can be characterized by the DPSI (see Eq. 6). The DPSI was normalized and calculated after landing with both feet in a time interval of three seconds. Figure 10 shows the observed frequencies in anterior-posterior (AP) as well as in the vertical direction in relation to the DPSI. The frequency in mediolateral direction was not considered due to the poor signal to noise ratio since the amplitudes are about two orders of magnitude less than the forces in vertical direction. However, it can be seen that the regression line for the vertical frequency has a positive slope, while there is a negative slope for the frequencies in AP-direction. This indicates that subjects with a higher DPSI react on the stimulation with a higher frequency in vertical direction and with a lower frequency in AP-direction.

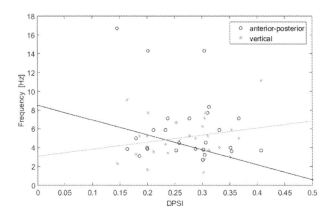

Fig. 10. Frequency in anterior-posterior, and vertical direction in relation to the DPSI.

In order to investigate the relation between frequency and balance ability, the participants are divided into subgroups with a good and a low balance ability. This was done based on the results of the DEMMI test item "tandem stand with eyes closed". If the participants were able to hold this position for 10 s, a good balance ability was assumed. Figure 11 shows the frequencies in relation to the DPSI for both subgroups.

The subgroup with good balance ability shows the similar slopes than in Fig. 10. The group with the lower balance ability shows inverse relationships between frequency and DPSI in both directions. Since a higher frequency indicates a faster reaction on a stimulation and a better dynamic quality an inverse relationship between DPSI and frequency was expected. The reason for the linear relation in vertical direction for the group with good balance ability might be due to the need of a greater compensation movement when jumping higher. This

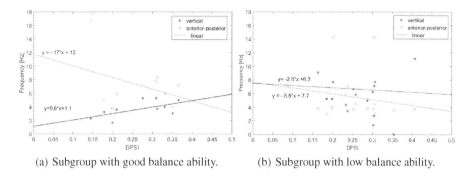

(a) Subgroup with good balance ability.   (b) Subgroup with low balance ability.

Fig. 11. Frequency in anterior-posterior and vertical direction in relation to the DPSI for a subgroup divided by their balance ability.

results in a higher DPSI, although the system can react with high frequencies and a good dynamic quality.

Linear regression analyses show that there is no significant relationship between DPSI and the frequencies for the whole study population and the subgroup with low balance ability. A significant correlation between DPSI and the frequency in vertical direction could only be found for the group with good balance ability. Considering the DPSI as observable element, we performed a stepwise model selection by the Akaike information criterion (AIC). The results of the linear regression are shown in Table 4.

Table 4. Influence of the frequencies on the DPSI for the subgroup with good balance ability. Significant results are marked by an asterisk.

	Estimation	SD	$p > |t|$
Frequency-vertical	0.0609	0.0204	<0.04*
Frequency-AP	−0.0183	0.0089	<0.1

However, further investigations are necessary to analyze the relationship between the natural frequency and balance ability.

7.4 Analyses of Spring Constant

As already mentioned before, the spring constant characterizes the stiffness of the muscles in a first approximation and is related to the damping. Therefore, a relationship between spring constant and muscle strength is expected. The spring constant can be calculated by following equation:

$$k = \frac{F}{\Delta x}, \tag{15}$$

with the force F and the displacement x (cf. Eq. 12 - Hooke's law). The spring constant is calculated at the point of maximum compression during the landing based on the acting force and the displacement of the COM (see Figs. 6 and 7).

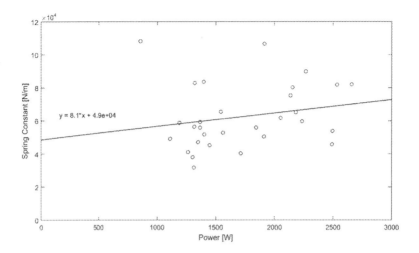

Fig. 12. Spring constant in relation to the jump power. A linear regression shows a significant relationship between these parameters.

The results for the spring constants of the participants regarding the jump power are shown in Fig. 12. A significant linear relationship can be found. Therefore, following correlation is given:

$$Strength \sim Jump\ Power \sim Jump\ Height \sim Spring\ Constant$$

Analog to Sect. 7.3, we considered the jump power as a clearly observable element and performed a stepwise model selection by the AIC. The results of the regression analyses are listed in Table 5. The frequencies have no significant influence on the jump power. But there is an influence of the spring constant and the jump height.

The changes of the jump power for a one unit change of the listed parameters are shown in Table 5. For example, the change of one unit in jump height (1 cm) has an influence of about 89.792 W. The change of 1 unit of the spring constant $(1\,Nm^{-1})$ results in a mean change of 0.009 W.

Table 5. Influence of the spring constant, the jump height, and the frequencies per axis on the jump power. Significant results are marked by an asterisk.

	Estimation	SD	$p > |t|$
Spring constant	0.0091	0.0028	<0.01*
Jump height	89.792	14.357	<0.01*
Frequency AP	−25.448	15.659	0.12
Frequency vertical	−2.372	24.492	0.92

7.5   Influences of Demographic Parameters

In order to clarify if body height, body weight, sex, and age influence the spring constant and the natural frequency, we investigated their correlations. The results of the linear regression are listed in Tables 6 and 7.

This analysis confirms that body height, age, and sex have no influence on the spring constant. Only the body weight has a significant influence, which could be expected due to the relation between spring constant and mass (see Eq. 14).

No influences of the demographic parameters were found for the frequencies in all three directions. The results for the frequency in the vertical direction are representative for all three directions listed in Table 7.

Table 6. Influence of demographic parameters on the spring constant. Significant results are marked by an asterisk.

	Estimation	SD	$p > |t|$
Body weight	1107.97	265.67	<0.01*
Body height	−628.54	477.04	0.19
Age	397.58	672.72	0.56
Sex	53.72	9636.79	0.99

Table 7. Influence of demographic parameters on the natural frequency in vertical direction. No significant influences could be found.

	Estimation	SD	$p > |t|$
Body weight	0.02	12.89	0.60
Body height	0.04	0.07	0.58
Age	−0.13	0.09	0.20
Sex	−1.71	1.49	0.26

8   Discussion

The main purpose of the present study was to develop a more robust analysis strategy than present methods, which is independent of measurement settings and applicable for different measuring devices. Therefore, we proposed to model the human lower extremities as an oscillating system and tried to describe this system by the parameters natural frequency and spring constant, which are the characterization variables (besides the damping ratio) in a transfer function. In order to investigate the suitability and sensitivity of our model, we conducted a prospective study with 30 probands aged 70 and above and analyzed the biomechanics of a jump as well as the resulting signals of our measurement systems. Besides the identification of the single jump phases, we focused on the oscillating behavior in the phase of landing and recovery after a vertical jump. The expected oscillating behavior could be observed in various degrees in all participants. Thus, the suitability and the general validity of our model could be confirmed.

In order to examine the applicability of our proposed model and the corresponding novel parameters for the description of the strength and balance ability, we have analyzed the spring constant and the natural frequency of each jump and investigated their correlation with the common parameters jump height and jump power as representing the strength and the DPSI as representing the balance. The found linear correlation between jump power and jump height are consistent with previous results in literature since they are sensitive indicators of the muscle performance and the muscle strength. A significant linear relation between jump power and spring constant was as well observed. Therefore, the spring constant can be assumed as an alternative and reliable parameter for strength and confirms our model's fundamental assumption that the spring constant characterizes the stiffness of the muscles in a first approximation and is related to the damping.

Between the natural frequency and the DPSI no significant correlation was found, except the relationship between frequency in the vertical direction and DPSI for the subgroup with good balance ability. Since the natural frequency of a system describes the dynamic quality and the ability how fast the system can react on stimulations, higher frequencies indicate a system of a higher quality, because it reacts faster on a stimulation to compensate the force. Therefore, an inverse relationship between DPSI and frequency was expected. An explanation for the linear relation might be the need of a greater compensation movement when jumping higher. This results in a higher DPSI, although the system can react with high frequencies and a good dynamic quality. However, since the oscillating behavior was observed in all jumps, the general validity of our approach could be confirmed.

Our findings confirmed also the independence of the natural frequency from influences of demographic parameters such as age, sex, body height, and body weight. The spring constant was only influenced by the body weight, which was expectable due to the relation between spring constant and mass.

In summary, our model is applicable for different measuring devices and independent of the system's sampling rate since the observed frequencies lie in a range below 20 Hz. Also, the trail length and the filter settings shouldn't influence the frequency. However, our investigations have been carried out on a limited study population (n = 30) and further examinations are necessary to analyze the relationship between frequency and balance ability and to make a systematic and more in-depth analysis regarding the influences of the measurement settings.

9   Conclusion

Counter movement jumps are well-suited to measure the essential parameters of functional ability (mobility, strength, and balance) within a single test. But current CMJ-based balance measures have been shown to be significantly prone to algorithmic and technical variations. Therefore, more robust alternatives are needed. In this article, a model-based approach for balance and strength analyses was introduced, which is based on the System and Control Technology and models the human lower extremities as an oscillating system. Thus, our model might provide the foundation for a new approach to characterize the strength and the ability of balance by the parameters spring constant and natural frequency. The findings of our conducted study with 30 participants (aged 70–87 years) confirmed the general validity of our model and verify the spring constant as a reliable parameter for strength. The significance of the natural frequency to evaluate the balance ability could not be finally found yet and requires further investigations to analyze the relationship between these parameters. Our model seems to be independent of measurement settings and devices since the observed frequency is not influenced by algorithmic and technical variations. In conclusion, a promising new reliable model for the characterization of strength and balance during jumps was presented and its suitability was confirmed in an initial evaluation study.

Acknowledgements. The study is funded by the German Federal Ministry of Education and Research (Project No. 01EL1422D).

References

1. Clegg, A., Young, J., Iliffe, S., Rikkert, M.O., Rockwood, K.: Frailty in elderly people. Lancet **381**(9868), 752–762 (2013)
2. Cruz-Jentoft, A.J., Baeyens, J.P., Bauer, J.M., Boirie, Y., Cederholm, T., Landi, F., Martin, F.C., Michel, J.P., Rolland, Y., Schneider, S.M., et al.: Sarcopenia: European consensus on definition and diagnosis report of the European working group on sarcopenia in older people. Age Ageing **39**, 412–423 (2010)
3. Elsawy, B., Higgins, K.E.: The geriatric assessment. Am. Fam. Phys. **83**(1), 48–56 (2011)
4. Guralnik, J.M., Simonsick, E.M., Ferrucci, L., Glynn, R.J., Berkman, L.F., Blazer, D.G., Scherr, P.A., Wallace, R.B.: A short physical performance battery assessing lower extremity function: association with self-reported disability and prediction of mortality and nursing home admission. J. Gerontol. **49**(2), M85–M94 (1994)
5. de Morton, N.A., Lane, K.: Validity and reliability of the de morton mobility index in the subacute hospital setting in a geriatric evaluation and management population. J. Rehabil. Med. **42**(10), 956–961 (2010)
6. Fried, L.P., Tangen, C.M., Walston, J., Newman, A.B., Hirsch, C., Gottdiener, J., Seeman, T., Tracy, R., Kop, W.J., Burke, G., et al.: Frailty in older adults: evidence for a phenotype. J. Gerontol. Ser. A: Biol. Sci. Med. Sci. **56**(3), M146–M157 (2001)
7. Siglinsky, E., Krueger, D., Ward, R.E., Caserotti, P., Strotmeyer, E.S., Harris, T.B., Binkley, N., Buehring, B.: Effect of age and sex on jumping mechanography and other measures of muscle mass and function. J. Musculoskelet. Neuronal Interact. **15**(4), 301 (2015)
8. Cooper, R., Kuh, D., Cooper, C., Gale, C.R., Lawlor, D.A., Matthews, F., Hardy, R., FALCon and HALCyon study teams: Objective measures of physical capability and subsequent health: a systematic review. Age Ageing **40**(1), 14–23 (2010)

9. Hellmers, S., Steen, E.E., Dasenbrock, L., Heinks, A., Bauer, J.M., Fudickar, S., Hein, A.: Towards a minimized unsupervised technical assessment of physical performance in domestic environments. In: Oliver, N., Czerwinski, M., Matic, A. (eds.) Proceedings of the 11th EAI Conference on Pervasive Computing Technologies for Healthcare, pp. 207–216 (2017)

10. Hellmers, S., Kromke, T., Dasenbrock, L., Heinks, A., Bauer, J.M., Hein, A., Fudickar, S.: Stair climb power measurements via inertial measurement units - towards an unsupervised assessment of strength in domestic environments. In: Fred, A., Gamboa, H., Zwiggelaar, R., Bermdez i Badia, S. (eds.) Proceedings of the 11th International Joint Conference on Biomedical Engineering Systems and Technologies, pp. 39–47 (2018)

11. Granacher, U., Gollhofer, A., Hortobágyi, T., Kressig, R.W., Muehlbauer, T.: The importance of trunk muscle strength for balance, functional performance, and fall prevention in seniors: a systematic review. Sports Med. **43**(7), 627–641 (2013)

12. Buehring, B., Krueger, D., Fidler, E., Gangnon, R., Heiderscheit, B., Binkley, N.: Reproducibility of jumping mechanography and traditional measures of physical and muscle function in older adults. Osteoporos. Int. **26**(2), 819–825 (2015)

13. Rittweger, J., Schiessl, H., Felsenberg, D., Runge, M.: Reproducibility of the jumping mechanography as a test of mechanical power output in physically competent adult and elderly subjects. J. Am. Geriatr. Soc. **52**(1), 128–131 (2004)

14. Dietzel, R., Felsenberg, D., Armbrecht, G.: Mechanography performance tests and their association with sarcopenia, falls and impairment in the activities of daily living-a pilot cross-sectional study in 293 older adults. J. Musculoskelet. Neuronal Interact. **15**(3), 249–256 (2015)

15. Kalyani, R.R., Corriere, M., Ferrucci, L.: Age-related and disease-related muscle loss: the effect of diabetes, obesity, and other diseases. Lancet Diab. Endocrinol. **2**(10), 819–829 (2014)

16. Hellmers, S., Fudickar, S., Büse, C., Dasenbrock, L., Heinks, A., Bauer, J.M., Hein, A.: Technology supported geriatric assessment. In: Wichert, R., Mand, B. (eds.) Ambient Assisted Living. ATSC, pp. 85–100. Springer, Cham (2017). https://doi.org/10.1007/978-3-319-52322-4_6

17. Hellmers, S., Fudickar, S.J., Dasenbrock, L., Heinks, A., Bauer, J.M., Hein, A.: Understanding jump landing as an oscillating system: a model-based approach of balance and strength analyses. In: van den Broek, E., Fred, A., Gamboa, H., Vaz, M. (eds.) HEALTHINF, pp. 159–168 (2017)

18. Palma, S., Silva, H., Gamboa, H., Mil-Homens, P.: Standing jump loft time measurement-an acceleration based method. In: Encarnao, P., Veloso, A. (eds.) Biosignals, no. (2), pp. 393–396 (2008)

19. Bui, H.T., Farinas, M.I., Fortin, A.M., Comtois, A.S., Leone, M.: Comparison and analysis of three different methods to evaluate vertical jump height. Clin. Physiol. Funct. Imaging **35**(3), 203–209 (2015)

20. Michaelis, I., Kwiet, A., Gast, U., Boshof, A., Antvorskov, T., Jung, T., Rittweger, J., Felsenberg, D.: Decline of specific peak jumping power with age in master runners. J. Musculoskelet. Neuronal Interact. **8**(1), 64–70 (2008)

21. Wikstrom, E., Tillman, M., Smith, A., Borsa, P.: A new force-plate technology measure of dynamic postural stability: the dynamic postural stability index. J. Athletic Training **40**(4), 305–309 (2005)

22. Meardon, S., Klusendorf, A., Kernozek, T.: Influence of injury on dynamic postural control in runners. Int. J. Sports Phys. Ther. **11**(3), 366 (2016)

23. Fransz, D.P., Huurnink, A., de Boode, V.A., Kingma, I., van Dieën, J.H.: Time to stabilization in single leg drop jump landings: an examination of calculation methods and assessment of differences in sample rate, filter settings and trial length on outcome values. Gait Posture **41**(1), 63–69 (2015)
24. Wikstrom, E., Tillman, M., Borsa, P.: Detection of dynamic stability deficits in subjects with functional ankle instability. Med. Sci. Sports Exerc. **37**(2), 169–175 (2005)
25. Choukou, M.A., Laffaye, G., Taiar, R.: Reliability and validity of an accelerometric system for assessing vertical jumping performance. Biol. Sport **31**(1), 55 (2014)
26. Elvin, N.G., Elvin, A.A., Arnoczky, S.P.: Correlation between ground reaction force and tibial acceleration in vertical jumping. J. Appl. Biomech. **23**(3), 180 (2007)
27. Milosevic, B., Farella, E.: Wearable inertial sensor for jump performance analysis. In: Proceedings of the 2015 Workshop on Wearable Systems and Applications, pp. 15–20 (2015)
28. Lawson, M., Webster, A., Stenson, M.: Effects of ankle bracing on the performance of the dynamic postural stability index. In: Conference Proceedings on International Journal of Exercise Science, vol. 12, p. 42 (2015)

Regression, Classification and Ensemble Machine Learning Approaches to Forecasting Clinical Outcomes in Ischemic Stroke

Ahmedul Kabir[1], Carolina Ruiz[1(✉)], Sergio A. Alvarez[2],
and Majaz Moonis[3]

[1] Worcester Polytechnic Institute, 100 Institute Road,
Worcester, MA 01609, USA
akabir@wpi.edu, ruiz@cs.wpi.edu
[2] Boston College, Chestnut Hill, MA 02467, USA
alvarez@bc.edu
[3] University Massachusetts Medical School, Worcester, MA 01655, USA
majaz.moonis@umassmeorial.org

Abstract. We applied different machine learning approaches to predict (forecast) the clinical outcome, measured by the modified Rankin Scale (mRS) score, of ischemic stroke patients 90 days after stroke. Regression, multinomial classification, and ordinal regression tasks were considered. M5 model trees followed by bootstrap aggregating as a meta-learning technique produced the best regression results. The same regression technique when used for classification after discretization of the target attribute also performed better than regular multinomial classification. For the ordinal regression task, the logit link function (ordinal logistic regression) outperformed the alternatives. We discuss the methodology used, and compare the results with other standard predictive techniques. We also analyze the results to provide insights into the factors that affect stroke outcomes.

Keywords: Ischemic stroke · mRS score · M5 model tree
Bootstrap aggregating · Ordinal regression

1 Introduction

Stroke is defined as the rapid loss of brain function caused by disturbances in the blood supply to the brain. It is one of the leading causes of death worldwide [1]. There are broadly two types of stroke – ischemic and hemorrhagic. The former occurs due to lack of blood flow to the brain, and the latter is caused by internal bleeding. Ischemic stroke, which accounts for almost 87% of all strokes [2], is the focus of this study. We consider different machine learning approaches that can build predictive models on the clinical data of ischemic stroke patients, with the aim of forecasting clinical outcomes 90 days after stroke. The data were collected retrospectively from the University of Massachusetts Medical School, Worcester, Massachusetts, USA and comprise demographic information, medical history and treatment records of 439 patients.

© Springer International Publishing AG, part of Springer Nature 2018
N. Peixoto et al. (Eds.): BIOSTEC 2017, CCIS 881, pp. 376–402, 2018.
https://doi.org/10.1007/978-3-319-94806-5_20

There are several reasons for wishing to predict how well a stroke patient will recover from stroke. If any such prediction can be made with a reasonable degree of confidence, it may assist medical experts manage stroke more effectively and allocate resources more efficiently. Furthermore, when the predictive models are built from the stroke data, they can reveal information on the factors that affect stroke outcome.

In this paper, the outcome of stroke patients is measured in terms of the modified Rankin Scale (mRS) score, an integer value between 0 and 6 measuring the degree of disability or dependence in daily activities of people who have suffered a stroke [3]. There are three approaches one may use to solve the problem of predicting this value. The first is to treat the target as a numeric attribute and apply some form of regression. The second approach would be to think of the several different mRS scores as different categories, in which case the problem becomes that of multinomial classification. The third approach is to note the ordered nature of the target attribute, and use ordinal regression techniques for prediction. We have addressed the prediction task from all three perspectives.

The outcome prediction of the patients is performed on the data we have about the patient at the time of discharge. The independent attributes in our study consist of demographic information, medical history and treatment records. The response or target attribute is mRS-90, the mRS score at 90 days following stroke onset (described in Table 1). Treating mRS scores as integer values, we perform regression analysis, in which we find that M5 model trees used in tandem with bootstrap aggregating (bagging) significantly outperforms other common regression methods such as linear regression. We then treat the target as a multinomial categorical attribute and apply several classification techniques such as logistic regression and C4.5 decision trees. Our studies show that classification using the aforementioned regression technique followed by translation of the target to a discrete value performs better than the standard classification methods mentioned. Finally, we treat mRS-90 as an ordered categorical variable, and use methods of ordinal regression using different link functions, of which the logit link function yield the best results. We visualize and analyze the models obtained through the different algorithms. The work presented in this paper is an extended and enhanced version of the work presented in a conference paper by the same authors [4].

In Sect. 2 of this paper, we present some background information on the different techniques used, and mention some related work from the literature. The methodology of our research is described in Sect. 3. That section deals with the steps that are taken to prepare and preprocess the data, and describes in full details the parameter choices we made in our prediction techniques. Section 4 presents a comparison of different prediction methods, and analyzes the results to gain more insights about the models discovered. Section 5 concludes with a summary of findings and directions for future work.

2   Background and Related Work

2.1   Modified Rankin Scale

The modified Rankin Scale (mRS) measure is the most widely used clinical outcome measure for stroke. It was first introduced by Rankin [3] and later modified to its current form by a group of researchers during the late 1980s [5]. The score is an integer between 0 and 6 signifying the various degrees of impairment caused by stroke, with 0 being the least amount of impairment and 6 being death. Table 1 presents a summary description of the different mRS scores. This study, for reasons described later, excludes patients with mRS scores = 6.

Table 1. Different mRS scores and their description [6].

Score	Description
0	No symptoms
1	No significant disability
2	Slight disability
3	Moderate disability: requires assistance
4	Moderately severe disability
5	Severe disability: patient bedridden
6	Death

Usually the score is assessed by a medical expert with the help of a questionnaire at various stages of stroke. Figure 1 depicts a simplified questionnaire developed by [7] that is used to assess mRS scores. In this study, the mRS scores are recorded in three different stages. The first is before admission, in which the degree of disability the patient had before the onset of stroke is retrospectively assessed. The next is at the time of discharge from the hospital after initial treatment of stroke. The last one is at 90 days after stroke onset, the score this study attempts to predict.

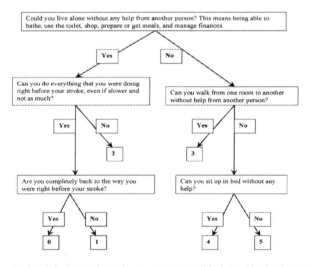

Fig. 1. A simplified questionnaire to assess modified Rankin Scale score [7].

2.2 M5 Model Trees

Among the regression methods we experimented with, the model trees built with the M5 algorithm was found to be very fruitful. We therefore provide some background on what they are and how they are constructed. A model tree is essentially a form of decision tree - a tree where each node represents a choice among several alternatives, and each leaf represents a decision that can be reached by following a series of choices at each node starting from the root of the tree [8]. The decision tree can perform both classification and regression. In classification, the leaf represents one of the classes the instance is to be categorized to. In regression, on the other hand, the leaf outputs a numeric value of the target attribute instead of a class [9]. A regression tree is simply a decision tree that performs regression. A model tree is a special form of regression tree where the decision in each leaf is a not a real number, but is itself a multivariate linear model. The numeric value predicted by the tree for a given test data instance is obtained by evaluating the linear equation in the leaf of the branch where the data instance belongs. Quinlan [10] described an algorithm, called M5, that is used to construct such a tree. Some improvements to the algorithm were made by [11].

According to the M5 algorithm, the construction of the model tree is a two-stage process. In the first stage, a decision tree induction algorithm is used which employs a splitting criterion that minimizes the intra-subset variability in the values down from the root through the branch to the node. The measure of variability is the standard deviation of the values that reach that node. The M5 algorithm examines all attributes and possible split points to choose the one that maximizes the expected reduction in standard deviation. The splitting process stops when the instances reaching a leaf have low variability or when fewer than a specified threshold number of instances remain [12]. In the second stage, the tree is pruned starting from the leaves upward. A linear regression model is computed for every interior node, including only the attributes tested in the sub-tree rooted at that node. As the final model for this node, M5 selects either this linear model or the model subtree built in the first stage, depending on which has the lower estimated error. If the linear model is chosen, pruning takes place and the subtree at this node is converted to a leaf containing this linear model [10].

Essentially the M5 model tree, like any decision tree, divides the problem space into several subspaces based on the branching decisions of the tree. It then fits separate linear models to the data points in each subspace. So, the model returned by the M5 algorithm is a piecewise linear model. Figure 2 illustrates this concept.

2.3 Bootstrap Aggregating

Our experiments show that using a meta-learning technique, called Bootstrap aggregating, greatly improves the prediction performance. Bootstrap aggregating, commonly known as "bagging", is an ensemble learning technique. Bagging relies on the aggregated predictions of multiple versions of a model rather than one single model. The first step in bagging is to create a bootstrap - a sample with replacements of the data instances drawn according to a uniform probability distribution. Each bootstrap is then fed separately to a predicting algorithm (can either be classification or regression) to build several predictor versions. When an unlabeled instance is given, each version of the predictor generates a separate prediction output. These individual outputs are then aggregated according to the type of task in question. For classification, a majority vote is taken. For the task of regression, the average of the predictor versions is taken [13]. Figure 3 summarizes the bagging process. Bagging improves generalization error by reducing the variance of the individual predictive models. If a base predictor is unstable - if it is not robust to fluctuations - the bagging process helps to stabilize it [8].

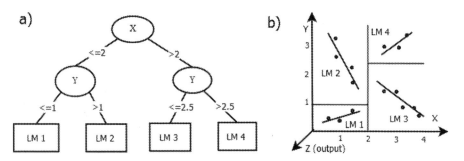

Fig. 2. (a) An example model tree built with the M5 algorithm with input attributes X and Y. Linear models LM 1 to LM 4 are built in the leaves. (b) The corresponding problem space showing separate subspaces defined by the tree and how each linear model fits points in the subspace. With permissions of both the authors and the publisher, this figure is adopted from [4].

The size and the number of the bootstraps are parameter that can be changed. In the most common case, the size of each bootstrap B_i is n, the same as that of the entire training set. In this case, on an average B_i contains approximately 63% of the original training data since each sample has a probability of $1 - (1 - 1/n)^n$ of being picked, which converges to about 0.63 for sufficiently large n [14]. This is because sampling is done with replacement, resulting in duplicate instances in each bootstrap.

2.4 Ordinal Regression

The different scores in the target attribute in our study clearly have an ordinal property. It is apparent that mRS-90 = 0 indicates a better outcome than mRS-90 = 1, which in turn indicates a better outcome than mRS-90 = 2, and so on. We can take advantage of this ordered nature of the target output by using ordinal regression, a prediction technique designed for ordered categories. This method was first introduced in [15]. The task of ordinal regression arises frequently in different domains, especially when human preferences play a major role [16].

Ordinal regression shares properties of both classification and regression. Like in classification, the output is a finite set. Like regression, there exists an ordering among the elements of the output attribute [16]. The ordinal regression algorithm assumes that the ordinal variable (the output attribute) is a manifestation of a latent continuous variable associated with the output, and the categories can be thought of as contiguous intervals on that continuous scale [17]. Ordinal regression uses a link function to transform the cumulative probabilities of the ordered variable to a continuous variable [18].

Some examples of link functions are: logit, probit and complementary log-log (cloglog). Ordinal regression with a logit link function is similar to logistic regression, so a comparison of the two may serve as a good explanation of how ordinal regression works.

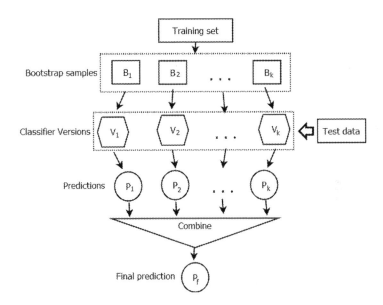

Fig. 3. Summary of the process of bagging. From the training set, k bootstraps are created. Each bootstrap B_1, ..., B_k is used to build predictor versions V_1, ..., V_k which make separate predictions P_1, ..., P_k. The final prediction P_f is a combination (average for regression, majority voting for classification) of all the predictions. With permissions of both the authors and the publisher, this figure is adopted from [4].

Let us first start with the binary logistic regression model. For consistency with the literature, we use in this subsection the term variable instead of attribute. The predictive attributes are referred to as independent variables and the target attribute is referred to as response variable. Let $X = \{X_1, ..., X_m\}$ be the vector of independent variable and Y be the response variable with possible outcomes 0 and 1. Let p be the probability that $Y = 1$. That is, $p = P(Y = 1)$. In logistic regression, it is assumed that there is a linear relationship between X and the logit transform of p:

$$logit = \ln\left(\frac{p}{1-p}\right) = \alpha + \beta_1 X_1 + ... + \beta_m X_m \qquad (1)$$

where α is a constant intercept and $\beta_{1...m}$ are coefficients of $X_{1...m}$.

If the response variable Y is discrete with more than two categories, then one of the categories is designated as a reference category, and a logit transform is calculated for each of the remaining categories. Suppose Y has k categories $1, ..., k$, and the probability of category i is given by $P(Y = i) = p_i$ for $i = 1, ..., k$. If k is the reference category, then logits for the other $k - 1$ categories are defined by

$$logit(Y = i) = \ln\left(\frac{p_i}{p_k}\right) = \alpha_i + \beta_{i1}X_1 + \ldots + \beta_{im}X_m, \quad i = 1, \ldots, k-1 \qquad (2)$$

Now let us examine the case in which the response variable Y is ordinal. The multinomial logistic regression model of Eq. 2 will not make use of the information about the ordering. One way to take advantage of the ordering is to use cumulative probabilities and cumulative logits. Considering k ordered categories the cumulative probabilities are defined by $P(Y \leq i) = p_1 +, \ldots, + p_i$ and the cumulative logits are defined by

$$logit(Y \leq i) = \ln\left(\frac{P(Y \leq i)}{1 - P(Y \leq i)}\right) = \ln\left(\frac{p_1 + \ldots + p_i}{p_{i+1} + \ldots + p_k}\right)$$

$$= \alpha_i + \beta_{i1}X_1 + \ldots + \beta_{im}X_m, \quad i = 1, \ldots, k-1 \qquad (3)$$

However, for ordered categories under certain conditions, the logistic coefficients do not depend on i, resulting in only one common β_{ij} for each covariate. In this case the cumulative odds are given by $e^{\alpha_i}e^{\beta_1 X_1 + \ldots + \beta_m X_m}$, which means that the k odds for each category i differ only with regards to the intercepts α_i. This means that instead of the $k-1$ different linear models of Eqs. 2 and 3 can be expressed by one linear model and the $k-1$ intercepts $\alpha_{1\ldots k-1}$. The $\alpha_{1\ldots k-1}$ can be thought of as the cut-off points in the underlying latent continuous variable. The equations and explanations in this subsection are adapted from [19].

Apart from the logit function shown in our example, other link functions following the same basic principles of ordinal regression may also be used. Table 2 shows a summary of the different link functions we experimented with.

Table 2. Different link functions used in the ordinal regression experiments in this paper. The formulae are given in terms of the probability p. For the probit function, φ is the cumulative distribution function for the normal distribution [18].

Link function	Formula
Logit	$\ln\left(\frac{p}{1-p}\right)$
Probit	$\varphi^{-1}(p)$
Complementary log log (cloglog)	$\ln(-\ln(1-p))$
Cauchit	$\tan(\pi(p - 1/2))$

2.5   Related Work

There have been numerous studies that focus on the outcome of stroke patients, using the mRS-90 score as a measure of stroke outcome. In most cases though, the mRS-90 score has been dichotomized so that the task of prediction becomes a case of binary classification. In clinical trials it is common to build a multivariate logistic regression model on the patients' data and analyze the results to understand the influence of different factors. Most of these studies focus on one particular treatment or condition, the effect of which on stroke outcome needs to be examined. The coefficients and odds ratios computed from the logistic regression model may lead to useful conclusions. We present here a selected few among such studies. [20] reported that using statins for treatment of ischemic stroke improved stroke outcome since the statins obtained an odds ratio of 1.57 in a logistic regression model predicting mRS-90 $\leq$ 2. This means that the patients who are administered statins have 1.57 times the probability of attaining mRS-90 $\leq$ 2 than those who are not treated with statins. A similar study with a different goal was done in [21] – the authors studied the effects of atrial fibrillation in stroke outcome. [22] studied hyperglycemia as a factor of stroke and concluded that it is associated with poor outcome. It was found in [23] that successful revascularization is associated with good outcome. [24] reported that leukoaraiosis is a factor influencing poor 90-day outcome of stroke. All the above studies dichotomized the mRS score to two levels – one consisting of mRS-90 $\leq$ 2 and the other of mRS > 2.

Some studies, however, have duly observed the ordinal nature of the measure of stroke outcome, and taken advantage of this by using ordinal regression. [25] used ordinal regression for their study on how comorbid conditions affect stroke outcome. In [26] it was observed that choosing an ordinal rather than a binary method of analysis allows trials of stroke outcome to have much smaller sample size for a given statistical power. [27] used ordinal logistic regression to study the effectiveness of angiotensin-receptor blocker in improving stroke outcome based on the modified Rankin score.

A point to note, however, is that the studies mentioned are concerned more with the details of the regression models – binary or ordinal, and less with the evaluation of the models' performance from a prediction perspective. There have not been many studies that focused solely on predicting the stroke outcome and employing machine learning models to assist in the prediction task. [28] aimed to predict stroke outcome using linear regression, but used the functional independence measure (FIM) which is a scale that measures stroke recovery in terms of activities of daily living [29]. A similar effort of predicting FIM was made by in [30]. Both these papers only used linear regression for the prediction task. To the best of our knowledge, there is no study that has methodically explored machine learning methods to predict the mRS-90 score as a measure of stroke outcome.

3   Methodology

3.1   Data Collection and Preparation

Our study was conducted on retrospective data obtained from medical records of 439 ischemic stroke patients admitted at the University of Massachusetts Medical School, Worcester, MA, USA between 2012 and 2015. The features relevant for stroke outcome prediction were identified and extracted to form our dataset. This process was a combination of domain expertise and empirical knowledge of machine learning procedures. In the first step, one of the authors of this paper, a clinical neurologist and expert on stroke, helped select a large set of attributes for extraction from the patients' medical records. The next step involved several data preprocessing measures. Attributes with a large amount of missing values were removed. Attributes with almost homogeneous values were also removed. The final set of attributes included demographic information (such as age and gender), medical history (such as diabetes and hypertension), habits history (such as smoking and drinking), subtype of stroke (such as large vessel and cardioembolic) [31], prescribed medication (such as anticoagulants), and mRS scores at different stages (before admission, at discharge and at 90 days). A measure of stroke severity determined by the National Institutes of Health Stroke Scale (NIHSS) score [32] were also included. Table 3 presents summary statistics of all the attributes of the stroke dataset used in this study. For the multivalued attribute stroke subtype, five binary attributes for the five possible values were created, with each attribute value specifying whether (1) or not (0) the patient had that particular subtype of stroke. This is done since there is no ordinal relationship among the different stroke types; so giving them numeric scores would make the model incorrect.

One important point to note is that patients who died within 90 days of stroke, therefore having a mRS score of 6, were excluded from this analysis. The reason is that patient death can occur for a combination of several reasons apart from stroke, such as advanced age or additional comorbid conditions. Therefore, for stroke outcome prediction, a decision was made to conduct experiments only with the patients who survived the stroke after 90 days. Prominent works on this area such as the Copenhagen Stroke Study [33] have also excluded dead patients in some of their models.

3.2   Regression

Algorithms and Parameters. We considered several regression techniques to predict stroke outcome. We used the machine learning tool Weka (version 3.8) [34] to run experiments with different regression methods. From our experiments, the most successful regression method was bagged M5 model trees. For bagging, the bootstrap size was kept equal to the size of the training set. 10 bootstraps were created from each training set. The model trees were pruned to reduce overfitting. This was done by requiring a minimum of 10 instances per leaf in the model trees. For every other parameter, the default values in Weka (version 3.8) were applied. For comparison with the bagged M5 model trees, we ran experiments with the most commonly used regression algorithm – linear regression. We used linear regression with and without bagging for performance comparison.

Evaluation Criteria. The performance of the regression models can be evaluated by measuring the degree of similarity between the actual values of the target attribute, and the predicted values returned by the models. 10-fold cross validation [35] was used to assess how well the models will generalize to an independent dataset. The training data set was pseudo-randomly partitioned into 10 subsets. Ten training and test rounds were then performed; on the i-th round, the union of all subsets except the i-th was used to train the regression model, which was then tested on the i-th subset. The reported performance value is the mean of the ten performance values obtained in this way. We measured three criteria for evaluation: the Pearson correlation coefficient, mean absolute error and root mean squared error.

Table 3. Summary statistics of the attributes of the stroke dataset. The total number of patients is 439. For continuous attributes, the mean and standard deviation are shown in a Mean ± Std. Dev. format. For categorical attributes the percentages of different values are given. For binary attributes, only the percentages of TRUE values are shown. For mRS scores at different stages, we summarize the overall mean and standard deviation along with the distribution of individual scores. For some of the attributes, shorter names are devised and shown in the rightmost column. These shorter versions of attribute names are used when describing the models in Sect. 4.

Attribute	Distribution of values	Short name (if applicable)
Stroke subtype	Small vessel: 12.3%, Large vessel: 23.7%, Cardioembolic: 31.4%, Cryptogenic: 23.7%, Others: 8.9%	Type = {SmVes, LgVes, Cardio, Crypto, Others}
Gender	Male: 57.4%, Female: 42.6%	
Age	67.2 ± 14.6, Range: 19–97	
NIHSS score at admission	7.2 ± 7.1, Range: 0–32	NIHSS-adm
Hypertension	74.7%	HTN
Hyperlipidemia	58.8%	HLD
Diabetes	29.8%	
Smoking	29.4%	
Alcohol problem	14.6%	Alcohol
Previous history of stroke	19.4%	Hist-stroke
Atrial Fibrillation	27.7%	AFib
Carotid Artery Disease	21.0%	CAD
Congestive Heart Failure	8.7%	CHF
Peripheral Artery Disease	6.4%	PAD
Hemorrhagic conversion	11.2%	Hem-Conv
tPA	20.5%	
Statins	47.4%	
Antihypertensives	62.9%	Anti-HTN
Antidiabetics	20.5%	
Antiplatelets	45.3%	
Anticoagulants	10.3%	Anti-Coag
Perfusion	8.7%	
Neurointervention	18.7%	NeuroInt
mRS before admission	0.41 ± 0.86 (0: 74.0%, 1: 15.0%, 2: 5.9%, 3: 2.1%, 4: 1.4%, 5: 0.5%)	mRS-adm
mRS at discharge	1.60 ± 1.63 (0: 35.3%, 1: 13.7%, 2: 15.3%, 3: 9.8%, 4: 11.6%, 5: 5.0%)	mRS-disch
mRS at 90 days	1.28 ± 1.46 (0: 46.9%, 1: 17.5%, 2: 14.4%, 3: 11.6%, 4: 6.2%, 5: 3.4%)	mRS-90

The Pearson correlation coefficient, R, is a measure of the linear dependence between $X = \{X_1,...,X_n\}$ and $Z = \{Z_1,...,Z_n\}$. It gives a value between -1 and $+1$ where -1 stands for total negative correlation, 0 for no correlation and $+1$ for total positive correlation. It can be defined as follows [36]:

$$R = \frac{\sum(X_i - \overline{X})(Z_i - \overline{Z})}{\sqrt{\sum(X_i - \overline{X})^2 \sum(Z_i - \overline{Z})^2}} \tag{4}$$

where $\overline{X}$ and $\overline{Z}$ are means of X and Z respectively.

When measuring the correlation coefficient for a prediction task, a higher value of the coefficient indicates more similarity between the actual and predicted outputs, and hence better prediction performance.

Mean absolute error (MAE) and root mean squared error (RMSE) are both widely used in prediction tasks to measure the amount of deviation of the predicted values from the actual values. The two are defined in the following way:

$$MAE = \frac{1}{n}\sum_{i=1}^{n}|z_i - \hat{z}_i| \tag{5}$$

$$RMSE = \sqrt{\frac{1}{n}\sum_{i=1}^{n}(|z_i - \hat{z}_i|)^2} \tag{6}$$

Where n is the number of predictions, $z_1,\ldots,z_n$ are the actual and $\hat{z}_1,\ldots,\hat{z}_n$ are the predicted values respectively [37]. Since MAE and RMSE measure differences between the actual and predicted outputs, lower values of these measures indicate better prediction performance.

3.3   Classification

Algorithms and Parameters. The best classification method found in this study is a technique where a classification is done based on the regression results obtained from bagged M5 model trees (as described in Sect. 3.2). When the numeric prediction is obtained from this regression method, we round it to the nearest integer and assign the instance to the class corresponding to that integer. For example, a regression output of 0.35 is assigned to class "0" and an output of 3.83 is assigned to class "4". We denote this approach here as *classification via regression*. For comparison, we consider two more widely used classification algorithms: logistic regression [15] and C4.5 decision tree [38]. The choice of logistic regression is motivated by the fact that it is the standard classification method used in clinical trial studies. As for decision tree, it gives a good diagrammatic representation of the prediction process as well as proving to be empirically successful in classification tasks. The machine learning tool Weka (version 3.8) [34] was used for our classification experiments as well. To reduce overfitting, the C4.5 Decision trees were pruned by requiring at least 10 instances per leaf. For every other parameter, the default values in Weka (version 3.8) were applied.

Evaluation Criteria. The main evaluation criterion for the classification algorithms used in this study is *accuracy* – the percentage of cases where the actual and the predicted classes are the same. But since there are six different classes with subtle variations between two adjacent mRS-90 scores, we may consider predictions that are close enough to the actual score to be fairly accurate as well. We therefore define "*near-accuracy*" to refer to the percentage of cases in which the classifier either makes an accurate prediction, or makes a wrong prediction which is either one more or one less than the correct mRS score. For example, if the correct class is 3, only a prediction of 3 will be correct in terms of accuracy, but a prediction of 2, 3 or 4 will be acceptable in terms of near-accuracy. Once again, 10-fold cross validation [35] (using the process described in Sect. 3.2) was used to assess how well the models will generalize to an independent dataset.

3.4   Ordinal Regression

Our experiments on ordinal regression were run in R using the R package *ordinal* [39]. We experimented with the five different link functions discussed in Sect. 2.4. The evaluation criteria used for ordinal regression is different from both classification and regression. This is because the ordinal scale leads to problems in defining an appropriate loss function [15]. The evaluation criteria used for conventional regression would not be applicable here because of the categorical nature of the target attribute. However, a simple hit-or-miss loss function does not reflect the ordering of the categories in the target attribute. We therefore use the Akaike Information Criterion (AIC) which offers an estimate of the relative information lost when a given model is used to represent the process that generates the data [40]. Smaller values of AIC indicate better fitted models. The other criterion we use is log-likelihood – a measure of the probability that the observed data is generated from a certain model. For this criterion, the higher values indicate better models.

4   Results and Discussion

4.1   Regression Models to Predict mRS-90

We performed supervised regression on the stroke data to predict the patient outcome after 90 days of stroke onset. The predictive and target attributes of the dataset are described in Table 3. We constructed models using M5 model tree and linear regression algorithms. We then applied bootstrap aggregating (bagging) using M5 model trees and linear regression models as respective base predictors. For comparison purposes, we constructed also the simple regression model whose prediction is always the average of the values of the dependent variable in the training set.

As described in Sect. 3.2, we experimented with several parameters of the algorithms to enhance performance of the models. In Table 4, we present the results of the best models achieved after experimentation with different parameter values. The comparison is in terms of the correlation coefficient (R), mean absolute error (MAE) and root mean squared error (RMSE).

Results show that bagging used in tandem with M5 model trees performs much better than all the other techniques. Even without bagging, the M5 model trees perform better than linear regression. The improvement in performance is most impressive when the mean absolute error is considered, but not so much when we consider the root mean squared error. This leads us to an important point.

Large errors have a relatively greater influence when the errors are squared. So, if the variance associated with the frequency distribution of the error magnitude increases, the difference between MAE and RMSE also increases [41]. From our observation of the relative MAE and RMSE values of the M5 model tree, we can conclude that there is a high variance in the prediction error of the M5 model tree. It therefore makes sense that a variance-reducing procedure like bagging should improve the performance of the model tree, as observed in Table 4. Note however that bagging does not have the same kind of effect in improving the performance of linear regression.

To see if any statistically significant improvement in performance is achieved, we performed paired t-tests in terms of correlation coefficient on each pair of the five methods considered. The difference between means for each pair are examined at a p-value of 0.05. The results of the tests are presented in Table 5. It shows that the performances of linear regression and M5 model trees (without bagging) are not statistically different from each other. When bagging is used with linear regression, it is unable to improve the performance significantly. However, when bagging is used with M5 model trees, the resulting regression model performs significantly better than the models of all the other methods.

Table 4. Comparison of different regression methods on stroke data in terms of R, MAE and RMSE. For R, higher values indicate better model fit, whereas for the MAE and RMSE metrics lower values are better. Table reused from [4].

Method	R	MAE	RMSE
Average prediction	−0.136	1.235	1.461
Linear regression	0.779	0.654	0.916
M5 model tree	0.785	0.577	0.905
Bagging with linear regression	0.783	0.649	0.908
Bagging with M5 model trees	0.822	0.537	0.832

Analysis of the Linear Regression Model. The linear regression model returns a linear equation delineating the amount of influence each predictive attribute has on the final outcome. Figure 4 shows the model obtained through linear regression. The attributes with a positive coefficient contribute to an increase in the mRS-90 score (worse outcome). The magnitude of the coefficient points to the degree of contribution. Note that the values of the continuous attributes *age* and *NIHSS* were scaled to a range between 0 and 1 before running linear regression. This allows comparison of their coefficients with those of all the other attributes.

From the linear regression model, we observe that older age, higher NIHSS at admission (more severe initial stroke) and higher mRS at discharge all have large positive coefficients. These implies that they are all predictive of a poor outcome.

Table 5. Results of statistical significance analysis on correlation coefficient with p-value of 0.05. Each cell represents the result of the paired t-test between a pair of algorithms. If the algorithm in the row is significantly better than the one in the column, a '≫' is shown. If it is significantly worse, a '≪' is shown. A '<->' indicates that there is no statistically significant difference. Table reused from [4].

	Average pred	Linear regression	M5 tree	Bagging lin. reg.	Bagging M5 trees
Average prediction	-	≪	≪	≪	≪
Linear regression	≫	-	<->	<->	≪
M5 model tree	≫	<->	-	<->	≪
Bagging with linear regression	≫	<->	<->	-	≪
Bagging with M5 model trees	≫	≫	≫	≫	-

Alcohol also has noticeable contribution towards a poorer outcome. All the stroke subtypes have a negative coefficient, so it is difficult to draw conclusions from these coefficients. Among the other attributes that have a negative coefficient, Perfusion is found to have fairly high contribution towards a better outcome.

```
mRS 90 days =
    -1.3935 * Type=LgVes +
    -1.6024 * Type=SmVes +
    -1.6628 * Type=Cardio +
    -1.5381 * Type=Crypto +
    -1.5945 * Type=other +
    0.786 * NIHSS-adm+
    0.2132 * mRS-adm +
    0.9537 * Age +
    -0.2473 * Smoking +
    0.3681 * Alcohol +
    0.2144 * Antidiabetic +
    -0.1012 * Antiplatelet +
    -0.3295 * Perfusion +
    0.6198 * mRS-disch +
    0.963
```

Fig. 4. Linear regression model to predict 90-days outcome of stroke from patients' data.

Analysis of the M5 Model Tree. We investigate the model returned by the M5 model tree algorithm to find insights about stroke outcome. Figure 5 shows the model tree where each leaf is a linear equation. The linear equations are shown alongside the tree. The sign and magnitude of coefficients of each predictive attribute in the equations give an indication of how the output attribute responds to changes in the given input attribute. The continuous variables age and NIHSS at admission are scaled to the range between 0 and 1, so that the magnitudes of these attributes are within the [0,1] range.

From the model tree of Fig. 5, it is clear that the tree divides the input space based on the mRS score at discharge, and builds linear models for different ranges of that score. By following the decision branches of the tree, we can see that the linear models LM 1 and LM 2 correspond to mRS discharge scores of 0 and 1 respectively. LM 3 is associated with mRS discharge scores of 2 and 3, and LM 4 with scores of 4 and 5.

Let us now take a closer look at each of the linear models. In LM 1, the y-intercept is a very small value and there is no other attribute that has a large enough coefficient to change the prediction substantially. This means that the mRS-90 prediction for almost all patients reaching this point of the tree will be close to 0. At LM 2, the mRS-disch value is 1 with a coefficient of 0.1265. Since the y-intercept is 0.3596, if all the other attributes are absent, the output is 0.4861. Let us call this the *baseline prediction* for this leaf. Other attributes will either increase or decrease this baseline prediction based on their coefficients. Older age, higher NIHSS at admission and antihypertensives contribute towards increasing the mRS-90 score. On the other hand, cardioembolic and cryptogenic strokes contribute significantly towards lowering the mRS-90 score. At LM 3, the mRS score can be either 2 or 3. In the former case, the baseline prediction is 2*0.0951 − 0.3414 = −0.1512 and in the latter case, it is 3*0.0951 − 0.3414 = −0.0561. However, there are several attributes in this model that may have a major impact on the final prediction, notably age, NIHSS at admission, diabetes, large vessel stroke subtype and mRS before admission. Higher values for some or all of the above attributes will result in increased mRS-90 score. For LM 4, the baseline prediction is either 2.6762 (for mRS discharge = 4) or 4.1181 (for mRS discharge = 5). If a patient reaches this leaf, the output mRS-90 prediction is likely to be quite high. Only neurointervention has a major effect of lowering the mRS-90 score.

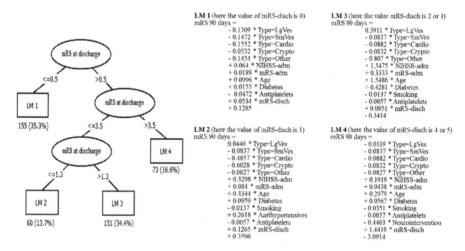

Fig. 5. The M5 model tree built on the stroke dataset with minimum 10 instances in each leaf. Each leaf is a linear model (LM1–LM4) predicting the target attribute mRS-90. The numbers under the leaves indicate how many instances are covered under that particular linear model. Each of the linear models are shown in detail alongside the tree.

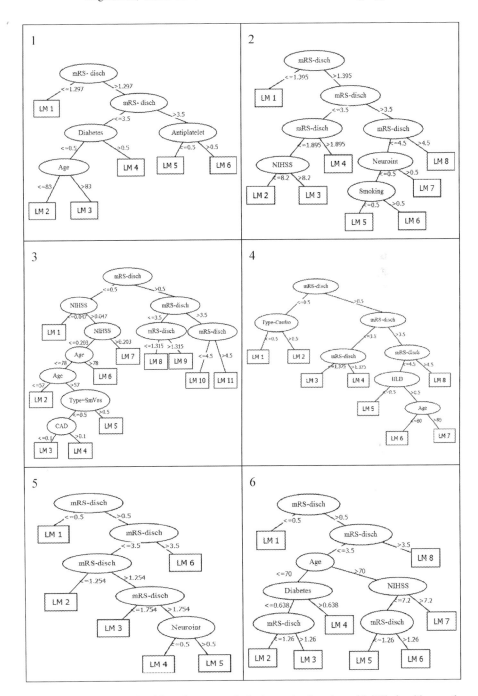

Fig. 6. Model trees obtained from bootstraps 1–6 when using bagging with M5 algorithm on the stroke data. Bootstrap numbers are shown alongside the tree for reference.

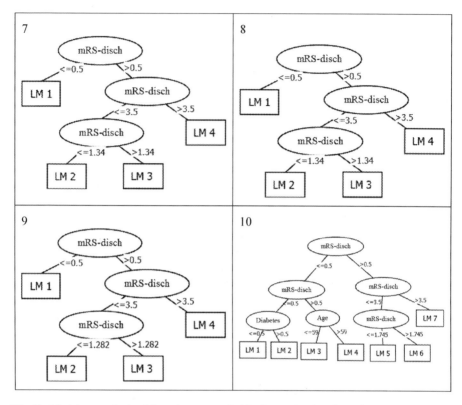

Fig. 7. Model trees obtained from bootstraps 7–10 when using bagging with M5 algorithm on the stroke data. Bootstrap numbers are shown alongside the tree for reference.

Analysis of the Bagged M5 Model Trees. In bootstrap aggregating, a number of bootstraps are created by sampling from the training data. Each bootstrap is used to build a model, which in our case is a M5 model tree. Since we used 10 bags, we obtained 10 model trees as shown in Figs. 6 and 7. Because of the huge number of linear models created in the trees, it is not possible to delineate all of them. So, we limit our discussion on the observations made from the structure of the trees and the internal nodes that were created.

The first glaring observation is the confirmation that mRS at discharge is the most influential attribute in the trees. In all 10 trees, it is the root of the tree, and in all but two trees it also acts as at least one of the children of the root. In several trees, the first linear model is formed by making a branch corresponding to mRS at discharge of 0. These linear models always evaluate to a very low mRS-90 score. Trees 7, 8 and 9 are almost identical to the single M5 tree we found using M5 model trees without bagging. Apart from mRS discharge, the other important attributes that occurred several times in the trees are: Age, diabetes, antiplatelet, NIHSS at admission and Neurointervention.

4.2   Classification Models to Predict mRS-90

We now consider the mRS-90 attribute as discrete multinomial (i.e., consisting of individual classes 0, 1, …, 5) instead of a continuous numeric attribute, and construct classification models to predict this discrete attribute. We used a classification via regression approach where the regression outputs from the bagged M5 model trees were discretized and treated as classification outputs. For comparison, we also applied two traditional multinomial classification techniques: C4.5 Decision tree and Logistic regression. We chose these two because the classification models induced by both of these algorithms are very expressive in nature. Moreover, Logistic regression is extensively used for multivariate analysis in medical literature. As the evaluation metrics, we chose accuracy and near-accuracy as described in Sect. 3.3.

Table 6 shows a comparison of the performance of classification via regression with those of multi-class classification using Logistic regression and C4.5 decision trees. For comparison purposes, we include also the majority class classifier which classifies any test instance with the mRS-90 value that appears most frequently in the training set. We experimented with different pruning parameters of the C4.5 decision trees, and show here the accuracies of the model that has the best generalization performance.

Table 6 shows that the classification via regression method performs better in terms of both accuracy and near-accuracy. To check whether this improvement is statistically significant, we performed paired t-tests on the classification accuracy for the four algorithms. The results, given in Table 7, show that classification via regression performs significantly better than logistic regression, but not significantly better than the C4.5 decision tree at a level of $p = 0.05$. The fact that we obtained significantly better results than logistic regression is noteworthy, since logistic regression is the default analysis method used in medical literature.

Table 6. Comparison of logistic regression, C4.5 and classification via regression (bagging with M5 model trees) on the stroke dataset in terms of accuracy and near-accuracy. Table reused from [4].

Method	Accuracy	Near-accuracy
Majority class	46.9%	64.4%
Logistic Regression	54.2%	83.6%
C4.5 (with pruning)	56.7%	86.8%
Classification via regression	59.7%	90.0%

In Table 8, we show the confusion matrix obtained from the best-performing classification model, i.e., the classification via bagged model tree regression. The diagonal of the matrix represents the correct predictions. One observation from the misclassifications is that there is a central tendency of prediction. For mRS-90 scores 0–2, the misclassifications tend to be on the higher side. That means, more predicted scores are overestimates rather than underestimates of the actual score. The opposite is true for mRS-90 scores of 3–5 where the predictions tend to err more by underestimating than overestimating.

Table 7. Results of statistical significance analysis on classification accuracy with p-value of 0.05. Each cell represents the result of the paired t-test between a pair of algorithms. If the algorithm in the row is significantly better than the one in the column, a '≫' is shown. If it is significantly worse, a '≪' is shown. A '<->' indicates that there is no statistically significant difference. Table reused from [4].

	Majority class	Logistic regression	C4.5 tree	Classification via regression
Majority class	-	≪	≪	≪
Logistic regression	≫	-	<->	≪
C4.5 tree	≫	<->	-	<->
Classification via regression	≫	≫	<->	-

Analysis of the C4.5 Decision Tree. For classification of mRS-90 values, we created a decision tree using the C4.5 algorithm. In order to avoid overfitting, we pruned the trees by imposing restrictions of having a minimum of 10 instances per leaf. The decision tree we obtained is shown in Fig. 8. The structure of the classification tree is similar to that of the regression trees we discussed before. The difference is that the leaf nodes of the classification tree are mRS-90 scores (0,...,5) rather than linear models to calculate the scores. Like the trees in our regression models, this tree also has mRS at discharge as the primary factor. Patients with mRS at discharge = 0 are predicted to have mRS-90 = 0. The same is true for patients with mRS at discharge = 1 unless they have a non-cryptogenic stroke and use antihypertensives, in which case the mRS-90 prediction is 1. Patients having mRS at discharge of 2 or 3 usually are predicted to end

Table 8. Confusion matrix for the method of supervised classification via regression using bagging with M5 model trees. The rows show the actual mRS scores while the columns show the ones predicted by the model. The diagonals (in darker gray) are the correct predictions. The cells adjacent to the diagonals (in lighter gray) are near-correct predictions missing the actual score by 1. Table adapted from [4].

Actual	Predicted					
	0	1	2	3	4	5
0	159	36	11	0	0	0
1	10	40	19	8	0	0
2	2	15	31	14	1	0
3	0	8	19	21	3	0
4	0	3	5	8	10	1
5	0	3	1	2	8	1

up with mRS-90 of 2. There are, however, exceptions in two cases: If the patients have low (0 or 1) mRS before admission, has a history of alcohol consumption and is younger than 87, they are predicted to do better and have mRS-90 of 1; On the other hand, if mRS before admission is higher than 1 and NIHSS at admission is higher than 5, they are predicted to do worse and have mRS-90 of 3. Patients having mRS at discharge of 4 have predicted mRS-90 of 2 or 3. Patients having mRS at discharge of 5 are predicted to have mRS-90 of 4 or 5.

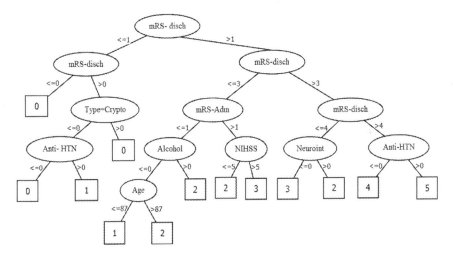

Fig. 8. C4.5 Decision tree constructed from the stroke data by treating the mRS-90 scores as multinomial categories.

Analysis of the Logistic Regression Model. Among the six categories of mRS-90, we chose the last category (mRS-90 = 5) as the reference category for multinomial logistic regression. Table 9 shows the coefficients that were obtained for each attribute/category combination. When analyzing this model, we need to consider the fact that all the coefficients are with respect to the reference category. So positive coefficients imply higher probability of being classified in that category than the reference category. A negative coefficient would imply the opposite. As a concrete example, diabetes has negative coefficients for all the categories, so a diabetic patient is less likely to have mRS scores 0–4 than mRS score of 5. We inspected the sign and magnitude of each attribute, and compared their coefficients across categories. The following attributes were found to have very high negative coefficients in all categories: age, NIHSS score at admission, and hypertension. In addition, several other attributes such as gender, diabetes and alcohol have negative coefficient across all categories. This means that all these attributes have a lower probability of being in the lower mRS scores (lower probability of better outcome). As for the different treatment methods, only perfusion has positive coefficients in all categories. Antidiabetics and antiplatelets also have positive coefficients for mRS scores of 0–3. This indicates that these methods of treatment improve the probability of going to a lower mRS score (better outcome).

4.3   Ordinal Regression to Predict mRS-90

We created ordinal regression models with different link functions, and recorded the Akaike Information Criterion (AIC) and log-likelihood for model comparison. Table 10 summarizes the results obtained. Since ordinal regression with the logit link function yields best result (lowest AIC and highest log-likelihood), we examine the model in more detail. Table 11 shows the coefficients and p-values obtained for that model.

In ordinal regression with the logit link function, the logit (or log of odds) of the final outcome is a linear combination of the independent attributes. The positive coefficients contribute to worse outcome. Two attributes – age and mRS at discharge – have high positive coefficients and are the only ones that have statistically significant

Table 9. Logistic regression coefficients for each category of the mRS-90 attribute for the stroke data. Here mRS-90 = 5 is used as the reference category.

Attribute	Coefficients for each category				
	0	1	2	3	4
Subtype = Large vessel	−0.886	1.652	−1.080	−13.28	−2.426
Subtype = Small vessel	−0.858	0.162	−2.960	−14.45	−4.619
Subtype = Cardioembolic	2.725	4.685	0.987	−12.24	−1.222
Subtype = Cryptogenic	−1.310	0.798	−1.758	−14.46	−4.119
Gender (female)	−3.200	−3.233	−3.076	−4.001	−3.098
Age	−19.60	−18.64	−16.43	−18.81	−13.25
NIHSS score at admission	−9.696	−9.376	−8.096	−6.668	−8.224
Hypertension	−29.73	−30.99	−31.28	−31.05	−30.68
Hyperlipidemia	2.869	2.598	2.882	2.735	2.670
Diabetes	−4.155	−4.010	−2.869	−3.472	−3.672
Smoking	4.538	4.680	4.029	4.353	2.530
Alcohol problem	−4.463	−5.363	−3.866	−4.179	−1.675
Previous history of stroke	−2.316	−2.018	−1.045	−1.331	−0.469
Atrial fibrillation	0.810	1.133	2.010	3.047	2.038
Carotid artery disease	−0.038	0.889	0.487	1.468	2.168
Congestive heart failure	−0.162	−0.007	−0.656	−1.405	−1.294
Peripheral artery disease	−1.909	−1.444	−0.274	−1.458	−2.282
Hemorrhagic conversion	−0.327	−1.130	−1.952	−1.029	−1.737
tPA	−0.641	−0.860	−0.565	−1.374	−1.289
Statins	−2.597	−2.323	−2.715	−2.057	−2.641
Antihypertensives	−1.595	−0.875	−1.052	−0.222	−1.340
Antidiabetics	0.030	0.658	0.478	1.194	−0.246
Antiplatelets	1.397	0.515	0.182	0.129	−0.244
Anticoagulants	−1.725	−1.295	−1.897	−1.797	−2.735
Perfusion	4.584	3.587	2.132	3.163	2.693
Neurointervention	−5.795	−6.002	−5.304	−6.513	−5.680
mRS before admission	−1.994	−1.222	−1.274	−0.636	−1.109
mRS at discharge	−3.754	−1.954	−1.133	−0.561	0.042

Table 10. Performance of ordinal regression on stroke data for different link functions. For AIC, smaller values indicate better performance whereas for log-likelihood, larger values (lower magnitude of negative values) indicate better performance.

Link function	AIC	Log-likelihood
Logit	651.96	−292.98
Probit	654.17	−294.09
Cloglog	663.71	−298.85
Cauchit	685.53	−309.77

Table 11. Ordinal regression (using the logit link function) coefficients for each attribute of the stroke data. The p-values are shown in the rightmost column, and the attributes with $p < 0.05$ are marked with asterisks.

Attribute	Coefficient	p-value
Subtype = Large vessel	0.438	0.461
Subtype = Small vessel	−0.259	0.738
Subtype = Cardioembolic	−0.062	0.918
Subtype = Cryptogenic	0.356	0.550
Gender	0.343	0.235
Age	4.164	0.001*
NIHSS score at admission	0.280	0.723
Hypertension	−0.545	0.201
Hyperlipidemia	0.118	0.730
Diabetes	0.426	0.289
Smoking	−0.396	0.199
Alcohol problem	0.407	0.297
Previous history of stroke	0.610	0.073
Atrial fibrillation	0.242	0.526
Carotid artery disease	0.378	0.319
Congestive heart failure	−0.037	0.939
Peripheral artery disease	0.553	0.253
Hemorrhagic conversion	−0.123	0.739
tPA	0.101	0.747
Statins	−0.096	0.776
Antihypertensives	0.388	0.289
Antidiabetics	−0.096	0.832
Antiplatelets	−0.302	0.164
Anticoagulants	0.347	0.406
Perfusion	−0.767	0.096
Neurointervention	−0.552	0.153
mRS before admission	0.269	0.089
mRS at discharge	2.002	<0.001*

(p < 0.05) impact. Other attributes having relatively strong impact according to the model are mRS before admission, history of previous stroke, and perfusion. The first two contribute to higher mRS scores whereas the last one contributes to lower mRS scores.

5 Discussion and Conclusions

This paper has presented the results of predicting the 90-day outcome of ischemic stroke patients based on the data consisting of their demographics, medical history and treatment records. The target attribute for prediction is the modified Rankin Scale score 90 days after stroke. The problem of prediction was approached from several angles: as a regression problem, as a multinomial unordered classification problem, and as an ordinal regression problem. For regression, a meta-learning approach of bootstrap aggregating (bagging) using M5 model trees as the base learner proved to be very effective, significantly outperforming the standard linear regression method. The same method, after translation of the target output from numeric to nominal, works successfully as a multinomial classification scheme, and significantly outperforms logistic regression, the most commonly used classification method in clinical trials. We also experimented with ordinal regression using different link functions, and obtained a useful model using the logit link function.

A model tree divides the input space into a number of subspaces defined around the attributes represented by internal nodes of the tree, and builds a model for each subspace. In our dataset, mRS at discharge proved to be an important attribute dominating the final outcome. Therefore, predictive algorithms that construct specialized models for different ranges of mRS score at discharge are likely to do well. This is exactly what we observed from our M5 model trees obtained by a single iteration of the M5 algorithm, as well as the many trees obtained by multiple iterations of bagging. By examining the model tree prediction errors for the stroke dataset considered, it is found that the variability of errors is much higher for model trees than for other regression methods such as linear regression. Since bagging is empirically known to reduce the instability and error variance of its base learners, it shows good performance for this particular dataset.

Through our experiments we obtained several predictive models that can take inputs in the form of patient data, calculate some function, and produce output in the form of the patient's 90-day stroke outcome. The regression models' output is a continuous real number estimating the numeric mRS score, and the classification models' output is a nominal value corresponding to the predicted category of the mRS score. For regression we analyzed the tree induced by the M5 model tree algorithm. We found that the internal nodes of the tree simply "direct" the decision towards linear models (at the leaves) based on the mRS score at discharge. By examining the individual linear models, we were able to identify different attributes that were associated with either improved or worsened outcome of stroke patients. For example, older age, more severe initial stroke, and presence of hypertension were associated with a poorer 90-day outcome even when their condition at the time of discharge was relatively good.

On the other hand, Neurointervention was found to be a procedure that was associated with improved outcome of patients who were in relatively poor condition at the time of discharge. We also analyzed the ten different model trees constructed when the bagging technique was applied to M5 model trees. Some of these trees were identical to the single tree discussed above, but there was a considerable amount of differences among the other trees. However, mRS at discharge was found to be the most important attribute in all of the trees. The other regression model that we observed was that of linear regression, which comes in the form of a linear equation. We analyzed the coefficients of the equation and found that, according to the model, older age, more severe initial stroke, higher mRS at discharge, and alcohol were correlated with poorer outcome, while the Perfusion procedure was correlated with better outcome.

As for the classification part of our study, we obtained models induced by the C4.5 Decision Tree and Logistic Regression algorithms. We also performed ordinal logistic regression and obtained a linear equation of the attributes that can be used to predict stroke outcome. The contributions of attributes towards a better or a worse outcome in these models were found to be similar to the ones observed in the regression models. To summarize some of the important observations made from both the regression and the classification models, we found that higher mRS score at the time of discharge, older age and more severe initial stroke are the most influencing factors that are associated with worsened stroke outcome. The presence of diabetes and hypertension also have some correlation with worse outcome. On the other hand, treatment procedures such as Perfusion and Neurointervention were shown to be associated with improved outcome of the patients.

There is room for future work to take this study forward. One limitation of the study is the exclusion of the patients who died within 90 days of stroke. As mentioned before, this is in line with other work in the literature (e.g., the Copenhagen Stroke Study [33]), but it would be interesting in future work to extend our approach to include these patients. We are also limited by a large amount of missing values in attributes that are part of the medical records but are not included in this study. By collecting data about more patients, and more data about each patient, we may be able to uncover some more useful patterns. Another future goal is to improve the process of classification via regression by discovering better ways to translate the numeric predictions to discrete classes. Future work includes also an in-depth analysis of the ordinal regression results and models that we obtained.

Acknowledgements. The authors thank Prof. Dr. Klaus Brinker for suggesting using ordinal regression as an additional technique in this research.

References

1. Raffeld, M., Debette, S., Woo, D.: International stroke genetics consortium update. Stroke **47** (4), 1144–1145 (2016). https://doi.org/10.1161/STROKEAHA.116.012682
2. Mozaffarian, D., Benjamin, E.J., Go, A.S., et al.: Heart disease and stroke statistics—2016 update. Circulation **133**(4), e38–e360 (2016). https://doi.org/10.1161/CIR.00000000000 00350

3. Rankin, J.: Cerebral vascular accidents in patients over the age of 60: II. Prognosis. Scott. Med. J. **2**, 200–215 (1957)
4. Kabir, A., Ruiz, C., Alvarez, S.A., Moonis, M.: Predicting outcome of ischemic stroke patients using bootstrap aggregating with M5 Model trees. In: van den Broek, E.L., Fred, A., Gamboa, H., Vaz, M. (eds.) 10th International Joint Conference on Biomedical Engineering Systems and Technologies, BIOSTEC 2017, Proceedings Volume 5: HealthInf, 21–23 February, Porto, Protugal, pp. 178–187 (2017)
5. van Swieten, J.C., Koudstaal, P.J., Visser, M.C., Schouten, H.J., van Gijn, J.: Interobserver agreement for the assessment of handicap in stroke patients. Stroke **19**(5), 604–607 (1988)
6. Banks, J.L., Marotta, C.A.: Outcomes validity and reliability of the modified rankin scale: implications for stroke clinical trials: a literature review and synthesis. Stroke **38**(3), 1091–1096 (2007)
7. Bruno, A., Shah, N., Lin, C., Close, B., Hess, D.C., Davis, K., Baute, V., Switzer, J.A., Waller, J., Nichols, F.T.: Improving modified rankin scale assessment with a simplified questionnaire. Stroke **41**(5), 1048–1050 (2010). https://doi.org/10.1161/STROKEAHA.109.571562
8. Tan, P.-N., Steinbach, M., Kumar, V.: Introduction to Data Mining. Addison-Wesley, Boston (2005)
9. Breiman, L., Friedman, J.H., Olshen, R.A., Stone, C.J.: Classification and Regression Trees. Wadsworth, Belmont (1984)
10. Quinlan, J.R.: Learning with continuous classes. In: Adams, A., Sterling, L. (eds.) 5th Australian Joint Conference on Artificial Intelligence, Hobart, Australia, pp. 343–348 (1992)
11. Wang, Y., Witten, I.H.: Induction of model trees for predicting continuous classes. In: van Someren, M., Widmer, G. (eds.) 9th European Conference on Machine Learning. University of Economics, Prague (1996)
12. Etemad-Shahidi, A., Mahjoobi, J.: Comparison between M5′ model tree and neural networks for prediction of significant wave height in Lake Superior. Ocean Eng. **36**(15–16), 1175–1181 (2009). https://doi.org/10.1016/j.oceaneng.2009.08.008
13. Breiman, L.: Bagging predictors. Mach. Learn. **24**(2), 123–140 (1996)
14. Aslam, J., Popa, R., Rivest, R.: On estimating the size and confidence of a statistical audit. USENIX/ACCURATE Electron. Voting Technol. Workshop **7**, 8 (2007)
15. McCullagh, P.: Regression models for ordinal data. J. R. Stat. Soc.: Ser. B (Methodol.) **42**(2), 109–142 (1980)
16. Herbrich, R., Graepel, T., Obermayer, K.: Regression models for ordinal data: a machine learning approach. Technische Universität Berlin, Fachbereich 13, Informatik, Berlin (1999)
17. Anderson, J.: Regression and ordered categorical variables. J. R. Stat. Soc.: Ser. B (Methodol.) **46**(1), 1–30 (1984)
18. Agresti, A.: An Introduction to Categorical Data Analysis. Wiley-Interscience, Hoboken (2007)
19. Bender, R., Grouven, U.: Ordinal logistic regression in medical research. J. R. Coll. Phys. Lond. **31**(5), 546–551 (1997)
20. Moonis, M., Kane, K., Schwiderski, U., Sandage, B.W., Fisher, M.: HMG-CoA reductase inhibitors improve acute ischemic stroke outcome. Stroke **36**(6), 1298–1300 (2005)
21. Marini, C., De Santis, F., Sacco, S., Russo, T., Olivieri, L., Totaro, R., Carolei, A.: Contribution of atrial fibrillation to incidence and outcome of ischemic stroke. Stroke **36**(6), 1115–1119 (2005)
22. Yong, M., Kaste, M.: Dynamic of hyperglycemia as a predictor of stroke outcome in the ECASS-II trial. Stroke **39**(10), 2749–2755 (2008). https://doi.org/10.1161/STROKEAHA.108.514307

23. Nogueira, R.G., Liebeskind, D.S., Sung, G., Duckwiler, G., Smith, W.S.: Multi MERCI writing committee: predictors of good clinical outcomes, mortality, and successful revascularization in patients with acute ischemic stroke undergoing thrombectomy: pooled analysis of the mechanical embolus removal in cerebral ischemia (MERCI) and multi MERCI trials. Stroke **40**(12), 3777–3783 (2009). https://doi.org/10.1161/STROKEAHA. 109.561431

24. Henninger, N., Lin, E., Baker, S.P., Wakhloo, A.K., Takhtani, D., Moonis, M.: Leukoaraiosis predicts poor 90-Day outcome after acute large cerebral artery occlusion. Cerebrovascular Diseases. **33**(6), 525–531 (2012). https://doi.org/10.1159/000337335

25. Kissela, B., Lindsell, C.J., Kleindorfer, D., Alwell, K., Moomaw, C.J., Woo, D., Flaherty, M.L., Air, E., Broderick, J., Tsevat, J.: Clinical prediction of functional outcome after ischemic stroke: the surprising importance of periventricular white matter disease and race. Stroke **40**(2), 530–536 (2008). https://doi.org/10.1161/STROKEAHA.108.521906

26. Optimising Analysis of Stroke Trials Collaboration: Calculation of sample size for stroke trials assessing functional outcome: comparison of binary and ordinal approaches. Int. J. Stroke **3**(2), 78–84 (2008). https://doi.org/10.1111/j.1747-4949.2008.00184.x

27. Sandset, E.C., Bath, P.M., Boysen, G., Jatuzis, D., Kõrv, J., Lüders, S., Murray, G.D., Richter, P.S., Roine, R.O., Terént, A., Thijs, V., Berge, E.: SCAST study group: the angiotensin-receptor blocker candesartan for treatment of acute stroke (SCAST): a randomised, placebo-controlled, double-blind trial. Lancet **377**(9767), 741–750 (2011). https://doi.org/10.1016/S0140-6736(11)60104-9

28. Gialanella, B., Santoro, R., Ferlucci, C.: Predicting outcome after stroke: the role of basic activities of daily living. Eur. J. Phys. Rehabil. Med. **49**(5), 629–637 (2013)

29. Granger, C.V., Hamilton, B.B., Keith, R.A., Zielezny, M., Sherwin, F.S.: Advances in functional assessment for medical rehabilitation. Top. Geriatr. Rehabil. **1**(3), 59–74 (1986)

30. Brown, A.W., Therneau, T.M., Schultz, B.A., Niewczyk, P.M., Granger, C.V.: Measure of functional independence dominates discharge outcome prediction after inpatient rehabilitation for stroke. Stroke **46**(4), 1038–1044 (2015). https://doi.org/10.1161/STROKEAHA. 114.007392

31. Adams Jr., H.P., Bendixen, B.H., Kappelle, L.J., Biller, J., Love, B.B., Gordon, D.L., Marsh 3rd, E.E.: Classification of subtype of acute ischemic stroke. Definitions for use in a multicenter clinical trial. TOAST. Trial of Org 10172 in Acute Stroke Treatment. Stroke **24** (1), 35–41 (1993)

32. Brott, T., Adams Jr., H.P., Olinger, C.P., Marler, J.R., Barsan, W.G., Biller, J., Spilker, J., Holleran, R., Eberle, R., Hertzberg, V., et al.: Measurements of acute cerebral infarction: a clinical examination scale. Stroke **20**(7), 864–870 (1989)

33. Nakayama, H., Jorgensen, H.S., Raaschou, H.O., Olsen, T.S.: The influence of age on stroke outcome. The Copenhagen Stroke Study. Stroke **25**(4), 808–813 (1994)

34. Frank, E., Hall, M.A., Witten, I.H.: The WEKA Workbench. Online Appendix for "Data Mining: Practical Machine Learning Tools and Techniques". Morgan Kaufmann, Burlington (2016)

35. Kohavi, R.: A study of cross-validation and bootstrap for accuracy estimation and model selection. In: Proceedings of the International Joint Conference on Artificial Intelligence (IJCAI), vol. 2, pp. 1137–1145 (1995)

36. Lee Rodgers, J., Nicewander, W.A.: Thirteen ways to look at the correlation coefficient. Am. Stat. **42**(1), 59–66 (1988)

37. Moore, D.S., Notz, W.I., Fligner, M.A.: The Basic Practice of Statistics. W.H. Freeman and Co., New York (2015)

38. Quinlan, J.R.: C4.5 - Programs for Machine Learning. Morgan Kaufmann, San Francisco (1992)

39. Christensen, R.H.B.: Regression Models for Ordinal Data [R package ordinal version 2015.6-28]. https://cran.r-project.org/web/packages/ordinal/index.html
40. Bozdogan, H.: Model selection and Akaike's Information Criterion (AIC): the general theory and its analytical extensions. Psychometrika **52**(3), 345–370 (1987)
41. Willmott, C.J., Matsuura, K.: Advantages of the mean absolute error (MAE) over the root mean square error (RMSE) in assessing average model performance. Clim. Res. **30**(1), 79–82 (2005). https://doi.org/10.3354/cr030079

Author Index

Printed in the United States
By Bookmasters